UNIVERSITY OF MEMPHIS LIBRARIES
P9-CFI-361

The Contemporary and Historical Literature of Food Science and Human Nutrition

A volume in the series

The Literature of the Agricultural Sciences

WALLACE C. OLSEN, series editor

Agricultural Economics and Rural Sociology: The Contemporary Core Literature
By Wallace C. Olsen

The Literature of Agricultural Engineering
Edited by Carl W. Hall and Wallace C. Olsen

The Literature of Animal Science and Health
Edited by Wallace C. Olsen

The Literature of Soil Science
Edited by Peter McDonald

The Contemporary and Historical Literature of Food Science and Human Nutrition
Edited by Jennie Brogdon and Wallace C. Olsen

THE CONTEMPORARY AND HISTORICAL LITERATURE OF FOOD SCIENCE AND HUMAN NUTRITION

EDITED BY

Jennie Brogdon and
Wallace C. Olsen

Cornell University Press

ITHACA AND LONDON

This book was typeset from disks supplied by the staff of the Core Agricultural Literature Project, Albert R. Mann Library, Cornell University. Nicole Kasmer Kresock prepared the machine-readable text begun by Jane Hunt. Nicole Kasmer Kresock, Sharon M. Van De Mark, and Eveline Ferretti made final corrections. The research was financially supported by Cornell Agricultural Experiment Station; National Agricultural Library, United States Department of Agriculture; and the Rockefeller Foundation.

First published 1995 by Cornell University Press.

Printed in the United States of America

♾ The paper in this book meets the minimum requirements of the American National Standard for Information Sciences—Permanence of Paper for Printed Library Materials, ANSI Z39.48-1984.

Library of Congress Cataloging-in-Publication Data

The contemporary and historical literature of food science and human nutrition / edited by Jennie Brogdon and Wallace C. Olsen.
p. cm. — (The Literature of the agricultural sciences)
Includes bibliographical references and index.
ISBN 0-8014-3096-8 (alk. paper)
1. Food. 2. Nutrition. 3. Food—Bibliography. 4. Nutrition—Bibliography.
I. Brogdon, Jennie. II. Olsen, Wallace C. III. Series.
TX357.C564 1995
613.2—dc20 94-46959

Contents

The Contemporary and Historical Literature of Food Science and Human Nutrition

1 Development and Trends in Food Science

JOSEPH H. HOTCHKISS

Food Science, Cornell University

Food science is the application of basic sciences and engineering such as chemistry, microbiology, biochemistry, and chemical engineering to food composition, production, manufacture, storage, distribution, and safety. It is related in many ways to nutrition but at the same time different. Nutrition deals largely with health and biochemical aspects of food components. Food science may involve nutritional issues, but more frequently it deals with the technology of food manufacture and processing, composition of foods, their storage, and safe distribution. For example, a nutritionist will have an interest in the effects of a food or food component (vitamin C) on health and well-being while a food scientist will be interested in the effects of processing or storage on the sensory and nutritional quality of the food, for example, how processing or storage affects vitamin C content. Nutritionists are interested in vitamin intake while food scientists are concerned with how to maintain or incorporate vitamins into foods.

Food scientists study the conversion of raw agricultural and fishery products, which are often not edible and have very short shelf lives in their raw form, into edible products which can be kept for longer periods and transported over distances. Food science has as one of its objectives the development of food products and technologies for food service industries such as hotels, restaurants, and institutions but is seldom directly involved in cooking and food preparation or large-scale feeding. These activities are more properly termed food service. Food scientists work in industry, government, and academia. Industry scientists are often involved in developing foods and processing raw agricultural commodities into finished products. Food scientists in government work to regulate the safety, quality, and value of foods and help the agricultural and food industries solve problems. Academic food scientists typically conduct basic research and teach food science subjects.

A. Developments before 1810

Food science is a new discipline. It officially started with the founding of the Institute of Food Technologists (IFT) in the United States in 1939. However, the provision of food has been a major human endeavor throughout recorded history. Unfortunately, this need has yet to be fully met for many populations. The best science and engineering of the times has always been applied to food production and preparation even when the best "science" of the day was little more than trial-and-error art or in some cases sorcery.

The shift from hunting and gathering food to domestication of plants and animals took place more than 8,000 years ago. One of the oldest human objectives was to preserve foods in order to be free of the seasonality of food production and the irregularities of nature. Early methods of preservation, many of which are used today, included drying, salting, smoking, and sugaring. The scientific basis for these preservation methods was unknown so they developed as arts rather than sciences. Nonetheless, these arts were important and their history is well documented.[1]

Fermentation is an example of applying the best science or art of the times to food manufacture and preservation. Fermented products have been known for millennia. The ancient Egyptians developed breadmaking 4,000 years ago. Beer and wine were made earlier, and fermented cheeses and other dairy products have been produced for nearly as long. These foods were important to ancient peoples as reflected in their legends and customs. The spontaneous generation of wine from grape juice was documented in mythology and literature which ascribed this conversion to gods such as Bacchus, the Greek god of wine. It was not until the 1860s that Louis Pasteur explained the real cause of fermentation. We now consider fermentation a science in its own right.

Until the nineteenth century dehydration (drying), salting, curing, and fermenting were still the only means of providing foods throughout the seasons. Spices were first added to foods as preservatives rather than flavorings. Most of these methods had their counterparts in nature, and even though based on art these early developments were the precursors of food science and technology.

Analysis of food was one of the earliest applications of chemistry. A number of components were isolated and identified from foods prior to 1800.[2] For example, F. Bartoletti (1586–1630) isolated lactose from milk,

1. (a) William J. Darby, Paul Ghalioungui and Loius Grivetti, *Food: The Gift of Osiris*, 2 vols. (London and New York: Academic Press, 1977). (b) Reay Tannahill, *Food in History* (New York: Stein & Day, 1973).

2. W. F. Shipe and C. O. Olentine, "Foods, 1. Survey" in *Ullmann's Encyclopedia of Industrial Chemistry*, 5th ed. (Weinheim: VCH Verlagsgesellschaft mbH, 1988), pp. 491–521.

J. R. Glauber (1604–1668) found fructose in honey, gluten was first isolated from wheat by F. M. Grimaldi (1618–1663), sucrose from beets by A.S. Marggraf (1709–1786), and citric acid was identified in lemon juice by C. W. Scheele (1742–1786).

B. Developments between 1810 and 1900

As science and technology developed in the eighteenth and nineteenth centuries so did food science and its literature. Food preservation moved from art and mythology to science and engineering. Early in the 1800s, science could seldom explain the reasons for many changes in foods such as the rising of bread or the curing of meats with saltpeter. Much of the literature of the period described food processing as an art (i.e., based on trial and error) rather than an area of scientific understanding.[3] If the process could not be explained, at least the means to achieve a desired result could be. This early literature took the form of cookbooks and preserving guides. Foods and its processing to convert raw products into edible foods became more refined; descriptions of this served as the beginning of modern food science literature.

The most notable discovery of this period was that of the French chef Nicholas Appert, published in 1810.[4] Napoleon was having trouble acquiring sufficient rations for his army so he offered a monetary prize for a solution. Appert found that food could be preserved indefinitely if it were sufficiently heated after being sealed in glass containers. The discovery of canning, which has no model in nature, has had profound effects. It meant that foods could be transported distances and held for a year or more without risk. Humans could be further removed from the seasonal vagaries of nature. This advancement was made not by a scientist but by a chef. This accomplishment and its results were quickly recorded in the cooking literature of that day; the process spread quickly and was used in the Americas within a decade. Roughly 14% of food consumed in the United States today is preserved by canning, making it the single most important food process.

Canning was not the only important development during this period. Other examples include the use of functional additives in foods, improve-

3. George F. Stewart and Maynard A. Amerine, "Evolution of Food Processing and Preservation," in *Introduction to Food Science and Technology*, 2d ed. (New York: Academic Press, 1982), pp. 1–32.

4. N. Appert, *L'Art de Conserver, Pendant Plusieurs Années, Toutes les Substances Animales et Végétales* (Paris: Patris, 1810), translated as *The Art of Preserving all Kinds of Animal and Vegetable Substances for Several Years*, 1st English ed. (London: Black, Perry and Kingsbury, 1811). (Available in English from Mallinckrodt Collection of Food Classics).

ments in drying, greater use of glass and metal for packaging, and increased use of heating processes such as pasteurization to improve or preserve foods. A. Coffey developed the continuous distillation still, and N. Rellieux the triple effect evaporator in 1830. The roller dryer and mill were developed shortly thereafter. G. Borden introduced evaporated (condensed) canned milk, which became a staple, and initiated a company that still bears his name. The retort, cream separator, and mechanical refrigerator were all invented between 1860 and 1900. Preservatives were also developed. The history of the use of potassium nitrate (saltpeter) as a preservative for meats and as means of preventing deadly botulism has been documented.[5] This additive may have been used before recorded history but when combined with sugaring and salting, nitrate became a major means of preserving meats in the eighteenth and nineteenth centuries.

Perhaps the most significant development was the application to food processing of the principles of mass production developed in the latter half of the nineteenth century. The growth of the Campbell's Soup Company is one of many examples. The technology for preserving foods thermally when sealed in cans (which is short for "canister") had been established in the late 1800s but Campbell and his associates looked at soup canning as a manufacturing process. They successfully produced a quality product at a reasonable cost. The company flourished and continues to do a large business in canned soups as well as other products. Others, such as William Underwood, made similar strides in thermal preservation in the nineteenth century. The automated manufacture of tin-coated cans helped reduce the cost of canned food. Before this, each can was handmade and expensive. Mass manufacture of inexpensive cans spurred mass manufacture of canned foods.

New scientific knowledge, such as Pasteur's discovery that microorganisms caused fermentation and spoilage in the 1860s, led to developments in the processing and preservation of foods and dairy products. Sanitation as a means of preventing or delaying spoilage and disease was being developed as a basic principle. Ammonia refrigeration showed that perishable foods, including milk, would keep longer if stored cold, again an application from nature. These changes had significant effects on the availability of foods as well as on public health. Milk is one of the safest foods available today, but in the days before pasteurization and refrigeration drinking milk was quite hazardous.

The expanding knowledge of nutrition stimulated food technology in the

5. E. F. Binkerd and O. E. Kolari, "The History and Use of Nitrate and Nitrite in the Curing of Meat," *Food and Cosmetics Toxicology* 13 (1975): 655.

late nineteenth and early twentieth centuries. While Appert's canning process had been discovered in the early nineteenth century, it wasn't until the discoveries of Pasteur that the scientific basis for the canning process was understood. Understanding that food played an important role in both causing and preventing major human diseases, scientists worked to develop processing and preservation methods so food could be delivered more widely to more people.

The scientific literature of the time reflected these changes in nutrition and in food science and technology.[6] Food processing began to be taught in universities, especially those with a strong emphasis on dairy or meat production or horticulture. For example, at both Cornell University and the University of Wisconsin, S. M. Babcock began applying the best science of the times to problems with dairy-based foods. In 1890 he developed a simple test for the butterfat content of milk, giving the industry a quality test upon which the economic value of milk could be based. This is still the basis for milk value today. Dairy science was taught at Cornell University from its very founding in 1869, as it was at most land-grant institutions.

The ability to produce foods at one location and consume them at a distance was a major factor in urbanization. Before 1850 most dairy products were made in the home or on the farm. In 1851 a dairy farmer named Jesse Williams opened a commercial cheese manufacturing plant in upstate New York. Cheese was transported to New York City for sale. Following this commercial and technical success, plants for bottling milk and manufacturing butter and other dairy products soon followed, and the dairy processing industry developed.

Food was commonly adulterated for economic gain in both Europe and the United States in the 1800s.[7] Science, particularly chemistry, was used to counter adulteration and chemically to define food composition, food quality, nutritional values, and safety. Application of scientific methods accelerated in the latter portion of the nineteenth century; Harvey Wiley, a U.S. Department of Agriculture (USDA) chemist, led the way. Wiley campaigned against the common practice of adulterating foods and published a number of articles and pamphlets on the subject.[8] He was in part responsible for the passage of food laws and the establishment of the U.S. Food and Drug Administration which to this day has responsibility for preventing

6. M. S. Peterson and D. K. Tressler, *Food Technology the World Over* (Westport, Conn.: AVI Publishing Co., 1963).

7. (a) F. C. Accum, *A Treatise on the Adulteration of Food, Culinary Poisons, Etc* (London: Longman, Hurst, Rees, Orme, and Brown, 1820). (b) L. C. Beck, *Adulterations of Various Substances Used in Medicine and the Arts* (New York: Samuel S. and William Wood, 1846).

8. H. W. Wiley, *An Autobiography* (Indianapolis, Ind.: Bobbs-Merrill, 1930).

adulteration of foods in the United States.[9] Similar movements were under way in Canada and Europe at the same time.

C. Developments between 1900 and 1945

The first forty-five years of the twentieth century saw tremendous advances in mass manufacturing of goods. The production of foods in the United States and the developed world was part of this trend. Advances in science and engineering were rapidly integrated into food processing technology. At the turn of the century, pioneering scientists began to study the canning process intensely.[10] S. C. Prescott at the Massachusetts Institute of Technology (MIT) conducted classical studies on the relationship between heat input and the death rate of microorganisms.[11] Out of this work as well as that of subsequent researchers such as C. O. Ball, C. R. Stumbo, W. D. Bigelow, and A. C. Richardson, was born the theoretical basis for canning.[12] The canning process and an understanding of thermal death of heat-resistant spores have produced one of the safest and most reliable food processes known.

Other technological developments of the period rank on a par with canning. The introduction and rapid expansion of mechanical refrigeration both on a commercial scale and in home refrigerators and freezers in the first decades of the twentieth century provided great opportunities in food technology. In the nineteenth century beef cattle had to be shipped live to large cities. The combination of the railroad and the refrigerated rail car allowed slaughter to take place closer to where cattle were raised, and only carcasses were shipped.

The importance of freezing as a method of food preservation was recog-

9. O. Anderson, *The Health of a Nation; Harvey Wiley and the Fight for Pure Food* (Chicago: University of Chicago Press, 1958).

10. (a) S. A. Goldblith, "A Condensed History of the Science and Technology of Thermal Processing, Part 1," *Food Technology* 25 (1971): 1256–1262. (b) C. O. Ball and F. C. W. Olson, *Sterilization in Food Technology* (New York: McGraw Hill Book Co., 1957). (c) Marcus Karel, Owen R. Fennema, and Daryl B. Lund, *Physical Principles of Food Preservation* (New York and Basel; Marcel Dekker, Inc., 1975). (*Principles of Food Science*, ed. by Owen R. Fennema, Part II)

11. (a) S. C. Prescott and W. L. Underwood, "Micro-Organisms and Sterilizing Processes in the Canning Industries," *Technology Quarterly* 10 (1) (1897): 183. (b) S. C. Prescott and W. L. Underwood, "Micro-Organisms and Sterilizing Processes in the Canning Industries; II: The Souring of Canned Sweet Corn," *Technology Quarterly* 11 (1) (1898): 6.

12. (a) W. D. Bigelow, G. S. Bohart, A. C. Richardson, and C. O. Ball, *Heat Penetration in Processing Canned Food* (Washington, D.C.: National Canners Association, 1920 [Research Laboratory, *Bulletin* no. 16–L]), 128 pp. (b) W. D. Bigelow and J. R. Esty, "The Thermal Death Point in Relation to Time of Typical Thermophilic Organisms," *Journal of Infectious Diseases* 27 (1920): 602–617.

nized in the early part of the twentieth century by an entrepreneur named Clarence Birdseye who, on the basis of experience in Canada, developed a process for freezing fish. A commercial operation was begun and became so successful that it was later sold to General Foods. The technology was rapidly expanded to other foods including meats, fruits, and vegetables. Several researchers including J. G. Woodroof and A. L. Arighi investigated the scientific basis of preservation by freezing during this period, and several scientific publications and texts appeared.[13]

In the 1800s most foods in commerce were shipped and sold in bulk form, often in wooden barrels. The first portion of the twentieth century saw the expansion of packaging in containers intended for direct sales to consumers, led by bottling of milk and canning of foods.[14] In the last years of the nineteenth century, the National Biscuit Company (later to become Nabisco) introduced Uneeda Biscuit in paperboard cartons. Other products were sold in "tins." Packaging gave foods protection during shipment and long shelf life, as well as allowing processing automation. Economic and technical ties formed between the packaging and food industries continue today.

In the latter half of the nineteenth century, the U.S. Congress established the state land-grant university system administered through the U.S. Department of Agriculture. Institutions began producing literature that mostly dealt with agricultural production on farms and ranches. In the first part of the twentieth century, the USDA and the land-grant schools began to recognize the importance of food processing and manufacture. A number of significant publications were produced by the university experiment stations which dealt with the theory and practice of food preservation and processing.[15]

The role of state and federal governments in assuring plentiful and safe food and preventing food fraud was rapidly expanded during the first half of the twentieth century. The first law in the United States intended to prevent adulteration was enacted in 1785 but it wasn't until the Pure Food and Drug Act of 1902 that the federal government began promulgating regulations.[16]

13. (a) J. G. Woodroof, *Microscopic Studies of Frozen Fruit and Vegetables* (Griffin, GA: Georgia Agriculture Experiment Station, 1938) [Bulletin no. 201]) 46 pp. (b) A. L. Arighi, M. A. Joslyn, and G. L. Marsh, "Enzyme Activity in Frozen Pack Vegetables" *Industrial & Engineering Chemistry* 28 (1936): 595–598.

14. T. W. Downes, "Food Packaging in the IFT Era: Five Decades of Unprecedented Growth and Change," *Food Technology* 43 (9) (1989): 228–240.

15. (a) Bigelow et al., *Heat Penetration in Processing Canned Food.* (b) H. L. Russell, *Gaseous Fermentation in the Canning Industry* (Wisconsin Agricultural Experiment Station, 1895 [12th Annual Report]. p.227.

16. R. D. Middlekauff, "Regulating the Safety of Food," *Food Technology* 43 (9) (1989): 296–307.

In 1927 the Food, Drug, and Insecticide Administration (renamed Food and Drug Administration in 1931) was formed within the USDA but later transferred to what is now the Department of Health and Human Services.[17] Regulating food composition and safety requires defining composition, and so considerable research and literature has resulted from government regulation.[18] The USDA since its inception in 1862 has had responsibility for promoting agriculture and food production. From its earliest days, USDA published broadly on food production, processing, and technology often in pamphlets or booklets (see data about government publications in Chapter 8 and Figure 8.2).

Several scientific organizations focusing on agriculture and food production were founded in the early part of the twentieth century, among them the Association of Official Analytical Chemists, the American Society of Cereal Chemists, the American Society of Agricultural Engineers, the American Dairy Science Association, and the Poultry Science Association. The Agricultural and Food Chemistry Division of the American Chemical Society was founded in 1908. These organizations had a significant effect on the development of the literature in food science and technology through their numerous journals, many of which continue today. Although the main focus of these organizations was on agricultural production, scientific papers and publications were also directed at products and processes.

Research on food science and its resulting literature were greatly expanded between 1920 and 1942. Scientific journals directed specifically at food science and agriculture were introduced; many of these journals still exist.

The founding of the Institute of Food Technologists (IFT) in 1939 stands as a watershed event in food science and technology.[19] Its beginnings can be traced back to the vision of a few people in the 1930s.[20] A conference on food technology organized by S. C. Prescott at MIT in 1937 was successful in bringing together 500 people with interests in food science and technology for the first time. A second meeting was organized by G. J. Hucker at the New York State Agricultural Experiment Station at Geneva. At this meeting the possibility of forming an organization dedicated to research in food science was explored, and a recommendation was brought before the

17. P. B. Hutt, "Development and Growth of the Food and Drug Administration," *Food Technology* 43 (9) (1989): 280–286.

18. P. B. Hutt, "Regulating the Misbranding of Food," *Food Technology* 43 (9) (1989): 288–295.

19. N. H. Mermelstein, "History of the Institute of Food Technologists: The First 50 Years," *Food Technology* 43 (1989): 14–16, 18, 30–32, 44–52.

20. R. L. Hall, "Pioneers in Food Science and Technology: Giants in the Earth," *Food Technology* 43 (9) (1989): 186–195.

600 attendees at the second conference at MIT in 1939. The group approved, and the IFT was created. The organization has grown to a membership of 25,000, and publishes a research journal (*Journal of Food Science*) and a more general main publication (*Food Technology*). Similar organizations have been formed elsewhere, including those in Canada, Australia, Mexico, Europe, and India. In all, there are nineteen IFT affiliate organizations around the world, fifty-five regional sections, and thirteen subject divisions with specific interests in food science and technology. Each of these organizations has promoted publications and held symposia which have been the basis for many monographs of significance.

A major impact on the literature of food science has been the teaching of agricultural chemistry and food science as disciplines, mostly, but not exclusively in land-grant universities.[21] Soon after their inception after 1862, several land-grant universities set up food-related departments, often aligned with a specific agricultural commodity such as meat, poultry, cereal, or dairy products, which would not be considered food science departments by today's definition. In the early part of this century, these commodity-based departments began to give way to broader programs with food science as a discipline; a trend that continues. The Institute of Food Science at Cornell University, which today encompasses two Food Science departments as well as faculty in other related fields had its start as part of general studies in agriculture in 1869. At the turn of the century it became the Department of Dairy Industry, and was so called until the 1960s when the name was changed to Food Science in recognition of its expanded role.

Four U.S. academic departments stand out as pioneers in the development of food science as a discipline early in the twentieth century. W. W. Chenowith, a faculty member in horticultural science at the University of Massachusetts, developed food processing courses in 1913. In 1926 the program was expanded when C. Fellers joined it which eventually led to the formation of a department. At about the same time, E. H. Wiegand at Oregon State University, who like Chenowith came from a horticulture department, established courses in fruit and vegetable processing which later became the department of food science. Both departments celebrated 75th anniversaries in 1993. About the same time, W. V. Cruess established food processing as part of the department of viticulture and enology in the College of Agriculture at the University of California, Berkeley. This later became food science and was transferred to the Davis campus. S. C. Prescott established the beginnings of food processing at MIT in 1913. Food

21. O. Fennema, "Education Programs in Food Science: A Continuing Struggle for Legitimacy, Respect, and Recognition," *Food Technology* 43 (1989): 170– 182.

science as a discipline was also being developed at the same time in Canada and Europe.

These four departments as well as programs at other universities had an early and strong influence on the literature of food science. Texts were required for courses as well as for practitioners in the industry, and while outdated, they still stand as pioneering efforts. Today there are sixty-nine institutions offering educational programs in food science, forty-two that meet IFT minimum standards.[22] These food science programs awarded over 800 undergraduate and graduate degrees in food science in 1985.

D. Selected Developments since 1945

Since World War II there has been a rapid and expanded application of science and technology to food production and processing.[23] The number of technological changes in food processing in the last five decades have perhaps been surpassed only by those in electronics. The changes have been led by innovations in the way foods are packaged and the integration of food processing and packaging.[24] Before 1945 packaging materials were largely limited to metal cans, glass jars, paperboard cartons, and cellophane wraps. Nearly all packages were made of single materials whose major function was to simply contain products. Packaging now must not only contain and preserve, but help prepare or use products, act as a marketing tool, increase convenience, and help process products. Combinations of dissimilar materials such as metal foils, plastics, and paper are common.

Perhaps the most innovative creation was aseptic packaging, using flexible materials developed by Tetra Pak of Sweden after World War II. This system integrated ultra-high temperature in the continuous thermal processing of liquids with a process that sterilized flexible packaging materials, formed those materials into packages, and filled and sealed the cartons without recontamination. This meant that perishable liquid products such as milk could be stored without refrigeration for several months. Aseptic packaging is an integration of food processing and packaging. This technology was declared by IFT to be the most significant food science innovation between 1939 and 1989.[25] The process deserves recognition for its contribu-

22. Ibid.

23. See S. A. Goldblith, "Fifty Years of Progress in Food Science and Technology: From Art Based on Experience to Technology Based on Science," *Food Technology* 43 (9) (1989): 88–107 & 286.

24. Downes, "Food Packaging in the IFT Era: Five Decades of Unprecedented Growth and Change."

25. IFT Staff Report, "Top 10 Food Science Innovations, 1939–1989," *Food Technology* 43 (9) (1989): 308.

tion to human nutrition since it has brought milk to many places where it was not available because of a lack of refrigeration.

The development of the microwave oven for commercial and home use has also spurred a considerable number of commercial innovations in food processing and packaging. Plastics which have sufficient barriers to protect foods for months at ambient temperatures yet are stable enough to be used in heating foods in microwave ovens are one product of this revolution. The commercial development of packaging materials which convert microwave energy into direct heat (susceptors) allowed the expansion of the microwave oven for use with new products.

Reducing the weight of glass and metal in packaging assured their continued use in spite of their large energy demands. New flexible materials such as metalized polypropylene, Saran, and EVOH which have high water vapor and oxygen barriers, have transformed entire industries such as the snack food business. Before such materials were introduced in the 1970s and 1980s, snack food manufactures had to be close to their markets because product shelf life was too short for long distance distribution. Increased shelf life meant that regional plants could be consolidated. The incorporation of barrier plastics into plastic bottles allowed many oxygen-sensitive products to be packaged in plastic containers.

Controlled atmosphere storage and modified atmosphere packaging have also been significant innovations. In the former technology, respiring fruit and vegetables are stored in warehouses in which the oxygen content has been lowered and the carbon dioxide raised. This slows the respiration of the produce and extends shelf life from weeks to months. A similar idea has been brought to distribution and consumer packaging. The atmosphere inside a package can likewise be altered to extend shelf life.

The challenge to packaging in the 1990s is to reduce the amount of materials used in order to reduce solid waste. Achieving this will require more innovation on the part of food processors and packaging manufacturers.

Further innovations in refrigeration and freezing have occurred. The introduction in the 1950s of whole frozen meals including TV dinners led the way to many new types of frozen foods. This trend continues along with improvements in the freezing process which provide a higher quality of frozen foods.

Other innovations in food processing have affected the U.S. diet.[26] For example, the ability to freeze orange juice concentrate has greatly affected juice consumption. The per capita consumption of orange juice in 1948 was about one glass per person per year. Now it's one glass per person every

26. See D. Lund, "Food Processing: From Art to Engineering," *Food Technology* 43 (9) (1989): 242–246.

other day. Aseptic packaging, which gained approval in the United States in 1981, has also greatly increased juice consumption. The use of membrane-based filter systems to separate even molecular components of foods is another innovation. The expanding use of microcomputers for process control and increased energy efficiency provides further examples of innovation in food processing.

New concepts and information in nutrition have led to substantial changes in food science and technology.[27] Several foods such as milk, flour, and salt are now fortified with specific nutrients.[28] This has nearly eradicated deficiency diseases in the United States. More recently, advances in knowledge about the role of diet in chronic diseases such as cancer and heart disease have led to changes in foods.[29] Interest in nutrition and chronic disease has led to new laws regulating food labeling. These laws have been enacted for the purpose of better informing consumers about the nutritional content of foods.

The desire to reduce the caloric content of the diet, principally by reducing fat and sugar consumption, has led to considerable innovation in ingredient technology. High intensity sweeteners with few or no calories have been developed. Particularly interesting are the current technological efforts to reduce the fat content of the diet while maintaining many of the desirable attributes of fats in foods. This has led to the development of many food substances that mimic fats. Food additives which inhibit chemical and biological deterioration have contributed to the quality and availability foods. These and other developments have brought food science and nutrition closer as complementary disciplines.

Concern for the safety of foods has also heightened during this period.[30] Scientists have come to understand that foods can have both positive and negative impacts on human health. The risks to health associated with foods can be classified as of microbial origin or stemming from naturally occurring toxicants, food contaminants, or intentional additives. There has been

27. See J. W. Erdman, "Nutrition: Past, Present and Future," *Food Technology* 43 (9) (1989): 220–227.

28. (a) American Medical Association, "The Mineralization and Vitaminization of Milk," *JAMA* 101 (1933): 1728. (b) M. C. Latham, "Nutritional Problems and Deficiency Diseases: General Principles," in G. T Strickland, ed., *Hunter's Tropical Medicine,* 7th ed. (Philadelphia: W. B. Saunders Co., 1991), pp. 911–914.

29. Catherine E. Woteki and Paul R. Thomas, ed. *Eat for Life: The Food and Nutrition Board's Guide to Reducing Your Risk of Chronic Disease* (Washington, D.C.: National Academy Press, 1992).

30. See R. L. Hall and S. L. Taylor, "Food Toxicology and Safety Evaluation: Changing Perspectives and a Challenge for the Future," *Food Technology* 43 (9) (1989): 270–279.

intense public debate over the last two decades about the size and severity of each of these risks. Often the public and regulatory agencies have demanded changes in the way foods are processed, treated, handled, or sold. Food safety has become a subdiscipline of food science with its own literature.

New basic disciplines have been applied to foods since the 1940s. For example, food scientists have drawn on statistics, psychology, and other cognitive sciences to understand how people perceive foods. This area of food science has become known as "sensory science." It is concerned with measuring responses to food taste, aroma, and appearance. Closely related is the study of food texture from a physical viewpoint as well as a sensory one.[31]

All of these changes have been reflected in an explosion in the literature of food science which can be seen by searching electronic bibliographic databases. *Current Contents* online (1990–1993) lists 33,805 records under "food or foods;" and *Food Science & Technology Abstracts*, 71,317. *AGRICOLA* retrieves 1,249 records for 1992 alone. These numbers are no doubt only a small portion of the literature in food science and technology since most articles and monographs would not be indexed by these simple keywords. For details on the size of literature output in food science see Chapter 3. S. A. Goldblith lists sixty-six "major" books in food science and technology published between 1939 and 1989.[32]

In those parts of the world where food is readily available, concerns are mostly about nutrition, safety, convenience, and enjoyment.[33] Unfortunately, food is not available in sufficient amounts for much of the world, and there the number one concern is the prevention of starvation and of nutrition-related diseases. Many parts of the world have not fully benefitted from food processing and preservation. It remains a major human challenge to supply adequate diet to all humans. Food science has provided much of the technology but this technology requires capital which is not available in all parts of the world.[34]

31. For a review of the major books in sensory science, see R. M. Pangborn, "The Evolution of Sensory Science and Its Interactions with IFT," *Food Technology* 43 (9) (1989): 248–256.

32. Goldblith, "Fifty Years of Progress in Food Science and Technology."

33. See F. M. Clydesdale, "Present and Future of Food Science and Technology in Industrialized Countries," *Food Technology* 43 (9) (1989): 134–144, 146.

34. See (a) R. Bressani, "Food Science and Technology in Developing Countries during the Past 50 Years," *Food Technology* 43 (9) (1989): 108–132. (b) G. F. Stewart and M. A. Amerine, *Introduction to Food Science and Technology* (New York, Longon: Academic Press, 1973).

E. Future Developments

Perusal of the current literature in food science suggests that the application of science and engineering to food and food processing will accelerate in the next two decades. Among the technologies which can be forecast from the literature are the application of biotechnology to food production and food ingredients.[35] For example, enzymes important in food processing or fermentation can be produced inexpensively in quantity by recombinant DNA technologies. Natural flavors can be enhanced by growing recombinant plant cultures. Biotechnology will also be increasingly used in detecting pathogenic microorganism in foods and food processing environments. Related initiatives in detecting pesticides and other contaminants in foods will also lead to increased food safety. Advances in the use of bio-electronic sensors will allow their use in monitoring food quality during processing as well as storage. Ionizing radiation, while still controversial, will find appropriate uses especially when combined with other technologies. Irradiation can, for example, inhibit the sprouting of fresh produce, thereby increasing shelf life. It can also be combined with modified atmosphere packaging to extend the shelf life and increase the safety of perishable foods. Aseptic systems to process particulate foods in a manner similar to the current liquid systems will find regulatory approval. This will lead to new combinations of products and packages and canned foods with improved quality. Further innovations in packaging, such as the use of molecule-thick coatings of glass on plastic flexible films to improve barrier properties, are currently being developed by the Japanese.

These and unforseen changes will be developed and documented. The challenge for both the food scientist and those responsible for making such literature available is to not be overwhelmed by the sheer mass of knowledge that will be published over the next two decades. Clearly the current system will not be able to deal with this mass of information, and changes in the way information is handled must be worked out.

35. S. Harlander, "Biotechnology: Yesterday, Today, and Tomorrow," *Food Technology* 43 (9) (1989): 196–206.

2. Knowledge and Changing Concerns in Human Nutrition

DAPHNE A. ROE*

Nutritional Sciences, Cornell University

*deceased 1993

Human nutrition, as a subject area, includes nutritional biochemistry, nutritional physiology, nutritional epidemiology, sociocultural aspects of eating behavior, dietetics, public health nutrition, clinical nutrition, and nutrition education.

In order to show how and why ideas and concerns about human nutrition have emerged since 1950, it is necessary to review earlier history. Here, earlier contributions of physiologists and of chemists are of special interest. Linkages between nutrition and public health also need to be examined in a longer historical context.

A. Major Developments, 1830 to 1950

From 1830 to 1900, anecdotal information on human nutrition was replaced with information obtained through scientific observation and experimentation. During this period, there were major advances in the knowledge of gastrointestinal function, of nutritional physiology, and of the need for food as an energy source. Also during these years, it was realized for the first time that specific diseases were clearly linked to diet and poverty.

The most important writings documenting this new information were those of William Beaumont who described changes taking place in the stomach in response to food consumption and changes in intestinal motility in response to dietary change,[1] and those of Claude Bernard who discovered the role of the liver in nutrient metabolism.[2] Later physiologists, working in

1. W. M. Beaumont, *Experiments and Observations on the Gastric Juice and the Physiology of Digestion* (Plattsburgh, N.Y.: F. P. Allen, 1833).

2. Claude Bernard, "Mémoire su le Pancréas, et sur le Role du Suc Pancréatique dans les Phénomènes Digestifs," *Supplément aux Comptes Rendus Hebdomadaires des Séances de l'Académie des Sciences* 1 (1856): 379–563.

England and France during the second half of the nineteenth century, contributed to basic knowledge of nutrition by defining the need for calories as well as nitrogen, during periods of adequate food intake as well as during starvation.

Those who made major discoveries in nutrition during the nineteenth century were either chemists, physiologists, or physicians. The science of physiological chemistry, or what we now call biochemistry, developed very largely as a result of the work of nineteenth-century German scientists. These included Karl Ludwig in Liepzig and Carl Voit and Max Rubner in Munich, who established centers of graduate and postgraduate training. These centers of learning attracted future nutritional scientists from the United States and from countries in Europe. It was largely in these centers that physiologists developed an understanding of human energy requirements and their measurement. It was also in these centers that German scientists realized the ability to analyze food and to study the composition of animal tissues. They then imparted their knowledge to their international graduate students. Several of the scientists who were trained in Germany established new centers for the education of nutritional scientists and nutrition research centers after returning to their own countries.

Pioneers in nutrition who were trained in Germany prior to 1900 include Lafayette Mendel, who subsequently developed the Sheffield School at Yale University as a research center for nutrition, and Charles Martin, who was responsible for the development of the Lister Institute in London. Others who were trained as physiologists in Germany include Ivan Pavlov, who later showed the importance of sensory inputs in the control of hunger, and Russell Chittenden, who later studied human protein requirements.

Within the first seventy years after human nutrition became established as a worthy area of scientific enquiry, caloric sources were defined, caloric needs were measured, and both the digestion of food and the absorption of nutrients were studied.

Between 1900 and 1950 researchers discovered vitamins, isolated them, determined their chemical structures, and demonstrated the relationships between these structures and biological activity. Progress in this area came about both from animal experiments and from the observation that individuals and populations who subsisted on cereal diets developed diseases that could be prevented and cured by dietary means. The recognition that laboratory animals required essential dietary factors other than protein, carbohydrate, fat and minerals for growth, health, and survival was largely due to the work of E. V. McCollum. In his book *The Newer Knowledge of Nutrition* (1918), however, McCollum acknowledges that he was influenced by the earlier work of Frederick Gowland Hopkins, who had demonstrated a need for "accessory food factors" in his studies of the effects of feeding purified diets.

Both before and after the work of Hopkins and McCollum, observations made it clear that human populations developed diseases when fed certain cereal-based diets. For example, the disease beri-beri was shown to occur in prisoners fed only a diet of polished rice. Once it was realized that such diets were somehow inadequate, studies were initiated to determine which foods contained preventive factors. These studies were then followed by chemical analyses aimed at isolating and characterizing the preventive factors. Casimir Funk, who successfully extracted an accessory food factor from rice polishings and from yeast, coined the term *vitamine* to describe these essential food factors. Another researcher whose discoveries contributed to our understanding of diseases caused by diets lacking in these essential nutrients was Conrad Eijkman, who advanced our knowledge of endemic beri-beri, a disease which was subsequently found to be due to vitamin B_1 (thiamin) deficiency.

Interestingly, eradication of nutritional deficiencies was successfully carried out by improvement in the diet of impoverished populations long before it became possible to cure such diseases by distribution of specific nutrients. Later, the idea of food fortification was developed and successfully put into practice to prevent goiter, associated with iodine deficiency. Bread and flour were fortified with B vitamins to prevent pellagra and deficiency of the vitamin riboflavin. This was also the first period in which nutritionists and economists cooperated for the purpose of solving the social causes of a nutritional deficiency disease. The great example of this cooperation was the work of Joseph Goldberger and Edgar Sydenstricker, who demonstrated that pellagra was caused not by eating moldy corn, as previously thought, but rather by consuming a sharecropper's meager rations, which lacked animal protein. It was also during this period that an international organization, the League of Nations, first developed a nutrition policy.[3]

Experiments carried out during the first forty years of this century resulted in the identification of both water- and fat-soluble vitamins. In 1912 Funk was successful in isolating an antineuritic fraction from rice polishings, later shown to contain the water-soluble vitamin B_1 (thiamin). In the following thirty years many of the other B vitamins were isolated. The properties of these vitamins were first isolated in crude extracts and later in

3. (a) Daphne A. Roe, *A Plague of Corn: The Social History of Pellagra* (Ithaca, N.Y.: Cornell University Press, 1973). (b) League of Nations, *The Problem of Nutrition*; *Vol 3, Nutrition in Various Countries (Series of League of Nations Publications*, 1936), pp. 17–68.

the purified preparations. Those contributing to our knowledge of the fat-soluble vitamins during this period include McCollum, E. Mellanby,[4] and M. Mellanby,[5] all in the United Kingdom.

Notable developments in nutritional science came from physiologists interested in the basic science of nutrition and from home economists and physicians interested in relationships between food consumption and human health. Publications which reflect a new ability of nutritionists to use findings of animal experiments to advise on human diets include McCollum's *The Newer Knowledge of Nutrition*, previously mentioned.

The basic science advances of the period include the ability to measure human energy expenditure, development of animal models with which to study nutritional physiology and the effects of nutritional deficiencies, the isolation of vitamins and the identification of their biochemical functions, new knowledge of the biochemical cause of diet-related diseases such as diabetes, and recognition that pathological states can be induced by nutrient excess as well as by deficiency.

Advances in Nutrition in Third World Countries Prior to 1950

Before 1950 studies in Third World countries focused on the differentiation of types of malnutrition in children. Pioneers include Cecily Williams, who described "kwashiorkor," a type of infant and early-childhood malnutrition associated with swelling of the face, reddish discoloration of the hair, and apathy. She recognized that this disease was a condition of children displaced from the breast and deprived of an alternate source of nourishment. Another form of malnutrition described during this period is beri-beri, observed in the Dutch East Indies. An anemia seen in pregnant women in Bombay was characterized by Lucy Wills as a macrocytic (large red cell) anemia, related to the consumption of cereal-based diets deficient in greens and meats. Later it was shown that this macrocytic anemia is caused by a deficiency of folic acid, normally obtained from dark green leafy vegetables.[6]

4. (a) Edward Mellanby, "The Part Played by an Accessory Factor in the Production of Experimental Rickets," *Journal of Physiology* 52 (1918): 11–12. (b) Edward Mellanby, *Experimental Rickets* (London: HMSO, 1921 [Medical Research Council Special Report no. 61]). (c) Edward Mellanby, *A Story of Nutritional Research: The Effect of Some Dietary Factors on Bones and the Nervous System* (Baltimore: Williams & Wilkins, 1950).

5. May Mellanby, *Diet and the Teeth III: The Effect of Diet and Dental Structure and Disease in Man* (London: HMSO, 1934 [Medical Research Council Special Report Series no. 191]).

6. (a) C. D. Williams, "Kwashiorkor, A Nutritional Disease of Children Associated with a Maize Diet," *Lancet* 2 (1935): 1151–1152. (b) C. Funk, "The Etiology of the Deficiency Diseases: Beri-Beri, Polyneuritis in Birds, Epidemic Dropsy, Scurvy, Experimental Scurvy in Animals, Infantile Scurvy, Ship Beri-Beri, Pellagra," *Journal of State Medicine* 20 (1912): 341–344. (c) L.

Another area of interest and progress was the identification of natural food toxins which cause fatalities. Although the toxic potential of certain plants and plant parasites was now recognized, uneducated and indigenous people in the Third World continued to believe that endemic food poisoning was a punishment from angry divine beings.[7]

B. Major Developments in Nutrition Knowledge since 1950

Linkages between Nutrition and Chronic Disease

Today, when people think about the relationship between nutrition and disease, the diseases which come to mind are the degenerative ones, such as coronary heart disease, hypertension, and maturity-onset diabetes. However, the relationship between nutrition and disease also includes the chronic diseases occurring in early life, which often have a genetic basis.

A connection between diet and these diseases was first made in the 1950s when two Dutch students, W. K. Dicke and Henri A. Weijers, presented a thesis and subsequently jointly published a report showing that intake of wheat flour aggravates celiac disease.[8] Not only were their findings subsequently confirmed, it was demonstrated that all sources of gluten have this effect and that the protein present in these foods, gliadin, triggers changes in the small bowel leading to nutrient malabsorption. The significance of these studies is that a disease which up to that time had led to malnutrition, stunting of growth, chronic anemia, and death in childhood became a condition which could be fully controlled by maintenance of a gluten-free diet.[9]

The 1950s and early 1960s were also the time when it became possible to use dietary measures to prevent the severe mental retardation associated with genetically determined diseases, such as phenylketonuria and galactosemia.[10]

Wills and M. M. Mehta, "Studies in Pernicious Anemia of Pregnancy," Part I "Preliminary Report," *Indian Journal of Medical Research* 30 (17) (1929): 777–779.

7. A. Van Veen, "Toxic Properties of Some Unusual Foods," in *Toxicants Occurring Naturally in Foods* (Washington D.C.: National Academy of Science/NRC, 1966), pp. 174–182.

8. (a) W. K. Dicke, *Investigation of the Harmful Effects of Certain Types of Cereal on Patients with Celiac Disease* (Utrecht: Thesis, 1950). (b) W. K. Dicke, H. A. Weijers, and J. H. Kamer, "Coeliac Disease," I, "Criticism of the Various Methods of Investigation," II, "The Presence in Wheat of a Factor Having a Deleterious Effect in Cases of Coeliac Disease," *Acta Paediatrica* 42 (1953): 24–42.

9. R. H. Barnes, "The Wheat Protein Effect in Celiac Disease," *New York State Journal of Medicine* 58 (1958): 1926–1927.

10. (a) M. D. Armstrong and F. H. Tyler, "Studies on Phenylketonuria," Part I, "Restricted Phenylalanine Intake in Phenylketonuria," *Journal of Clinical Investigation* 34 (1955): 565–568. (b) D. Y Hsia, *Inborn Errors of Metabolism*, 2d ed., Part I, *Clinical Aspects* (Chicago: Year Book Medical Publisher, 1966). pp. 180–184.

Since 1950, major changes in emphasis and concern in human nutrition have included a new awareness of diseases linked to caloric and nutrient excess and the development of new interventions aimed to get people to adopt a diet which is less likely to lead to chronic disease and premature mortality. Advances in this area are explained by changes in the age structure of the population, with a greater proportion being in an older age group, and the cost of health care associated with effects of diet-related diseases.

The relationship between heart disease and the intake of fats and cholesterol is another example of the linkage between diet and chronic disease. Interest in this subject first arose in the period before 1950. In 1910 A. Windaus reported a finding he obtained from the chemical analysis of cadavers: the cholesterol content of aortas with the pathology of atherosclerosis was higher than that of aortas without atherosclerotic changes. Anitschkoff subsequently demostrated that atherosclerotic lesions could be produced in rabbits by feeding them cholesterol. In the 1950s more interest was generated in the role of cholesterol in the development of atherosclerosis when it was recognized that the process of atherogenesis (that is, the development of plaques of cholesterol-laden cells in the walls of arteries) was the precursor lesion for later coronary artery blockage.[11] The knowledge that coronary arteries blocked with cholesterol-laden plaques are associated with heart attacks led the way to the development of drugs that inhibit cholesterol synthesis. Earliest of the released drugs was triparanol. This was initially heralded as a product with the capacity to reduce the risk of cardiovascular disease. The side effects of this drug necessitated its withdrawal, however. Following this initial therapeutic failure, research proceeded more cautiously. The aim was to produce a drug that would lower the risk of cholesterol deposition in arteries while producing fewer and more tolerable side effects.[12]

Epidemiological evidence showed associations between high-fat, high-cholesterol diets and coronary heart disease and between high intake of saturated fat and cardiovascular risk.[13] Public health recommendations for reduction of dietary fat, saturated fat, and cholesterol began in the 1970s. The evidence that a fat-controlled diet would be beneficial was discussed at

11. S. M. Grundy, *Lipids and Cardiovascular Disease* (Bethesda, Md.: LSRO/Federation of American Societies for Experimental Biology, 1991 [FDA Contract no. 223-88-2124. Task Order 9]), pp. 1–38.

12. J. Avigan, D. Steinberg, H. E. Vroman, M. J. Thompson, and E. Mosettig, "Studies of Cholesterol Biosynthesis: The Esterification of Desmosterol in Serum and Tissues of Animals Treated with MER-29," *Journal of Biological Chemistry* 235 (1960): 3123–3126.

13. *Surgeon General's Report on Nutrition and Health* (Washington, D.C.: U.S. Government Printing Office, 1988 [US DHHS Publ (PHS) no. 88–50210]), pp. 1–20.

the 1981 International Congress on Nutrition.[14] The advice that people reduce their fat and cholesterol intake has since been given national recognition in the *Surgeon General's Report on Nutrition and Health* of 1988, in *Dietary Guidelines for Americans*, and in *Diet and Health*, a 1989 publication by members of the Food and Nutrition Board of the National Academy of Sciences.[15]

Throughout the 1960s and 1970s attention was given to the chronic disease risks related to consumption of a low-fiber diet. A number of chronic diseases including constipation, diverticulitis, and bowel cancer were found to be more common in industrialized countries, where people have low-fiber diets, than in Third World countries, where people eat more high-fiber foods. Denis Burkitt concluded that fiber in the diet has a protective effect.[16] Interestingly enough, this was a revival of an idea promulgated in the 1830s by the great physiologist William Beaumont, that ingestion of "innutritious substance" is essential to human health and freedom from chronic disease. In the early 1970s H. C. Trowell defined fiber in the diet as "the skeletal remains of plant cells that are resistant to digestion by enzymes of man."[17] Later bran became the term for the fiber that Burkitt had extolled as a preventive of constipation and other gastrointestinal problems including diverticular disease.[18] In the 1980s physicians and nutritionists became interested in other plant materials originally classified as fiber, including pectins and gums, as bulking agents. Psyllium gum became popular as a substance that would induce early satiety and therefore reduce appetite in the obese. It is now also widely recommended as a treatment of constipation. The brans, on the other hand, have gained a new popularity as a means of reducing blood cholesterol levels. Oat bran is more sought after than others because it seems to have a special efficacy in lowering blood cholesterol levels. It is dubious whether all the claims about the health advantages of fiber can be substantiated. Right or wrong, the advocates of fiber and its proponents in the food industry have convinced much of the public, especially the middle class public, that their health will be improved if they eat bran muffins and bran breakfast cereals.

14. S. B. Hulley, "Diet-Heart Policy: Tailoring to Individual Needs;" in A. E. Harper and G. K. Davis, eds., *Nutrition in Health and Disease and International Development: Symposium of the XII International Congress on Nutrition* (New York: Alan R. Liss Inc., 1981).

15. *Diet and Health: Implications for Reducing Chronic Disease Risk* (Washington, D.C.: National Academy Press, 1989).

16. D. P. Burkitt, A. R. P. Walker, and N. S. Painter, "Effect of Dietary Fibre on Stools and Transit Times and Its Role in the Causation of Disease," *Lancet* 2 (1972): 1408–1410.

17. (a) H. C. Trowell, "Guide Fibre, Dietary Fibre and Atherosclerosis," *Atherosclerosis* 16 (1972): 138. (b) H. C. Trowell, "Definitions of Fibre," *Lancet* 1 (7856) (1974): 503.

18. J. H. Cummings, "What Is Fiber," in G. A. Spiller and R. J. Amen, eds., *Fiber in Human Nutrition* (New York: Plenum Press, 1976), pp. 1–30.

The basic chemical studies of fiber sources and the roles of different fiber sources in human health as perceived in the 1970s are well described in the 1976 book *Fiber in Human Nutrition*.

Other linkages between diet and the development of chronic disease have been emphasized more recently. These include the role of mutagens, formed in meats by processing and broiling, as potential causal factors in the development of bowel cancer. *Diet, Nutrition and Cancer*, the proceedings of a meeting on dietary factors and cancer risk, stresses the innovative approach of linking basic research to policy decisions.[19] Since 1980 other studies have shown that a high-fat diet leads to a higher risk of cancer and that the carotenoids (yellow-orange pigments in yellow and dark green vegetables) help protect against lung and bowel cancer.[20]

Studies of the association between obesity and chronic disease have been carried out since the 1970s. It has become increasingly evident that obesity is a risk factor for non-insulin-dependent diabetes as well as hypertension.[21] Critical discussions of the associations between diet and chronic disease are found in the 1989 book *Diet and Health.* A series of monographs commissioned by the Food and Drug Administration in connection with food-labeling claims convey current knowledge about the linkages between diet and disease, including findings from animal and human studies.[22]

Most recently, diets that lack certain antioxidant nutrients including vitamin C, vitamin, E and the carotenoids have been considered particularly undesirable relative to the risk of heart disease and cancer.[23] Diets that lack yellow, orange and dark green vegetables and orange fruits are deficient in carotenoids; diets lacking fruits and vegetables, including potatoes, are deficient in vitamin C. Extensive studies of the need for antioxidant nutrients made since the mid 1980s have demonstrated that carotenoids and vitamin E stimulate immune function and that the carotenoids additionally possess cancer-protective properties.

19. P. B. McCay, "Dietary Fat and Cancer: An Overview," in D. A. Roe, ed., *Diet, Nutrition and Cancer: From Basic Research to Policy Implications* (New York: Alan R. Liss Inc., 1983).

20. (a) K. K. Carroll, *Lipids and Cancer* (Bethesda, Md., 1991 [LSRO/Federation of American Societies for Experimental Biology FDA Contract No.223-88-124]), pp. 1–29. (b) N. V. Dimitrov, "Beta-Carotene: Biological Properties and Applications," in J. Bland, ed., *A Year in Nutritional Medicine* (New Canaan, Conn.: Keats Publishing Inc., 1986), pp. 167–202.

21. (a) H. Keen, and J. M. Ekoe, "The Geography of Diabetes Mellitus," *British Medical Bulletin* 40 (1984): 359–365. (b) E. R. Buskirk and S. Puhl, "Adipose Tissue Distribution and Metabolic Consequences," in O. A. Levander, ed., *AIN Symposium Proceedings on Nutrition* (Rockville, Md.: AIN, 1987), pp. 97–102.

22. *Evaluation of Publicly Available Scientific Evidence Regarding Certain Nutrient-Disease Relationships* (Bethesda, Md.: LSRO/Federation of American Societies for Experimental Biology, 1991 [FDA Contract no. 223-88-2124]).

23. L. J. Machlin, "Protective Role of Vitamins against Free Radical Tissue Damage," in Levander, *AIN Symposium*, pp. 51–54.

Dietary, Lifestyle, and Health Interventions Designed to Prevent Degenerative Conditions

Since 1950 there has been a new emphasis on interventive programs designed to improve public health and to retard degenerative processes linked to aging. Major effort has been put into educating the public about how to decrease the risk of chronic health problems by making changes in both diet and lifestyle. In attempts to apply research findings to the betterment of public health, nutritional scientists have promoted increased calcium intake as a means to decrease the risk of osteoporosis, exercise and low-fat diets to lower the risk of cardiovascular disease, reduction in sugar intake to lower calories and cancer risk, fluoridation of water supplies and preventive dentistry to prevent caries, and reduced intake of laxatives and antacids to prevent risks of drug-induced malnutrition.[24] Their efforts have been supported by United States federal agencies including the National Institutes of Health, by British and European funding agencies, and by such industry-based organizations as the National Dairy Council in the United States. Outcomes of such programs indicate a differential acceptance by the public. Those who consider health maintenance a priority and who are better educated have made more dietary and lifestyle changes than those who believe that their health destiny will remain unchanged, no matter what modifications they make. The inequalities of health status and nutritional status in the United Kingdom and the United States and the underlying social, economic, and cultural explanations are detailed in *The Black Report, The Health Divide*,[25] and *Aging and Health*.[26]

New Knowledge of the Outcomes of Nutritional Deficiencies

The years from 1950 to 1980 were also associated with new understandings of the impact of nutritional deficiencies on tissues during periods of maximal growth and development.[27] It was in this period that Lucille Hurley

24. (a) E. Newbrun, "Criteria Indicative of Cariogenicity or No-Cariogenicity of Foods and Beverages," in *Health and Sugar Substitutes: Proceedings of the ERGOB Conference, Geneva*. (S. Basel: Karger, 1978), p. 253. (b) E. Newbrun, "Systemic Use of Fluorides: Assessment of Cost/Benefit Features and Practicality," in *Relative Efficiency of Preventive Procedures in Dental Public Health* (Ann Arbor, Mich.: University of Michigan School of Public Health, 1978). (c) Daphne A. Roe, *Drug-Induced Nutritional Deficiencies*, 2d ed. (Westport, Conn.: AVI Publ. Co., 1985), pp. 1–318.

25. Sir Douglas F. B. Black et al., *Inequalities in Health: The Black Report*, ed. P. Townsend and N. Davidson (London: Penguin Books, 1988). Includes Margaret Whitehead, *The Health Divide* (originally published in 1987).

26. James R. Bayne, *Aging and Health* (Ottawa: Canadian Welfare Council, 1965). (Prepared as a background paper for the Canadian Conference on Aging; Toronto, January 1966.)

27. E. M. Widdowson, "Body Composition and Energy Metabolism before and after Birth," in L. A. Cioffi, W. P. T. James, and T. B. Van Itallie, eds., *The Body Weight Regulatory System* (New York: Raven Press, 1981).

and others investigated the effect of trace element deficiencies on the developing fetus.[28] In the same period, the effects of nutritional deficiencies on immune function were discovered, as well as the effects of protein-energy malnutrition on the behavioral development of the infant.[29] The last fifty years have also been a period of research advances in nutritional biochemistry. We have learned of metabolic pathways that, if blocked due to genetic aberrations or to the effects of drugs, can cause life-threatening health problems.[30] Importantly, this new knowledge has permitted the development of drugs and diets for disease management, such as drugs which reduce cholesterol levels in those at high risk of coronary artery disease.[31]

Research has also advanced our knowledge of the adverse nutritional affects of alcohol. The research in this area, conducted by C. S. Lieber and his colleagues, has been at the cellular and tissue level as well as in clinical studies.[32]

Between 1950 and 1970 there was little awareness of malnutrition as a risk factor for infection, slow wound healing, and hospital-based mortality, although a few surgeons drew attention to the problem in the mid-1950s. Few physicians were aware of the importance of nutritional support relative to a good prognosis in hospital patients. This may be explained by the assumption, common at the time, that the demise of certain previously endemic forms of malnutrition such as pellagra meant that malnutrition in hospital patients was of concern only in skid-row alcoholics and cancer patients. During the 1970s physicians came to realize that malnutrition caused by an inadequate diet might arise during hospitalization. New interest in hospital-based malnutrition was largely the work of B. R. Bistrian and his colleagues,[33] who not only heightened the awareness of malnutrition among physicians and nurses but also developed methods for rapid diagnosis and nutritional support.[34]

Knowledge of the effects of malnutrition on immune function arose in

28. L. S. Hurley, *Developmental Nutrition* (Englewood Cliffs, N.J.: Prentice Hall, 1980).

29. (a) R. K. Chandra, "Nutritional Regulation of Immunity: An Introduction," in R. K. Chandra, ed., *Nutrition and Immunology* (New York: Alan R. Liss Inc., 1988), pp. 1–8. (b) V. Reddy, "Protein-Energy Malnutrition: An Overview," in Harper and Davis, *Nutrition in Health and Disease* . . .

30. Roe, *Drug Induced Nutritional Deficiencies.*

31. M. C. Linder, "Nutrition and Atherosclerosis," in M. C. Linder, ed., *Nutrition, Biochemistry, and Metabolism with Clinical Applications*, 2d ed. (New York: Elsevier, 1991), pp. 449–474.

32. (a) M. A. Korsten and C. S. Lieber, "Nutrition in the Alcoholic," in *Medical Clinics of North America* 63 (1979): 963–972. (b) E. Newbrun, "Systemic Use of Fluorides."

33. B. R. Bistrian, J. Vitale, and G. Blackburn, "Prevalence of Protein-Calorie Malnutrition in General Medical Patients," *JAMA* 235 (1976): 1567.

34. B. R. Bistrian, "Interaction of Nutrition and Infection in the Hospital Setting," *American Journal of Clinical Nutrition* 30 (1977): 1228–1232.

part from hospital studies which showed the effects of protein-energy malnutrition on patients' immune functions. This was derived both from observation and from laboratory studies of zinc deficiency, both as an endemic disease and as developed in patients with inflammatory bowel disease. Two other new discoveries were that certain antioxidant nutrients given in pharmacological amounts will boost immune function and may indeed reduce the decrement in immune function associated with aging, and that carotenoids, one of the antioxidant nutrients that protect immune function, have cancer-protective properties.[35]

New Technologies Leading to Better Understandings

Technological advances have led to new areas of nutrition information including the development of radioisotope and stable isotope methods for studying nutrient absorption and metabolism.[36] Chromatographic methods, including thin-layer chromatography, gas chromatography, and high-performance liquid chromatography, have permitted the isolation of nutrients and their metabolites in plasma and tissues as well as in body secretions and urine. Modern methods of isolating subcellular tissue components have allowed the characterization of nutrient-binding protein, such as cellular retinol-binding proteins important in the regulation of vitamin A metabolism.[37] Cell and tissue culture methods have recently been used to investigate the growth of tumor cells and the effects of nutrients on growth processes. A recent application of in vitro culture methods has been used in the study of the effect of cellular antioxidant status on HIV virus replication.[38]

The development of new animal models and the breeding of mutant strains of rats, mice, and chickens have allowed studies of the interplay of genetic factors, diet, and environmental toxins on survival and chronic disease development. For example, rats bred for spontaneous hypertension have been used to examine the roles of different nutrients in modulating blood pressure.[39]

Newer physiological techniques, including endoscopy and intubation

35. (a) Machlin, "Protective Role of Vitamins." (b) A. Bendich, "Antioxidant Vitamins and Immune Responses," in Chandra, *Nutrition and Immunology*, pp. 125–147.

36. P. R. Flanagan, "New and Traditional Methods of Assessing Mineral Interactions," in Levander, *AIN Symposium*, pp. 41–45.

37. G. Wolf, "Cellular Retinol-Binding Protein Functions in the Regulation of Retinoid Metabolism," *Nutrition Reviews* 50 (1992): 197–199.

38. D. H. Baker and R. J. Wood, "Cellular Antioxidant Status and Human Immunodeficiency Virus Replication," *Nutrition Reviews* 50 (1992): 15–18.

39. H. P. Schedl, "Calcium, Vitamin D and Hypertension in Animal Models," in Levander, *AIN Symposium*, pp. 115–118.

with sampling of intestinal contents through triple lumen tubes, have permitted us to gain new knowledge of relationships between gastrointestinal hormone secretion and nutrient absorption in humans. The technique of using triple lumen tubes has also been employed to examine the effects of disease, alcohol, and therapeutic drugs on the absorption of vitamins such as folic acid.[40] New methods for measuring human body composition and energy expenditure in humans have permitted better understanding of food-energy requirements of people of different age groups in health and under disease conditions.[41]

Most recently, the tools of endocrinology, biotechnology, and gene transfer have led to the development of farm animals whose meat contains less fat and is thus more desirable for health maintenance.[42]

Nutrition Societies and Their Journals

The development of nutrition societies has provided a means of communication between nutrition scientists. The proceedings of these societies document nutrition scientists' concerns over time, as regards public welfare and scientific relevance.

In 1939 several prominent nutritional scientists in the United Kingdom formed the Nutrition Society. These include Sir Charles Martin, Sir John Boyd Orr, Stanislas Kon, and Leslie Harris. The history of this society was written by its well-known archivist, Alice Copping.[43] Further information on this society can be obtained from Elsie Widdowson's account of its presidents and honorary members.[44] Publications of the Nutrition Society include its *Proceedings*, which include symposia and the *British Journal of Nutrition*. Leslie Harris, the first secretary of the Society, also played a major role during 1946–1960 in the development of the International Union of Nutritional Scientists (IUNS). The IUNS has been responsible for plan-

40. C. H. Halsted, "Intestinal Absorption of Dietary Folates," in M. F. Picciano, E. L. R. Stokstad, and J. F. Gregory, eds., *Folic Acid Metabolism in Health and Disease* (New York: Wiley-Liss, 1990), pp. 23–45.

41. (a) S. B. Heymsfield, "Human Body Composition: Analysis by Computerized Axial Tomography and Nuclear Magnetic Resonance," in Levander, *AIN Symposium*, pp. 92–96. (b) D. A. Schoeller, E. Ravussin, Y. Schutz, K. J. Acheson, P. Baertschi, and E. Jequier, "Energy Expenditure by Doubly Labelled Water: Validation in Humans and Proposed Calculation," *American Journal of Physiology* 250 (1986): R823–R830.

42. B. A. Crooker, M. A. McGuire, W. S. Cohick, M. Harkins, D. E. Bauman, and K. Sejrsen, "Effect of Dose of Bovine Somatostatin on Nutrient Utilization in Growing Dairy Heifers," *Journal of Nutrition* 120 (1990): 1256–1263.

43. A. Copping, "History of the Nutrition Society," *Proceedings of the Nutrition Society* 37 (1978): 105–138.

44. E. M. Widdowson, comp., *The Nutrition Society, 1941–1991: Presidents and Honorary Members, Their Stories and Recollections* (Wallingford, Oxon, U.K.: CAB International, 1991).

ning international nutrition congresses as well as promoting international research.

The first nutrition journal to appear in the United States was the *Journal of Nutrition*, which began in 1928. This is the official publication of the American Institute of Nutrition, which was founded the same year. Major changes in format came about when Lucille Hurley was editor. Hurley started the current system of dividing groups of papers by subject matter. In the 1990s this journal broadened its scope to afford more coverage of studies in human nutrition.

Nutritional societies formed in the United States since 1950 include the American Society for Clinical Nutrition, the Society for Nutrition Education, and the Society for Parenteral and Enteral Nutrition. Each of these societies has a professional journal with a different reading public. The *Journal of the American Society for Clinical Nutrition*, which first appeared in 1954, is mainly read by nutritionists in academic institutions, including those working in medical schools. Membership in the society includes physicians and clinical nutritionists working in hospitals. The *Journal of Nutrition Education*, begun in 1969, is read by nutritionists interested in conveying nutrition concepts to students and practical information to the public, including those in low literacy groups. The *Journal of Parenteral and Enteral Nutrition*, begun in 1977, is read by clinical nutritionists, dietitians, and clinical pharmacists associated with nutrition support teams in hospitals.

Awards Recognition in Nutrition

The landmarks in nutritional discoveries are well documented by key papers in journals, by symposia, and by citations concerning awards made to nutritional scientists. Scientific breakthroughs made by nutritionists in the United States are recorded by the prizes awarded by the American Institute of Nutrition (AIN). Awards made from the time of founding of the AIN until 1978 are recorded in the *Proceedings of a Symposium Commemorating the Fiftieth Anniversary of the Journal of Nutrition* (1978). More recent prize winners are documented in later volumes of the journal. Some of them received their awards a number of years after they made their discoveries. Changing trends of research direction become apparent when prizes are examined decade by decade.

1950–60. Studies of vitamin deficiencies, their causation and treatment
William Castle received the Mead Johnson award for his studies of pernicious anemia; Henry Steenbock received the Borden Award in nutrition for his

studies of the preventive effects of ultraviolet light against rickets. Both of these prizes were for work accomplished much earlier than the time of award. However, during the same period an award was given to Grace Goldsmith for her more current work on B vitamins, notably her studies of the interrelationships of the amino acid tryptophan and niacin. Other important discoveries in the area of B vitamin research, including work by Max Horwitt on riboflavin, were also acknowledged by prizes.

1961–1970. Studies on relationships between malnutrition and behavioral development

Richard Barnes received the Borden Award for his work on the effects of protein-energy malnutrition on mental development.

It is important to note that many major recent advances in nutrition are linked to advances in technology over the last fifty years. Other awards, granted for the development of new concepts in nutritional epidemiology and nutritional anthropology during the last forty years, are largely dependent on earlier pioneering efforts in the social sciences. Many scientific efforts now bearing fruit were initiated by the mentors of those who now lead the field.[45]

1971–1980. Studies of the active forms of nutrients

A number of awards went to nutritional scientists who identified the active nutrients formed by metabolic changes occurring after absorption. These studies were of particular scientific relevance in that they also showed sites of nutrient action. Among the nutritional scientists whose work was carried out and acknowledged during this period were Hector DeLuca on vitamin D metabolites and Donald McCormick on B vitamins.

1981–1992. Studies of trace element deficiencies, immune function, and nutritional interventions

A number of awards have been made to nutritional scientists who have been responsible for the identification of trace element deficiencies in man and in animals. This category includes the important work of Marian Robinson of the University of Otago, New Zealand, on selenium deficiency. Other areas receiving major awards are studies of the biochemical changes in lipid metabolism responsible for atherogenesis and coronary heart disease. Among the scientists receiving major awards for this work are J. L. Goldstein and Donald Zilversmit. Awards have also been given for work linking loss of immune function to dietary deficiency. In 1990 Ranjit Chandra received the McCollum Award for his pioneering work. Recognition of his many contributions reinforced a special and unique contribution of nutritional science, namely the linking of clinical observations and laboratory studies to advances made in

45. (a) M. K. Horwitt, O. Kreisler, and P. Wittman, "Investigations of Human Requirements for B-Complex Vitamins," *Bulletin of the National Research Council*, no. 116 (1948), pp.1–106. (b) D. M. Hegsted, "Balance Studies," *Journal of Nutrition* 106 (1976): 307–311.

industrialized and Third World countries. Awards for work conducted in the Third World have also gone to Barbara Underwood for her work in the prevention of vitamin A deficiency.

International Organizations Concerned with Food, Nutrition, and Health Promotion

Within the United Nations the major international organizations concerned with food, nutrition, and public health are the World Health Organization (WHO), the Food and Agricultural Organization (FAO), and UNICEF. The goals and nutrition-related work of these organizations have been described both in monographs and at international meetings.[46]

WHO is particularly concerned with the health of populations and with the prevention and controlling of epidemic and endemic diseases. It has been involved in programs aimed at eradicating or controlling infectious diseases. Since the risk of infectious disease is heightened by malnutrition, and since infection is a cause of malnutrition, WHO has provided resources for nutrition intervention programs aimed at decreasing the incidence of infectious disease. It has also supplied expertise to control endemic nutritional diseases such as scurvy and pellagra in refugee camps.

The eradication of world hunger by improving the food supply is an avowed aim of the FAO. This organization has also been highly concerned with surveys of the prevalence of nutritional diseases in different countries.

UNICEF's special role has been to decrease infant mortality and to promote child health. Its major concerns have been the promotion of breastfeeding and the reduction of protein-energy malnutrition among children.

The World Bank and the World Food Program have been important for the support of international nutrition research and for the supply of food aid to hungry nations.[47] All these organizations share the view that food aid to needy countries, while necessary in the short term, must be supplemented by programs for boosting food production.[48]

46. (a) T. G. Taylor and N. K. Jenkins, eds., *Proceedings of the XIII International Congress of Nutrition* (London and Paris: John Libbey, 1986), esp.: A. Pradilla, "The Contribution of the World Health Organizations to Nutrition," pp. 32–36; (b) F. Ronchi-Proja, "The Contribution of FAO to Nutrition," pp. 36–39; (c) R. Jolly, "The Work of UNICEF in Relation to Nutrition," pp. 44–48. (d) R. Jolly and G. A. Cornia, eds., *The Impact of World Recession on Children* (Oxford: Pergamon Press, 1984).

47. D. J. Shaw, "The Contribution of the World Food Program to Nutrition," in Taylor and Jenkins, *Proceedings of the XIII Congress*, pp. 39–44.

48. A. Berg, "Nutrition and the World Bank," in Taylor and Jenkins, *Proceedings of the XIII Congress*, pp. 48–52.

Nutrition Advances in the Third World since 1950

Progress in nutrition survey methodology allowed better definition of the prevalence of endemic forms of malnutrition in the Third World. Before 1950 it was widely believed that lack of protein was the major cause of malnutrition in infants and young children. As a result, high-protein weaning foods were developed and tested in nutrition intervention programs in Central America. This preoccupation with protein continued until the 1960s, when awareness of caloric deficit as the major problem in early childhood malnutrition became more generally accepted.

Field research has advanced our knowledge of nutrition problems in the Third World, uncovering close links between malnutrition in infants and bottle-feeding and between high death rates in children suffering from protein-energy malnutrition and dehydration associated with diarrheal disease. Intervention programs have focussed on the promotion of breast-feeding and oral rehydration.[49] These programs have been implemented in many countries by training community health workers how to encourage uneducated women not to bottle-feed their infants. Community health workers have also been taught oral rehydration procedures, which they pass on to mothers in rural and urban communities.

Studies carried out by Joachin Cravioto and his group in Guatemala have identified deficits in behavioral development that commonly follow chronic protein-energy malnutrition in early childhood.[50] Most recently, a report on the Third World nutrition situation concluded that protein-energy and micro-nutrient malnutrition continues to affect a large number of people.[51]

The work of many distinguished nutritional scientists from the Third World has been fostered by nutrition institutes, national governments, and international organizations. An institute of particular note is the National Institute of Nutrition in Hyderabad, India, where medical doctors Cam Gopalan, Vinodini Reddy, Mahtab Bamji, and Kamala Krishnaswami have conducted their work. Their areas of expertise and interest include childhood malnutrition in India, B vitamin deficiencies, and the disposition of drugs in malnourished children and adults. Their work has been widely

49. M. C. Latham, "Nutritional Problems and Deficiency Diseases: General Principles," in G. T. Strickland, ed., *Hunter's Tropical Medicine,* 7th ed. (Philadelphia: W. B. Saunders Co., 1991), pp. 911–914.

50. B. Robles, G. R. Ramos, and J. Cravioto, "Evaluation of the Behavior of the Child with Advanced Malnutrition and of Its Modifications During Recovery: Preliminary Report" (in Spanish), *Boletin Medico del Hospital Infantil de Mexico* 1959; 16 (1984): 317.

51. United Nations Administrative Committee on Coordination, Subcommittee on Nutrition, *Second Report on the World Situation*, 2 vols. (Geneva: United Nations, 1992). Prepared in collaboration with the International Food Policy Research Institute, Washington, D. C.

published, but it is most accessible in the proceedings of the international congresses of nutrition sponsored by the International Union of Nutritional Scientists.

The development of centers for field investigations of nutritional diseases in the Third World has also permitted the advanced training of students from local areas as well as those coming from other parts of the world. Nutrition units of this kind include one developed by John Waterlow in Kingston, Jamaica,[52] and the Institute of Nutrition of Central America and Panama (INCAP) in Guatemala. The work conducted in Kingston includes investigations of protein-energy malnutrition. INCAP has played a fundamental role in studies of the long-term impacts of early malnutrition, and also in the training of nutritional scientists from industrialized and Third World countries. The work of these and other nutrition institutes has been described in the *Proceedings of the International Congresses on Nutrition.* The combination of research and training in Third World countries has meant that major nutritional problems occurring there can be studied in their ecological settings. Despite research progress, nutritional interventions, and evaluations of the outcomes of interventions, however, the problems of widespread hunger and malnutrition remain as major causes of infant and early-childhood morbidity and mortality. In many Third World countries, such as India, Kenya, and Caribbean countries, more men and women are surviving into old age; Western foods, considered prestigious, have entered the diet. The result is that these countries now have problems of diet-related chronic disease. Diabetes and hypertension have emerged as major problems in the cities. The geography of these diseases within Third World countries has been the central theme of a number of scientific meetings with published proceedings.

Collaborative International Studies of Recent Development

Nutritional surveillance has been developed by Jean-Pierre Habicht, John Mason, and others for use in the Third World to provide early warning of famine, so that steps may be taken to avert catastrophe. Nutritional surveillance methods have also been used to evaluate the effectiveness of nutrition intervention programs in the Third World and to modify program efforts in the light of findings. These surveillance programs have required the close cooperation between central and regional governmental agencies and those

52. J. C. Waterlow, *Fatty Liver Disease in Infants in the British West Indies* (London: HMSO, 1948 [MRC Special Report Series No 263]), p. 84.

who implement programs at the local level. It has also been necessary to provide training manuals for surveillance personnel.[53]

Collaborative studies of the effects of diet and environmental toxins on the risk of chronic disease are being carried out by investigators from the United States and other developed countries, from Third World countries, and from industrialized countries that have regional nutritional problems of special interest. For example, the Chinese Institute of Preventive Medicine and Cornell University are conducting collaborative studies of the relationship between consumption of regional foods and localization of site-specific cancer.[54]

Also in progress are cross-cultural studies of nutrition and aging with the aim of identifying eating and lifestyle patterns associated with healthy living to an advanced age. These studies are linked historically to the earlier studies of nutrition of the elderly in the United Kingdom conducted by Exton-Smith and his colleagues.[55]

International collaboration has been achieved in defining nutrient requirements and setting dietary standards. This effort is based on the pioneer work of McCance, Widdowson, and Hollingsworth.[56] Data sharing is carried out using recent methods of communication including FAX, computer diskettes, and INTERNET or other computer networks. Publication of completed studies in hard-copy journals and books remains the system of choice for dissemination of information, however. The maintenance and expansion of nutrition literature in libraries accessible to nutritionists in the industrialized and Third World countries is therefore of the utmost importance.

Conclusion

It may be asked what disciplines and what body of nutrition knowledge have led to the advances in nutrition made since 1950. The disciplines are a diverse group including biochemistry, physiology, radiobiology, pharmacology, toxicology, immunology, epidemiology, human ecology, anthropology, and medical science. The body of nutrition knowledge is the

53. J. Mason and J. P. Habicht, "Nutritional Surveillance," in Harper and Davis, *Nutrition in Health and Disease . . .* , pp. 539–547.

54. J. Chen, R. Peto, J. Li, and T. C. Campbell, "Nutritional Status and Cancer Mortality in China," in Taylor and Jenkins, *Proceeding of the XIII Congress*, pp. 127–129.

55. A. N. Exton-Smith, "Nutritional Deficiencies in the Elderly," in A. N. Howard and I. McLean Baird, eds., *Nutritional Deficiencies in Modern Society* (London: Newman Books, 1973), pp. 82–97.

56. (a) R. A. McCance and E. M. Widdowson, *The Composition of Foods*, 3d ed., (London: HMSO, 1960 [Special Report Series Medical Research Council no. 297]). (b) D. F. Hollingsworth, "Dietary Standards," in R. E. Olson, ed., *Present Knowledge in Nutrition*, 5th ed. (Washington D.C.: Nutrition Foundation Inc., 1984), pp. 711–723.

accumulated work of earlier nutritionists and physiologists. This knowledge was transmitted not only through books and scientific papers but, as R. E. Olson points out,[57] through nutrition training and research, through the teaching of graduate students, and through the dissemination of nutrition knowledge in the meetings of nutrition societies and in journals.

As this examination of the evolution of nutrition knowledge and practice has demonstrated, information accumulates and consolidates not only through observations, experiments and interventions, but through documentation. It is essential that the earlier nutrition literature be preserved.

The author of this chapter appreciates the suggestions and comments made by Dr. D. H. Hegsted.

57. R. E. Olson, "Clinical Nutrition: An Interface between Human Ecology and Internal Medicine," in W. O. Atwater, ed., *Nutrition Reviews* 36 (1978): 161–178.

3. Determining the Core Publications and Characteristics of Food Science and Human Nutrition Literature

JENNIE BROGDON
Rockville, Maryland

Food science and human nutrition constituted one of seven subject areas studied by the Core Agricultural Literature Project, Albert R. Mann Library, Cornell University.[1] The purpose of the project was to identify the core literature for teaching and research in academic institutions. The results can be used in the evaluation of academic library collections, in the selection of titles for preservation, and in the building of academic agricultural research libraries in the Third World.

Study of the food science and human nutrition literature for the Core Project was conducted in two phases:

1. Core literature from 1950 through 1993; methodology and results of this phase are presented in this chapter and in the two following.
2. Historical literature from 1850 through 1949; methodology and results are in Chapter 8.

This chapter uses the information gained in the citation analysis of the literature of food science and human nutrition, and compares it when possible with data from other sources.

A. Analysis Structure and Scope

Scientific study of food science and human nutrition is relatively recent. Nutrition was not recognized as a separate discipline until the beginning of

1. Wallace C. Olsen and Jan Kennedy-Olsen, "Determining the Current Core Literature in the Agricultural Sciences," in *Quarterly Bulletin of the International Association of Agricultural Information Specialists* 36 (1–2) (1991): 122–127.

the twentieth century, and food science was not firmly recognized until after World War II. These late developments have been attributed to their heavy reliance on methodologies or results from earlier sciences. Samuel Thier has discussed the many sciences comprising nutrition, and Syd Green has done so for food science and technology.[2] Early studies appeared in the literature of the established fields of chemistry, physiology, and medicine.

Food science and human nutrition are usually viewed as two distinct disciplines which became interrelated through an overlap in interests: food scientists strive to conserve or enhance nutrients during processing, and nutritionists determine the biological effects of the types and amounts of nutrients in the food consumed. Each has a basic research side and an applied area, as well as social, cultural, economic, and educational aspects. There are numerous definitions for each discipline, and boundaries are difficult to establish. The most basic definition is that food science is the study of changes in food occurring during its production, harvesting, processing, preservation, storage, and preparation. Human nutrition is the study of the relationship between food and health.

To aid the Core Agricultural Literature Project, a Food Science and Human Nutrition Steering Committee composed of recognized scientists in both disciplines established the subject parameters and provided recommendations for source documents to be analyzed. The membership was:

Owen R. Fennema
University of Wisconsin

Cutberto Garza
Cornell University

Joseph H. Hotchkiss
Cornell University

Michael C. Latham
Cornell University

Nevin S. Scrimshaw
Harvard Center for Population Studies

The committee established the following subject categories which were used in the selection of source documents and the review of monographic lists.

1. General Food and Nutrition; Intervention; Planning and Policy; Psychology and Research; Anthropology
2. Food Chemistry, Composition, and Biotechnology; Flavors and the Senses

2. (a) Samuel O. Thier, "The Sciences of Nutrition," *Food Technology* 44 (8) (1990): 26–34. (b) Syd Green, *Keyguide to Information Sources in Food Science and Technology* (London and New York: Mansell, 1985).

3. Food Processing, Engineering, Packaging, Storage
4. Food Microbiology, Toxicology, Protection, and Regulation
5. Food Management and Dietetics
6. Nutrition Biochemistry and Metabolism
7. Human and Clinical Nutrition; Assessment; Body Composition; Physical Activity

Source documents were selected to provide several approaches to a subject and thereby avoid potential skews. Earlier as well as more recent publications have been included, although the steering committee agreed that the more recent a publication, the more likely it is to be up-to-date and useful. Books or articles that are classics and of long-lasting importance were not overlooked. The subject scope of the books to be analyzed had to be weighed carefully to ensure that all major aspects were covered adequately and that more recent subject areas were covered. Authorship of individuals had to be balanced to include authors from Britain, Japan, and other developed countries as well as those from the Third World. Similarly stringent representation of literature in the Third World had to be adequate to the scope of the work in those countries. The aim was to provide so broad an analysis of literature that all vital educational and research points of views and all geographic influences were registered. The steering committee was invaluable in identifying these important source documents and counseling on subject or geographic skews. Fifty monographs were analyzed: twenty-eight for food science, seventeen for human nutrition, and four that overlapped both disciplines. In addition, monographic titles only were taken from sixteen additional publications and two journal articles. These were placed in a master monographic list with all other monographs obtained from the citation analysis. This list was then used for peer evaluation. All the source documents are listed.

Sources of Citations in Food Science and Human Nutrition

*items were not analyzed, but monographs were extracted for inclusion in peer evaluation.

MONOGRAPHS

Amerine, Maynard A., Rose Marie Pangborn, and Edward B. Roessler. *Principles of Sensory Evaluation of Food*. New York and London; Academic Press, 1965. 602p.

Bailey, Alton E., and Daniel Swern, eds. *Bailey's Industrial Oil and Fat Products . . .* by Marvin W. Formo, et al. 4th ed. New York; Wiley, 1979–1985. 3 vols. (Select chapters in vol. 1 analyzed; vols. 2 and 3 were fully analyzed.)

Bauernfeind, J. Christopher, ed. *Vitamin A Deficiency and Its Control*. Orlando, Fla.; Academic Press, 1986. 530p.
Becher, Paul, ed. *Encyclopedia of Emulsion Technology*. New York; M. Dekker, 1983. 3 vols. (Selected analysis)
Birch, Gordon G. *Analysis of Food Carbohydrate*. London and New York; Elsevier Applied Science Publishers, 1985. 311p.
*Birch, Gordon G., Allan G. Cameron, and Michael Spencer. *Food Science*. 3d ed. Oxford and New York; Pergamon Press, 1986. 175p.
*Bodwell, C. E., J. S. Adkins, and D. T. Hopkins, eds. *Protein Quality in Humans: Assessment and in Vitro Estimation*. Westport, Conn.; Avi Pub. Co., 1981. 435p.
Branen, A. Larry, P. Michael Davidson, and Seppo Salminen, eds. *Food Additives*. New York; M. Dekker, 1990. 736p. (*Food Science and Technology* No. 35)
*Briggs, George M., and Doris H. Calloway. *Nutrition and Physical Fitness*. 11th ed. New York; Holt, Rinehart, and Winston, 1984. 623p.
Brown, Myrtle L., ed. *Present Knowledge in Nutrition*. 6th ed. Washington, D.C.; International Life Sciences Institute-Nutrition Foundation, 1990. 532p.
Brun, T. A., and M. C. Latham, eds. *World Food Issues: Maldevelopment and Malnutrition,* (Volume 2) Ithaca, N.Y.; Cornell Program in International Agriculture, 1990. 126p.
Chandra, Ranjit K., ed. *Nutrition and Immunology*. New York; Liss, 1988. 342p.
Chen, Lincoln C., and Nevin S. Scrimshaw, eds. *Diarrhea and Malnutrition: Interactions, Mechanisms and Interventions*. New York; Plenum Press, 1983. 318p.
Concon, Jose M. *Food Toxicology*. New York; M. Dekker, 1988. 2 vols. 1371p.
Davidek, Jiri, Jan Velisek, and Jan Pokorny, eds. *Chemical Changes During Food Processing*. Amsterdam and New York; Elsevier, 1990. 448p.
**Davidson and Passmore Human Nutrition and Dietetics*. 8th ed., by R. Passmore, M. A. Eastwood, et al. Edinburgh and New York; Churchill Livingstone, 1986. 666p.
Diehl, Johannes F. *Safety of Irradiated Foods*. New York; M. Dekker, 1990. 345p.
Dreher, Mark L. *Handbook of Dietary Fiber: An Applied Approach*. New York; Dekker, 1987. 468p.
Eskin, N. A. M. *Plant Pigments, Flavors and Textures; The Chemistry and Biochemistry of Selected Compounds*. New York; Academic Press, 1979. 211p.
FAO/WHO Expert Consultation, 1977, Rome. *Dietary Fats and Oils in Human Nutrition: Report* . . . jointly organized by the Food and Agriculture Organization and the World Health Organization, Rome, September 1977. Reprinted, with corrections. Rome; FAO, 1980. 102p. (*FAO Food and Nutrition Series* No. 20)
*Fellows, Peter. *Food Processing Technology: Principles and Practice*.
Chichester, Eng.; E. Horwood; New York; VCH, 1988. 505p.
Fennema, Owen R., ed. *Food Chemistry*. 2d ed., rev. and expanded. New York; M. Dekker, 1985. 991p.
*Ferrando, R. *Traditional and Non-Traditional Foods*. Rome; Food and Agriculture Organization, 1981. 156p. (*FAO Food and Nutrition Series* No. 2)
*Gibson, Rosalind S. *Principles of Nutritional Assessment*. New York and Oxford; Oxford University Press, 1990. 691p.
Gittinger, J. Price, Joanne Leslie, and Caroline Hoisington, eds. *Food Policy: Integrating Supply, Distribution, and Consumption*. Baltimore; Published for the World Bank by Johns Hopkins University Press, 1987. 567p.
Gormley, T. R., G. Downey, and D. O'Beirne. *Food, Health and the Consumer*. London and New York; Elsevier Applied Science, 1987. 317p.

Gruenwedel, Dieter W., and John R. Whitaker, eds. *Food Analysis: Principles and Techniques*. New York; M. Dekker, 1984–1987. 8 vols. Analyzed: Vol. 1, Physical Characterization; vol. 2, Physicochemical Techniques; vol. 3, Biological Techniques.
*Gunstone, Frank D., and Frank A. Norris. *Lipids in Foods: Chemistry, Biochemistry, and Technology*. 1st ed. Oxford and New York; Pergamon Press, 1983. 170p.
Hetzel, Basil S. *The Story of Iodine Deficiency: An International Challenge in Nutrition*. Oxford and New York; Oxford University Press, 1989. 236p.
Himes, John H., ed. *Anthropometric Assessment of Nutritional Status*. New York; Wiley-Liss, 1991. 431p.
*Hultin, Herbert O., and Max Milner, eds. *Postharvest Biology and Biotechnology; Symposium Papers,* Philadelphia, June 1977, sponsored by the Institute of Food Technologists and International Union of Food Science and Technology. Westport, Conn.; Food and Nutrition Press, 1978. 462p.
Institute of Medicine (U.S.). *Nutrition during Lactation*. Subcommittee on Lactation, Committee on Nutritional Status During Pregnancy and Lactation, Food and Nutrition Board, Institute of Medicine, National Academy of Sciences. Washington, D.C.; National Academy Press, 1991. 309p.
Jagtiani, Jethro, Harvey T. Chan, Jr., and William S. Sakai, eds. *Tropical Fruit Processing*. San Diego, New York, etc.; Academic Press, 1988. 184p.
Jay, James M. *Modern Food Microbiology*. 3d ed. New York; Van Nostrand Reinhold, 1986. 642p.
Jelliffe, Derrick B., and E. F. Patrice Jelliffe, in collaboration with Alfred Zerfas and Charlotte G. Newmann. *Community Nutritional Assessment: With Special Reference to Less Technically Developed Countries*. Oxford and New York; Oxford University Press, 1989. 633p.
Jerome, Norge W., Randy F. Kandel, and Gretel H. Pelto, eds. *Nutritional Anthropology: Contemporary Approaches to Diet and Culture*. Pleasantville, N.Y.; Redgrave Pub. Co., 1980. 433p.
Kadoya, Takashi, ed. *Food Packaging*. San Diego; Academic Press, 1990. 424p.
*Kilgour, O. F. G. *Mastering Nutrition*. Houndsmills, Eng.; Macmillan, 1985. 321p.
Knight, John B., and Lendal H. Kotschevar. *Quantity Food Production, Planning, and Management*. 2d ed. New York; Van Nostrand Reinhold, 1989. 445p.
Knorr, Dietrich, ed. *Food Biotechnology*. New York; M. Dekker, 1987. 613p.
Kramer, Donald E., and John Liston, eds. *Seafood Quality Determination; Proceedings of the International Symposium* . . . coordinated by the University of Alaska Sea Grant College Program, Anchorage, November 1986. Amsterdam and New York; Elsevier, 1987. 677p. (*Developments in Food Science* No. 15)
*Kritchevsky, David, Charles Bonfield, and James W. Anderson, eds. *Dietary Fiber: Chemistry, Physiology, and Health Effects; Proceedings of the George Vahouny Fiber Conference* . . . April 1988, Washington, D.C. New York; Plenum Press, 1990. 499p.
Larsson, Kare, and Stig E. Friberg, eds. *Food Emulsions*. 2d ed., rev. and expanded. New York and Basel; Marcel Dekker, 1990. 510p.
Lawrie, Ralston A. *Meat Science*. 4th ed. Oxford and New York; Pergamon Press, 1985. 267p.
Lorenz, Klaus J., and Karel Kulp, eds. *Handbook of Cereal Science and Technology*. New York; M. Dekker, 1991. 882p. (*Food Science and Technology* No. 41) (Select chapters analyzed)
Maarse, Henk, ed. *Volatile Compounds in Foods and Beverages*. 1st ed. New York; M. Dekker, 1991. 764p. (*Food Science and Technology* No. 44)

Macrae, R. *HPLC in Food Analysis*. London, New York, etc; Academic Press, 1982. 340p.
Manoff, Richard K. *Social Marketing: New Imperative for Public Health*. New York; Praeger, 1985. 293p.
Manson-Bahr, Philip E. C., and D. R. Bell. *Manson's Tropical Diseases*. 19th ed. London; Bailliere Tindall, 1987. 1557p. (1st ed., 1898. by Sir Patrick Manson) (Two sections analyzed)
Matz, Samuel. *The Chemistry and Technology of Cereals as Food and Feed*. 2d ed. McAllen, Tex.; Pan-Tech International, 1991. 751p.
*McWilliams, Margaret. *Foods: Experimental Perspectives*. New York; Macmillan Pub. Co., 1989. 584p.
*Muller, Hans G. *An Introduction to Tropical Food Science*. Cambridge and New York; Cambridge University Press, 1988. 316p.
Patwardhan, Vinayak N. *The State of Nutrition in the Arab Middle East*. Nashville, Tenn.; Vanderbilt University Press, 1972. 308p.
Potter, Norman N. *Food Science*. 4th ed. Westport, Conn.; Avi Pub. Co., 1986. 735p.
Rao, M. A., and S. H. H. Rizvi. *Engineering Properties of Foods*. New York; M. Dekker, 1986. 398p.
*Rechcigl, Miloslav, Jr., ed. *CRC Handbook of Nutritional Requirements in a Functional Context*. Boca Raton, Fla.; CRC Press, 1981. 2 vols. (Analyzed Vol. 1, pp. 427–37, Nutrition and Reproduction; Man, by D. H. Woollam; pp. 495–501, Nutrition and Lactation; Human, by D. B. Jelliffe and E. F. P. Jelliffe.)
Robinson, David S. *Food: Biochemistry and Nutritional Value*. Harlow, Eng.; Longman Scientific & Technical; New York; Wiley, 1987. 554p.
Shils, Maurice E., and Vernon R. Young, eds. *Modern Nutrition in Health and Disease*. 7th ed. Philadelphia; Lea & Febiger, 1988. 1694p.
*Simko, Margaret D., Catherine Cowell, and Judith A. Gilbride, eds. *Nutrition Assessment: A Comprehensive Guide for Planning Intervention*. Rockville, Md.; Royal Tunbridge Wells, 1984. 396p.
Solms, J., D. A. Booth, R. M. Pangborn, and O. Raunhardt, eds. *Food Acceptance and Nutrition*. London, etc.; Academic Press, 1987. 490p.
Somogyi, J. C., and H. R. Muller, eds. *Nutritional Impact of Food Processing; Proceedings of the 25th Symposium of the Group of European Nutritionists on Nutritional Impact of Food Processing, Reykjavik, Sept. 1987*. Basel; Karger, 1989. 346p. (*Bibliotheca "Nutritio et Dieta"* Vol. 43)
Stephenson, Lani. *Impact of Helminth Infections on Human Nutrition*. London; Taylor and Francis, 1986. 233p.
Stone, Herbert, and Joel L. Sidel. *Sensory Evaluation Practices*. Orlando, Fla.; Academic Press, 1985. 311p.
*Tomkins, Andrew, and Fiona Watson. *Malnutrition and Infection; A Review . . . with discussions by N. S. Scrimshaw*. London; Clinical Nutrition Unit, London School of Hygiene and Tropical Medicine, 1989. 136p. (At head of title: United Nations, Administrative Committee on Coordination/ Subcommittee on Nutrition.)
Walstra, Pieter, and Robert Jenness. *Dairy Chemistry and Physics*. New York; Wiley, 1984. 467p.
Weichmann, J., ed. *Postharvest Physiology of Vegetables*. New York; M. Dekker, 1987. 597p. (*Food Science and Technology* No. 24)

JOURNAL ARTICLES

**Nutrition Abstracts and Reviews (Series A)*

Vol. 61:74–11 (Feb. 1991) J. N. Johnston and G. P. Savage, "Mercury Consumption and Toxicity with Reference to Fish and Fish Meal."
Vol. 60:827–842 (Oct. 1990) International Life Sciences Institute Europe, Nutrition Working Group. "Recommended Daily Amounts of Vitamins & Minerals in Europe."

During the citation analysis, each monographic, journal, and report title cited in the source documents was recorded and a tally made each time it was cited again. The year of publication was recorded and, for monographs, data was collected on places of publication and types of publishers. Additional details on methodology and the results of the analysis are presented in Chapters 4 and 5. Some results of this analysis along with pertinent information from other sources are used in the following section.

B. Selected Literature Characteristics

As part of the Core Agricultural Literature Project, select characteristics of the literature were studied. These characteristics are: (1) subject concentrations within each discipline and changes over time, (2) language concentrations, and (3) types of publications. Data were obtained through literature reviews, analyses of bibliographic databases, literature studies, and the Core Project analysis of more than 60,000 citations. The results on language concentrations and types of publications were compared to results obtained for four other agricultural subject areas studied in the Core Project. Those interested in detailed surveys of published literature are referred to the guides already published.[3]

Subject Concentrations in Food Science and Human Nutrition

Only one article was located that specifically dealt with changes in subject emphasis. In this work, citations in each category of the *Food Science and Technology Abstracts* database were determined for each of twenty years and trends were identified.[4] Of interest because of the Third World

3. (a) Green, *Keyguide*. (b) Paula Szilard, *Food and Nutrition Information Guide* (Littleton, Colo.: Libraries Unlimited, 1987). (c) Richard J. Blanchard and Lois Farrell, eds., *Guide to Sources for Agricultural and Biological Research* (Berkeley: University of California Press, 1981). (d) Robyn C. Frank, Frank Berry, and Holly Berry Irving, eds., *Directory of Food and Nutrition Information for Professionals & Consumers*, 2d ed. (Phoenix: Oryx Press, 1992).

4. Chen Yon-Rong and Qi Gu-Yun, "Utilization of FSTA—Analysis of Trends and Develop-

aspects was an article comparing the subject emphases in food science articles published in India with those published in the United States during a one-year period.[5] Further details from these studies are presented later.

Changes in subject emphasis can be determined by searching bibliographic databases. This is the only comprehensive, efficient, and relatively reliable method for determining subject concentrations in the literature. Comparisons can be made between databases and general trends can be observed.

Citations to the literature of these subjects are widely distributed in bibliographic databases. M. Henninger listed eighteen databases (two are actually subsets) with citations on food science and technology; Natalie Updegrove discussed twenty databases useful to nutrition professionals; and Paula Szilard listed seventeen databases to search for topics in these subjects.[6] Some of the databases are specific to food science: *Food Science and Technology Abstracts*,[7] *Foods Adlibra*,[8] or *FROSTI*;[9] others, like *Nutrition Abstracts and Reviews, Series A, Human and Experimental*, are specific to human nutrition.[10] *Nutrition Abstracts and Reviews* is a file within the *CAB Abstracts* database, one of the three major agricultural databases.[11] The other two, *AGRIS* and *AGRICOLA*, contain citations to both food science and human nutrition.[12]

---

ments in Food Science and Technology," in Jozsef Vago, Udo Schutzsack, Laszlo Labancz, and Peter Horvath, eds., *Proceedings of the Third International Conference on Food Science and Technology Information*, Budapest, October 1989 (AGROINFORM—IFIS Gmbh, 1990 [FSTAS Reference Series No. 10]), pp. 151–166.

5. K. A. Ranganath and B. Ramanna, "Information for Food Industry—Indian Experience," in M. R. Raghavendra Rao, ed., *Proceedings of the Second International Food Convention*, Mysore, February 1988, (Central Food Technological Research Institute [India], 1989), pp. 804–811.

6. (a) M. Henninger, "Bibliographical Search Online and with CD-ROM," in *Informatics in Food and Nutrition* (Stockholm: Royal Swedish Academy of Science, November 1991), pp. 44–50. (b) Natalie A. Updegrove, "Database Searching: Information Retrival for Nutrition Professionals," *Journal of Nutrition Education* 22 (5) (1984): 241–247. (c) Szilard, *Food and Nutrition Information Guide*.

7. *Food Science and Technology Abstracts* (Shinfield, England: International Food Information Service, 1969—).

8. William J. Mayer and Joel T. Komp, "Foods Adlibra—A Highly Current Database for the Food Industry," *Database* 2 (3) (1979): 10–23.

9. *FROSTI* (Food RA Online Scientific and Technical Information), is published in Leatherhead, England, by the Leatherhead Food Research Association (LFRA). Begun in 1974 it appears weekly and is available as an abstract journal and online.

10. *Nutrition Abstracts and Reviews, Series A, Human and Experimental* (Aberdeen, Scotland: Commonwealth Agricultural Bureaux International, Int. 1977—).

11. *CAB Abstracts* is the composite tape indexing product of CAB International. Begun in 1973, it was preceded in several agricultural subject areas by its printed abstracting publications which are currently produced from the tape database. The composite database is available from commercial sources online and in compact disk format.

12. (a) *AGRIS* is the tape indexing product of the FAO, begun in 1975. Citations are available from commercial sources online, printed, and in compact disk format. (b) *AGRICOLA* (Agricultural

Table 3.1. Subject concentrations in *AGRIS*

Food science	Publication years:	1975–80	1985	1990	Average
Food science & technology		5.7%	3.5%	2.0%	5.0%
Food processing, preservation & microbiology		36.3	26.6	25.1	33.5
Food contamination & toxicology		20.5	14.5	16.5	19.2
Food additives		2.7	25.5	27.1	8.9
Food packaging		6.7	2.1	2.3	5.6
Food composition		27.9	27.4	27.1	27.7
	Citation totals	74,201	13,721	12,548	100,470
					Average 12,559

Human nutrition		1986	1988	1990	Average
Human nutrition—general aspects		19.4	18.9	19.6	19.3
Physiology of human nutrition		26.2	24.3	22.5	24.3
Diet and diet-related diseases		45.4	49.5	51.6	49.0
Nutrition programs		9.0	7.3	6.3	7.4
	Citation totals	2,858	2,828	3,338	9,024
					Average 3,008

In addition, because of the multidisciplinary nature of the subject areas, citations appear in the bibliographic databases of related sciences such as chemistry,[13] biochemistry,[14] and medicine.[15]

For this Core Project study, subject concentrations within each discipline were determined in four major databases: *AGRICOLA*, *AGRIS*, *Food Science and Technology Abstracts,* and *Nutrition Abstracts and Reviews, Series A*. The subject categories in these databases were not sufficiently similar to permit direct comparisons across all files.

AGRIS, produced by the Food and Agriculture Organization, covers all aspects of agriculture including human nutrition, and contains over 1.5 million citations submitted by 135 cooperators around the world. In the case of human nutrition it includes all aspects related to food and agriculture, but it does not include some medical and clinical aspects. Data from *AGRIS* are shown in Table 3.1.

Online Access), the indexing product of the United States National Agricultural Library, has been issued on machine readable tape since 1970. The citations are available from commercial sources online, printed, and in compact disk format.

13. *Chemical Abstracts* (Columbus, Ohio: Chemical Abstract Services, 1907—).

14. *Biological Abstracts* (Philadelphia: Bio Science Information Service of Biological Abstracts, 1926—).

15. *Medline* (Bethesda, Md.: National Library of Medicine, 1970—).

The most striking change in *AGRIS* food science is the increase in citations relating to food additives—from 2.7% in 1975–1980 to 27.1% in 1990. The major decline during the same fifteen-year period, 11.2%, was in food processing, preservation, and microbiology. This category and food composition are the two highest ranking citation subjects. The most notable change in human nutrition was the 6.2% increase in diet and diet-related diseases from 1986 to 1990. It is of interest to note that the average number of food science citations per year was four times higher than the human nutrition citations during the same period.

AGRICOLA, produced by the U.S. National Agricultural Library, contains over 2.6 million citations covering all aspects of agriculture. *AGRICOLA* and *AGRIS* use almost identical subject schemes. Food science and human nutrition citation concentrations are presented in Table 3.2. The total number of citations for each year shows that fewer entries are being added to the database since 1985, when *AGRICOLA* began to concentrate on U.S. literature. In general, percentages of food science entries were similar for all time periods with only two categories showing changes greather than 2%: food storage entries declined 2.3%; food contamination and toxicology

Table 3.2. Subject concentrations in *AGRICOLA*

Food science	Publication years:	1980	1985	1990	Average
Food science & food products (general)		7.3%	7.6%	8.8%	7.8%
Food processing (general)		21.9	19.1	19.3	20.4
Food storage		8.1	7.2	5.8	7.2
Microbiology of food processing		5.3	6.6	6.4	6.0
Food contamination & toxicology		16.7	17.8	19.3	17.7
Food packaging		1.8	2.1	1.9	1.9
Food additives		3.4	3.1	2.9	3.2
Food composition & quality		35.5	36.5	35.6	35.8
	Citation totals	12,002	8,374	6,779	27,155
					Average 9,052

Human nutrition		1980	1985	1990	Average
Human nutrition		16.7	13.1	15.3	14.9
Nutrition & health education		13.8	6.0	6.1	8.7
Food service management		5.9	4.8	4.2	5.0
Physiology of human nutrition		20.7	29.4	24.5	25.0
Diet & diet-related diseases		42.9	46.8	49.9	46.4
	Citation totals	5,283	5,781	4,543	15,607
					Average 5,202

entries increased by 2.6%. These figures show a remarkedly unchanging pattern of subject concentration. The percentage of human nutrition entries showed a marked decrease in nutrition and health education from 13.8% in 1980 to 6.1% in 1990. There was a 7% increase in entries for diet and diet-related diseases.

Whereas *AGRIS* shows three times as many citations to food science as to human nutrition, *AGRICOLA* shows fewer than twice as many. Since both databases have the same subject coverage, the likely explanation is that *AGRICOLA* concentrates on human nutrition literature more than on food science as a result of a policy or management decision. It also could represent a decline in the developed world's literature in food science as compared to human nutrition. *AGRIS* represents input from most Third World countries, where food science has a greater emphasis than human nutrition. In both databases nearly half of all nutrition literature is concerned with diet and diet-related diseases (47.9% and 46.4%).

The 2.5 million citation database produced by CAB International (CABI) contains food science and nutrition-related citations in various subsets of the database. Food science citations appear in *Dairy Science Abstracts, Horticultural Abstracts,* and *Nutrition Abstracts and Reviews, Series A, Human and Experimental*. In addition, nutrition citations also appear with dairy science and economics subsets of CABI. For this study, only *Nutrition Abstracts and Reviews, Series A* was searched recognizing that some additional nutrition citations are in other subfiles. Subject concentrations are presented in Table 3.3. The only consistent trend was a decline in disease and therapeutic nutrition (from 31.1% in 1977 to 26.5% in 1990). The very different subject categories in Table 3.3 do not allow for exacting comparisons with *AGRICOLA* and *AGRIS*.

The *AGRICOLA* and *CAB Abstracts* data in this chapter were verified with the individual database creators.

Food Science and Technology Abstracts, begun in 1969 by the Interna-

Table 3.3. Subject concentrations in *Nutrition Abstracts and Reviews; Series A*

Categories	1977	1980	1985	1990	Average
Techniques	11.7%	11.4%	12.3%	9.3%	11.2%
Foods	11.7	9.2	9.5	12.7	10.7
Physiology & biochemistry	36.4	39.7	37.4	38.9	38.1
Human health & nutrition	8.1	10.2	13.0	12.6	11.1
Disease & therapeutic nutrition	31.1	29.5	27.8	26.5	28.9
Citation totals	9,628	9,316	8,604	7,456	35,004
					Average 8,951

Table 3.4. Subject concentrations in *Food Science and Technology Abstracts*

Categories / Publication years:	1975	1980	1985	1990	Average
Basic food science	4.5%	5.9%	4.8%	8.9%	5.9%
Food microbiology (changed to Biotechnology in 1990)	0.7	0.8	1.4	9.5	2.9
Food hygiene and toxicology	3.0	3.4	3.2	8.8	4.5
Food engineering	2.6	3.4	3.9	2.1	3.0
Food packaging	3.8	3.4	4.4	1.5	3.4
Alcoholic and non-alcoholic beverages	12.6	11.9	13.0	9.4	11.8
Fruits, vegetables, and nuts	12.4	12.2	11.7	13.5	12.4
Cocoa and chocolate products	0.6	0.7	0.7	0.4	0.6
Sugars, syrups, starches, and candy	6.7	5.7	5.8	2.2	5.1
Cereals and bakery products	9.3	9.0	10.3	9.4	9.5
Fats, oils, and margarine	3.8	3.8	3.6	3.3	3.6
Milk and dairy products	18.6	15.1	11.6	9.9	13.8
Eggs and egg products	1.3	1.3	0.9	1.1	1.1
Fish and marine products	4.6	4.5	5.7	4.5	4.9
Meat, poultry, and game	11.4	14.5	14.7	12.1	13.2
Additives, spices, and condiments	4.0	4.4	4.2	3.4	4.0
Citation totals	15,415	15,239	17,294	14,528	62,476
					Average 15,619

tional Food Information Service, contains more that 412,000 abstracts covering literature from approximately ninety-two countries in forty languages. The abstracts are divided into sections representing subject and commodity areas. These concentrations from online searching are presented in Table 3.4. The categories with the highest percentages of entries for all four years are milk and dairy products (13.8%), meat, poultry, and game (13.2%); fruits, vegetables, and nuts (12.4%); alcoholic and non-alcoholic beverages (11.8%); and cereals and bakery products (9.5%). Although in slightly different order, these are the same top five categories reported in an analysis of abstracts in the database for 1969 to 1988.[16] In that study, the highest category was milk and dairy products (12.42%), followed by meat, poultry, and game (11.55%), alcoholic and non-alcoholic beverages (11.45%), fruits, vegetables, and nuts (11.04%), and cereals and bakery products (8.53%). These five categories constituted 55.2% of all citations. In this same study, category percentages were plotted by computer for each year from 1969 to 1988. A general rising trend in papers on basic food science was noted.

The data in Table 3.4 were obtained from the online file of *FSTA* (Dialog

16. Chen and Qi, "Utilization of FSTA."

is the vendor) and sent for verification to the International Food Information Service (IFIS) in Reading, United Kingdom, where the file was searched in CD-ROM format. The online citation totals in Table 3.4 are 0.1% lower than those in the *IFIS* search. The insignificant difference appears to come from *IFIS*'s more recent datafile with additional 1990 data.

The first five categories in Table 3.4 deserve clarification. Unlike other agricultural databases, where multiple subject code entries are not uncommon, *FSTA* citations are given one subject code only. Citations listed under headings such as food engineering or food microbiology deal with these concepts in broad general terms and hence are coded into this category. Conversely, works on fruits, fats, or cereals, which may only touch on microbiology or package engineering, will be coded by the commodity.

Particular note is called to the surge in biotechnology in 1990, resulting from work in this relatively new area and from the merger with the food microbiology category.

Table 3.5. Top food science areas in the literature of India and the United States, 1981

Rank	India		United States	
1	Milk and dairy products	18.6%	Meat and poultry	33.5%
2	Fruits and vegetables	17.4	Fruits and vegetables	14.8
3	Oil, oilseeds, nuts	16.1	Oil, oilseeds, nuts	11.2
4	Cereals and millet	10.4	Seafood	7.1
5	Meat and poultry	9.5	Milk and dairy products	6.2
Total number of papers		242		384

Table 3.5 summarizes an interesting comparison that was made in 1981 between the food science priority areas of a developed country (the United States) and that of a developing or periphery country (India).[17] Analysis of 242 food science papers published in India showed that 18% were on dairy products, 17% were on fruits and vegetables, 16% were on oils and oilseeds, and 10% were on cereals and millet. The second and third ranks are the same in a study of 384 articles published in the *Journal of Food Science*, which has a U.S. emphasis almost exclusively. In the United States, however, the top-ranked area of interest was meat and poultry, and the fifth-ranked was milk and dairy products, directly the reverse of the results for India.

17. Ranganath and Ramanna, "Information for Food Industry."

Language Concentrations

Three studies, two on food science and one on human nutrition,[18] provided information on language. Additional data were obtained from *Food Science and Technology Abstracts* and *Nutrition Abstracts and Reviews, Series A*. Because of their worldwide coverage, these databases reflect the languages of concentration. The two food science studies are displayed in Table 3.6 along with data from the 1990 *Food Science and Technology Abstracts* database.

Table 3.6. Languages in food science and technology literature

	1969–1984[18a]	1965[18b]	1990[c]
English	52.15%	39.6%	71.7%
German	14.87	20.4	8.7
Russian	9.82	13.6	3.6
French	4.98	5.6	4.0
Japanese	4.31	2.6	2.8
Italian	2.74	3.7	2.2
Polish	2.12	3.7	0.7
Other	9.01[a]	10.8[b]	6.3
Total analyzed	270,336	12,077	15,657

[a]35 languages and source [b]16 languages and source [c]*FSTA* data

English is growing as the major language of food science and technology, followed by German, Russian, French, and Japanese. The 1965 comparison study is from papers in journals only.[19] The number of different languages increased from twenty-three in 1965 to forty-two in 1984. This reflects the development of this field around the world as well as the improved coverage in the database.

English is decidedly influential in the literature of human nutrition, with 85.8% of all citations (Table 3.7). German, French, Spanish, and Russian are the next most used languages.

In a study of 762 citations from two journals, Grybowski reported that only 14 (1.8%) were to languages other than English.[20] Nine of these were

18. (a) E. J. Mann, "Dissemination of Food Science and Technology Research and Development Information," *IAALD Quarterly Bulletin* 29 (4) (1984): 75–90. (b) E. J. Mann, *Evaluation of the World Food Literature* (Farnham Royal, England: Commonwealth Agricultural Bureaux, 1967). (c) Helen Grybowski, "Human Nutrition," in T. D. Wilson and Esther Herman, eds., *Fundamentals of Documentation: Students' Papers* (College Park, Md.: School of Library and Information Services; University of Maryland, 1973), pp. 138–156.

19. Mann, *Evaluation of the World Food Literature*.

20. Grybowski, "Human Nutrition."

Table 3.7. Languages in human nutrition literature

	1984–1992[a]
English	85.8%
German	3.5
French	2.4
Spanish	1.6
Russian	1.1
Polish	0.7
Japanese	0.3
Other	4.6

[a]Analysis of 71,636 entries from online file of *Nutrition Abstracts and Reviews, Series A, Human and Experimental*

to articles in German, French, and Spanish. The small number of citations to languages other than English is probably biased, since the two journals surveyed were both published in the United States.

The major languages in food science and in human nutrition are similar to the major languages in agricultural economics, agricultural engineering, animal science, and soil science, as analyzed in the Core Agricultural Literature Project (Table 3.8).

Table 3.8. Percentages of literature in English and second languages in six subject areas

Subject	English	Second language	
Agricultural economics and rural sociology[d]	87.6%[a]	French	2.5%[a]
	64.1[b]	German	8.0[b]
Agricultural engineering[d]	88.4[a]	Russian	5.0[a]
	70.9[b]	German	8.9[b]
Animal science and health[d]	73.0[a]	German	4.9[a]
	67.0[b]	German	7.1[b]
Soil science[e]	86.8[a]	German	5.6[b]
	79.6[b]		
Food science	52.2[c]	German	14.9[c]
Human nutrition	85.8[b]	German	3.5[b]

[a]Data from *AGRICOLA* online. [b]Data from *CAB Abstracts* online. [c]*Food Science & Technology Abstracts* online. [d]For more information see: Wallace C. Olsen, *The Literature of Animal Science and Health* (Ithaca, N.Y.: Cornell University Press, 1993). [e]Peter McDonald, ed., *The Literature of Soil Science* (Ithaca, N.Y.: Cornell University Press, 1994).

Types of Publication

Types of publications were discussed in two recent articles on food science and an older one on human nutrition.[21] Data were also obtained from the bibliographic entries in the *Food Science and Technology Abstracts* database, which are coded so that the type of document can be identified. Similar data can be determined for the CABI bibliographic entries, which are coded as numbered parts (journal articles), numbered wholes (mostly reports in a series), unnumbered parts, and unnumbered wholes. The last three categories match the monograph and report definitions as used in this volume.

According to the indexes of *Food Science and Technology Abstracts*, journals are the major form of publication for food science and technology, followed by patents (Table 3.9). These percentages are similar to those reported by Mann from the same abstracting service as shown in the second column of Table 3.9.[22] It must be remembered that very limited report literature is included in *FSTA*, and that almost no books are indexed at the chapter level which would be analogous to indexing journal articles.

Table 3.9. Type of publication indexed in *Food Science and Technology Abstracts*

	1969–1992[a] N=424,772	1969–1984[b] N=270,336
Journal articles	79.75%	80.27%
Reviews	NS[c]	2.58
Books	1.61	1.80
Standards	NS	3.16
Patents	11.2	12.19
Conference proceedings	1.23	NS[c]

[a]Derived from online files [b]Mann, "Dissemination of Food Sciences Information."
[c]NS = Not searched

Sue Hill, a researcher with IFIS, searched the *FSTA* CD-ROM datafile and provided the data in Table 3.10, which provides slightly greater detail. The percentages are essentially the same, however.

An analysis of 4,570 citations from three food science journals published in 1980 likewise found that journals ranked first (74.46%), but it recorded a much higher percentage of books (14.46%) and far fewer cited patents

21. (a) Mann, "Dissemination of Food Science Information." (b) B. S. Maheswarappa and K. Surya Rao, "Journal Literature of Food Science and Technology: A Bibliometric Study," *Annals of Library Science and Documentation* 29 (3) (1982): 126–134. (c) Grybowski, "Human Nutrition."
22. Mann, "Dissemination of Food Science."

Table 3.10. Type of publication recorded in *FSTA* CD-ROM database

	1969–1992 N=412,224	1969–1984 N=269,985
Journal articles	80.3%	78.5%
Reviews	2.6	2.6
Books	1.5	2.1
Standards	3.3	3.2
Patents	11.1	12.2
Conference proceedings	1.1	1.4
Theses	0.1	0.1

(0.90%) and standards (0.15%).[23] Conference proceedings and workshops were reported at 4.81%. The low percentage of cited patents and standards indicates that scientific authors are not citing these formats as frequently as abstracting services index them, perhaps because patent and standards literature is more closely allied with direct applications literature.

Journal literature is even more important in the human nutrition literature (Table 3.11), judging from the CABI service.

A study of 600 citations from two nutrition journals published in 1968 reported that 80% were references to journal articles, 14% were to books and technical reports, and 1% were to standards. The remainder were references to conference reports (6%) and theses (1%).[24] As part of the Core Project analysis, 197 nutrition classics reprinted in *Nutrition Reviews* from 1973 through 1990 were analyzed. *Nutrition Reviews* described nutrition classics as publications that redefined or initiated a field of scientific inquiry. Of these classics, 189 publications (95.9%) appeared in journals, 3.6% in books. The time spread was from 1593 to 1980 with a median age of 1941.

In the citation analysis study of the Core Agricultural Literature Project reported in this book, 61,875 citations were analyzed as to format of pub-

Table 3.11. Type of publications indexed in *Nutrition Abstracts and Reviews, Series A*

	1977–1992 N=129,350
Journal articles	90.9%
Government reports and documents	2.5
Monographs, thesis, proceedings	6.6

23. Maheswarappa and Rao, "Journal Literature of Food Science."
24. Grybowski, "Human Nutrition."

lication. Journal literature compromised 75.6%, followed by monographs at 22.7% (see Table 4.1).

Journal citations, represented as percentages of all literature in the four studies of food science cited in this chapter and in Table 4.1, are fairly consistent and confined to a seven point spread: 72.8%, 74.5%, 79.8%, and 80.3%. In the human nutrition literature the spread is greater, and the percentage of journal literature is higher: 79.0%, 80.0%, and 90.9%. The lowest figure in each set is from the Core Project analysis (see Table 4.1), which includes instructional and research literature. The extremely high 90.9% figure, for journals in *Nutrition Abstracts and Reviews, Series A* (Table 3.11), is not fully representative of the literature published in the nutrition field and may represent a management decision to concentrate on research/journal literature. The percentage of journal literature in food science is similar to that reported for other disciplines analyzed in the Core Agricultural Literature Project, while the percentage for human nutrition journal literature is higher (Table 3.12).

Table 3.12. Journals as a percent of agricultural literature

All agriculture	74%–85%[a]
Agricultural economics and rural sociology	54.8[a]
Agricultural engineering	58.1[b]
Animal science and health	75.0[b]
Soil science	72.9[c]
Food science and technology	72.8
Human nutrition	79.0

[a]Wallace C. Olsen, *Agricultural Economics and Rural Sociology; The Contemporary Core Literature* (Ithaca, N.Y.: Cornell University Press, 1991).

[b]Wallace C. Olsen, *The Literature of Animal Science and Health* (Ithaca, N.Y.: Cornell University Press, 1992) (Table 5.1).

[c]Peter McDonald, ed., *The Literature of Soil Science* (Ithaca, N.Y.: Cornell University Press, 1994).

One type of publication which does not appear in these analyses but which is becoming increasingly important is the presentation of data in electronic format. A major area in this format is food composition data, where printed tables are being superseded by computer databases from which computations can be made and tables can be printed.[25] Other databases cover food consumption and adulteration. Detailed discussions of these databases are presented in Chapter 6.

The importance of this format is demonstrated by several recent publica-

25. John C. Klensin, "Infoods An Overview," in *Informatics in Food and Nutrition*.

tions: (1) a special issue of *Trends in Food Science and Technology* (vol. 2, no. 11) devoted to online information resources; (2) an entire issue of *World Review of Nutrition and Dietetics*, vol. 68 [1992] entitled *International Food Data Bases and Information Exchange Concepts, Principles and Designs*; and (3) a conference on informatics in food and nutrition held at the Royal Swedish Academy of Sciences in 1991.[26]

Additional Selected References

Directory of Online Databases. 2 vols. Santa Monica, Calif.: Cuadra Associates, 1992.

Ensor, Pat. *CD-ROM Research Collection: An Evaluative Guide to Bibliographic and Full-Text CD-ROM Databases*. Westport, Conn.: Meckler, 1991.

Nixon, J. M. "Online Searching for Human Nutrition: An Evaluation of Databases." *Medical References Services Quarterly* 8 (Fall 1989): 27–35.

Van der Veer, O. and J. P. Kooger. "Evaluation of Abstract Journal and Other Sources Consulted for 75 Literature Searches on Food Science and Food Technology." *Aslib Proceedings* 30 (8) (1975): 302–311.

26. *Informatics in Food and Nutrition* (Uppsala, Sweden: 1991).

4. Core Monographs in Food Science and Human Nutrition

JENNIE BROGDON
Rockville, Maryland

WALLACE C. OLSEN
Mann Library, Cornell University

One objective of the Core Agricultural Literature Project was identification of monographic titles published in the past forty years which are still useful in academic study and research. These titles would be the core monographic literature of each discipline. A second objective was to determine whether the titles judged to be of highest merit in the academic community of developed countries differed from such titles in Third World countries. The resulting lists can be used in the evaluation of library collections and in the preparation of full-text compact disk products for use in establishing or improving academic and research libraries in the Third World. The list will also guide decisions on which older materials are most worthy of preservation.

A. Citation Analysis Methodology

The monographs presented in this chapter were identified through analysis of citations from a selected number of broad-based source documents (see Chapter 3). The citation analysis of fifty source documents was a laborious and time-consuming task. Every citation within a volume or selected chapter was examined. Each monograph or chapter in one, each report and its series, was identified and tallied in this process. Additional information was also gathered concerning publishers, dates of publication, place of publication, and other extraneous information. As each monograph was identified, it was placed in a list; and each time it was cited again by any author, this was counted as another citing. Detailed explanations of the methods used were reported in the first volume of this series[1].

Three criteria were used in selecting of monographic titles from the source documents: the monographs cited must be distinct works, usually with an author or editor; the title must be specific to the work; and the work must be complete in itself. Works published within a series in which each work has a separate author, a specific subject matter, and a distinct title were analyzed as monographs. Proceedings were also counted as monographs when there was a separate editor, a specialized subject, and a unique title. Proceedings of a society or conference which met yearly and published consistently on the same subject were classed with journals.

Previous work in citation analysis, done to locate primary teaching and research monographs, indicated that some types of materials could automatically be excluded from peer review. Such materials accounted for about 30% of all monographic items. Excluded from selection were

1. Pamphlet-like materials of fifty pages or fewer which were cited only once or twice
2. Local and national government documents which covered site-specific topics
3. Titles well outside the scope of these disciplines
4. Specialized works which were highly site-specific
5. Publications prior to 1950, unless cited more than five times

B. Characteristics of Publications Cited in Source Document Analyses

In the analysis process 61,875 citations were examined, and data were recorded for each. This large number of citations is twice or three times higher than the number analyzed in all but one earlier subject areas of the Core Agricultural Literature Project. This was partially a result of dealing with what are essentially two disciplines, food science and human nutrition. The two subjects are combined into a single department at twelve land-grant universities in the United States, whereas ten universities have split departments; but this difference is not reflected in the literature.[2] Information concerning the monographic citations from the analysis is summarized in this section.

1. (a) Wallace C. Olsen, "Citation Analysis," in *Agricultural Economics and Rural Sociology; The Contemporary Core Literature* (Ithaca, N.Y.: Cornell University Press, 1991), pp. 39–52. (b) Wallace C. Olsen, "Citation Analysis for Creation of Core Lists," in *Agricultural Economics and Rural Sociology*, pp. 53–66.

2. *1991–92 Directory of Professional Workers in State Agricultural Experiment Stations and Other Cooperating State Institutions* (Washington, D.C.: U.S. Dept. of Agriculture, 1992).

Analysis included calculations of the median year, or half-life, of the monographs cited. The half-life is a measure of how long publications remain relevant. It is the median age of fifty percent of the publications cited, calculated from the year the source document was published. This provides a relative guide of the currency of literature, based on its use and citation by authors. The half-life of all the monographs and reports in series analyzed in the source documents was 8.8 years. This means that half of all the citations recorded were more than 8.8 years old and getting close to being of little value. Data was also gathered for those documents which concentrated on food science. Here the half-life was 10.1 years. The human nutrition literature has a much faster turnover, with a half-life of 6.2 years. For each monographic title selected from the citations, the following information was noted:

Author, editors
Title
Date of publication
Type of publisher (e.g., commercial, governmental, organizational)
Publisher by name
Country of publication (the first one listed if more than one)

During this process, the titles were entered in a computerized list. Each time the same title or chapter in it was cited, a tally was made. Early editions were combined with the latest edition. A tally was made for each data element listed above, and the data were analyzed.

Format of Literature Cited

Table 4.1 provides data on the format of the literature cited. Citations to journals account for 75.6% of the total citations for food science and human nutrition combined. This figure and the 22.7% for monographs differ from

Table 4.1. Food science and human nutrition literature citation analysis results

Format	Both subjects combined N=61,875		Food science N=34,324		Human nutrition N=27,551	
Journals	46,760	75.6%	24,989	72.8%	21,771	79.0%
Monographs	14,033	22.7	8,394	24.5	5,639	20.5
Dissertations	252	0.4	168	0.5	84	0.3
Patents	830	1.3	773	2.2	57	0.2

the figures recorded in the agricultural and food science databases, where journals constitute 80–90% of the citations (see Tables 3.9 and 3.10). This discrepancy occurs because the bibliographic databases concentrate nearly exclusively on research as reported in journals, whereas the Core Project data reflect instructional and research literature in nearly equal proportions. But in any event, with a range of 76–90% the journal literature is clearly paramount in this subject field.

Monographic Publishers

The publishers of monographic titles in the citation analysis are heavily dominated by commercial presses (Table 4.2)

Table 4.2. Publishers of monographs

(N = 11,739)	
Commercial	60.7%
Governments (incl. UN & FAO)	19.0
Societies & organizations	12.5
University presses & departments	7.8

The top-ranked commercial publishers from the Core Project citation analysis are given in Table 4.3. Six of the publishers appear on all three lists, with Academic Press being first on each. Springer-Verlag, W. B. Saunders, McGraw-Hill, and Interscience do not appear in the combined ranking but are in either the food science or human nutrition top ten. These

Table 4.3. Primary commercial publishers in food science and human nutrition

Rank	Combined subjects	Food science	Human nutrition
1	Academic	Academic	Academic
2	AVI	AVI	Plenum
3	Wiley	Wiley	Elsevier
4	Elsevier	Elsevier	Raven
5	Plenum	Applied Science Publ.	Wiley
6	M. Dekker	M. Dekker	W. B. Saunders
7	Applied Science Publ.	CRC	CRC
8	CRC	Plenum	M. Dekker
9	Raven	Pergamon	McGraw-Hill
10	Pergamon	Interscience	Springer-Verlag

publishers were eleventh through fourteenth in the combined ranking. AVI, Applied Science, and Pergamon Press appear on the food science list but not on the human nutrition list, whereas the opposite is true for Raven, W. B. Saunders, and McGraw-Hill.

Governments or governmental agencies, the second largest group of publishers, were represented by seventy-three different governmental bodies. This demonstrates the tremendous scope of the literature, which comes from or pertains to nearly all portions of the world. This diversity of countries is primarily the result of human nutrition literature. The United States government was by far the major publisher, with 50.8% of all citations in the government group, followed distantly by the Food and Agriculture Organization, with 7.4%, and by the United Kingdom with 7.3%. These are the top three publishers of literature of concern either to the developed world or to the Third World. The primary additional players are the World Health Organization, the governments of Canada and the Netherlands, and the United Nations.

The third largest group of publishers identified in the analysis are societies, associations, and independent organizations. Table 4.4 identifies the top ten of the seventy-two organizations cited.

The top six publishers were represented in the analyzed literature of both disciplines, although more heavily in food science than in human nutrition. This clearly shows a commingling of the scientific literature in these two fields.

The relative weak influence of monographs or reports published by universities is rather surprising. The top six organizations in ranked order are Oxford University Press, Cornell University (Press and departments), Mas-

Table 4.4. Society and organizational publishers in ranked order

American Chemical Society
American Oil Chemists Society
American Association of Cereal Chemists
International Food Policy Research Institute
World Bank
American Organization of Agricultural Chemists
Nutrition Foundation[a]
Society of Chemical Industry[b]
American Society for Testing Materials[b]
Pan American Health Organization[a]

[a] = All citations from nutrition literature
[b] = All citations from food science literature

sachusetts Institute of Technology, Johns Hopkins University Press, Harvard University, and Cambridge University Press. These top six constitute 41.4% of all university monographs cited. A total of 121 individual universities were cited in the analysis.

C. Peer Evaluation of Monographic Lists

Members of the Steering Committee (see Chapter 3) reviewed the compiled monograph list before it was sent for peer review. All reviewers, whether from developed or Third World countries, had teaching and research experience and a minimum of fifteen years professional experience. Reviewers were instructed to evaluate the academic or instructional value of those titles or authors with which they were familiar and to rank those titles with regard to their importance for academic libraries in developed countries and for institutions in the Third World. They were encouraged to recommend titles for evaluation.

One list was compiled for the developed countries and a second for Third World countries. The developed countries list was divided into these categories before being sent for review:

1. General food and nutrition, intervention, planning and policy, psychology and research, anthropology, and general topics
2. Food chemistry, composition, and biotechnology; flavors and the senses
3. Food processing, engineering, packaging, storage
4. Food microbiology, toxicology, protection and regulation
5. Food management and dietetics
6. Nutrition biochemistry and metabolism
7. Human and clinical nutrition, assessment, body composition, physical activity

All evaluators received the list of titles in the first category along with other lists to match their subject specialty. Reviewers were sent instruction sheets and explanations of the project and asked to rank each title on a three point scale: 1 for a vital core title, one of the 500 most significant books including the graduate level; 2 for a significant title, one of the 1,000 most needed books; and 3 for a title of marginal interest or value.

Reviewers of the Third World list of monographs received a single list divided into three categories:

1. General food and nutrition, intervention, planning and policy
2. Food science
3. Food management and human nutrition

A composite list with three subdivisions was used because it held 50% fewer titles than the developed countries lists. It was also felt that because the transfer of advanced knowledge to the Third World was great, individuals might be able to rank titles in all three sections of the list. A two point scale was used: 1 for an important title which should be available in a Third World academic library, and 2 for a title of marginal value.

Each iteration of a list was reviewed, with titles being dropped and added through the citation analysis process and upon reviewers' recommendations. There were eleven valid reviews of the developed countries lists and fifteen of the Third World lists. This valuable effort of the reviewers is greatly appreciated.

Reviewers of Third World Monographs

Jose M. Aguilera
Universidad Catolica de Chile
Santiago, Chile
Luiz Eduardo Carvalo
Rio de Janeiro, Brazil
Jorge Chirife
Ciudad Universitaria, Nunez
Buenos Aires, Argentina
Rodolfo Florentino
Food and Nutrition Research Institute
Manila, Philippines
Peter Heywood
University of Queensland
Brisbane, Australia
Shi Huang
Scientific Research Institute,
Food Fermentation Industries
Beijing, China
Benny Kodyat
Directorate of Community Nutrition
Ministry of Health
Jakarta, Indonesia
P. R. Kulkarni
University of Bombay
A. O. Oguntunde
University of Ibadan
Ibadan, Nigeria
O. Paredes-Lopez
Unidad Irapuato, CIEA-IPN
Irapuato, Gto., Mexico
Bulan Phithakpol
Institute of Food Research & Product Development
Bangkok, Thailand
Antoni Rutkowski
Dept. of Food Technology
Warsaw, Poland
A. T. Shehata
University of Alexandria
Alexandria, Egypt
Prakash Shetty
St. John's Medical College
Bangalore, India
Noel W. Solomons
CeSSIAM
Hosp. Ojos y Oidos Dr. Rodolfo
Robles V Guatemala City, Guatemala

Reviewers of Developed Countries Monographs

Jiri Davidek
Institute of Chemical Technology
Prague, Czechoslovakia
Owen Fennema
University of Wisconsin

John E. Kinsella
University of California, Davis
Tai Wan Kwon
Korea Food Research Institute
Kyongki-Do, Korea
Jurg Solms
Swiss Federal Institute of Technology
Zurich, Switzerland
Lindsay H. Allen
University of Connecticut
John L. Beard
Pennsylvania State University
Stewart Truswell
University of Sydney
Sydney, Australia
Cutberto Garza
Cornell University
Michael C. Latham
Cornell University
Sue Hill
International Food Information Service
Reading, United Kingdom

D. Weighting the Monograph Lists

Several procedures were followed in ranking the titles:

1. Each time a monograph or a chapter of a monograph was cited in a source document, a count was made and coded into the working lists. Reviewers were unaware of the counts. These hits were given the weight of one per citing.
2. Rankings by reviewers were coded for each of the two top rankings. These were scored 2 or 1 and multiplied times the number of recommendations in each category. A statistical equalization of the seven developed countries lists was required because the first, the general list, was sent to each reviewer, resulting in a greater number of evaluations than for the six specialty lists.
3. If a title was reprinted, it was given a score of one.
4. If a title went through more than one edition, it was given a score of two.

The equation for the computation is:

$$(\text{hits} \times 1) + (\# \times 2 + \# \times 1) + (\text{Reprint} \times 1) + (\text{Edition} \times 2)$$

This formula was used for both developed and third world lists of monographs, which were then ranked separately. Using this equation, the peer evaluations accounted for between 73.4% and 73.5% of all the scores in the two lists.

Within each list the scores were broken into three logical ranks based on accrued value. In both lists the first rank (for the most important monographs) held the fewest titles; the greatest number of titles grouped around the middle rank or median. Numbers and percentages of titles in each list by rank are:

Developed countries list			Third World list	
N=927			N=495	
16.0%	148	FIRST ranking	16.3%	81
52.5	487	SECOND ranking	45.0	222
31.5	292	THIRD ranking	38.7	192

The total list has 1,063 unique titles. There are 362 titles common to both lists, an overlap of 34.1%.

Readers are reminded that all the titles in this Core List are valuable monographs for instruction and research today. Many monographs of lesser value were never submitted to reviewers or were removed by peer-evaluation (52% of all titles were dropped). Therefore, all the monographs in the two lists should be viewed as important. Rankings in three categories within each list are provided to assist in making decisions for purchase, preservation, or collection assessment.

Core List of Monographs for Food Science and Human Nutrition, 1950–1993

Developed countries ranking		Third World ranking
	A	
Second	Abelson, Philip H., ed. Food: Politics, Economics, Nutrition, and Research. Washington, D.C.; American Association for the Advancement of Science, 1975. 202p. (AAAS Miscellaneous Publication no. 75–7)	Third
Third	Abraham, S., ed. Carcinogenesis and Dietary Fat. Boston; Kluwer Academic Pub., 1989. 492p.	
	Achaya, K. T., ed. Interfaces Between Agriculture, Nutrition and Food Science; Proceedings of a Workshop, Hyderabad, India, Nov. 1981. Tokyo; United Nations University, 1984. 408p. (Food and Nutrition Bulletin, Supplement no. 9)	Second
Second	Adamson, Arthur W. Physical Chemistry of Surfaces. 5th ed. New York; Wiley, 1990. 777p. (1st ed., published by Interscience Pub., 1960. 629p.)	

Developed countries ranking		Third World ranking
Second	Aebi, Hugo E., and Roger Whitehead, eds. Maternal Nutrition during Pregnancy and Lactation; A Nestle Foundation Workshop, Lutry/Lausanne, April 1979. Bern; Huber, 1980. 354p. (Nestle Foundation Publication Series no. 1)	Second
First	Ajl, Samuel J. et al., eds. Microbial Toxins. New York; Academic Press, 1970–1980. 8 vols.	Third
Second	Alberts, Bruce et al. Molecular Biology of the Cell. 2d ed. New York; Garland Pub., 1989. 1219p. (1st ed., 1983. 1146p.) (Available in Spanish: Biología Molecular de la Célula. Barcelona; Omega. 1312p.)	
	Alcock, P. A. Food Hygiene Manual. London; H. K. Lewis, 1980. 339p.	Third
Third	Alfin-Slater, Roslyn B., and David Kritchevsky, eds. Cancer and Nutrition. New York; Plenum Press, 1991. 491p. (Human Nutrition: A Comprehensive Treatise, Vol. 7)	Third
Third	Alfin-Slater, Roslyn B., and David Kritchevsky, eds. Nutrition and the Adult: Macronutrients. New York; Plenum Press, 1980. 290p. (Human Nutrition: A Comprehensive Treatise, Vol. 3A)	Third
Second	Alfin-Slater, Roslyn B., and David Kritchevsky, eds. Nutrition and the Adult: Micronutrients. New York; Plenum Press, 1980. 424p. (Human Nutrition: A Comprehensive Treatise, Vol. 3B)	Second
Second	Alleyne, G. A. O. et al. Protein-Energy Malnutrition. London; E. Arnold, 1977. 244p.	First
Third	Alpers, David H., Ray E. Clouse, and William F. Stenson. Manual of Nutritional Therapeutics. 2d ed. Boston; Little, Brown, 1988. 486p. (1st ed., 1983. 457p.)	Second
Second	Altschul, Aaron M., ed. New Protein Foods. New York; Academic Press, 1974–1985. 5 vols. (Vols. 3–5 edited by A. M. Altschul and H. L. Wilcke.)	
Second	Amdur, Mary O., John Doull, and Curtis D. Klaasen, eds. Carett and Doull's Toxicology: The Basic Science of Poisons. 4th ed. New York; Pergamon Press, 1991. (1st ed., edited by Louis J. Cassarett and John Doull, New York; Macmillan, 1975. 768p.)	Third
Second	American Academy of Pediatrics. Committee on Nutrition. Pediatric Nutrition Handbook . . . edited by Gilbert B. Forbes and Calvin W. Woodruff. 2d ed. Elk Grove Village, Ill.; American Academy of Pediatrics, 1985. 421p. (1st ed., Evanston, Ill.; American Academy of Pediatrics, 1979. 472p.)	Second
Third	American Association of Cereal Chemists. Approved Methods of the American Association of Cereal Chemists. 8th ed. St. Paul, Minn.; AACC, 1983–. (Editions kept up to date by supplementary and replacement pages. Title varies. 1st ed. as Methods for the Analysis of Cereals and Cereal Products, Reference Tables. Lancaster, Pa.; Lancaster Press, 1928. 180p.)	Third

Developed countries ranking		Third World ranking
First	American Oil Chemists' Society. Official Methods and Recommended Practices of the American Oil Chemists' Society; David Firestone, editor of analytical methods. 4th ed. Champaign, Ill.; AOCC, 1989–. (looseleaf) (Earliest ed., as Official and Tentative Methods of the American Oil Chemists' Society, 1937. 1 vol.)	First
First	American Physiological Society. Handbook of Physiology; A Critical, Comprehensive Presentation of Physiological Knowledge and Concepts. Rev. ed. Edited by S. R. Geiger. Bethesda and Baltimore; American Physiological Society, 1977 to the present, and under constant revision. Currently in 23 vols. divided into 6 sections. (Supersedes original ed., 1959–1976, 39 vols.)	Second
Second	American Public Health Association. Technical Committee. Compendium of Methods for the Microbiological Examination of Foods . . . edited by Marvin L. Speck. 2d ed. Washington, D.C.; American Public Health Association, 1984. 914p. (1st ed., 1976. 710 p.)	
Second	American Society of Brewing Chemists. Methods of Analysis . . . 7th ed., rev. St. Paul, Minn.; ASBC Executive Secretary, 1976, 1981. 1 vol. (First published in 1937 as Official and Tentative Methods of Analysis.)	
Second	Amerine, M. A., and Rose Marie Pangborn. Principles of Sensory Evaluation of Food. New York; Academic Press, 1965. 602p.	Second
Third	Andersen, Jean E., and Aree Valyasevi, eds. Effective Communications for Nutrition in Primary Health Care; Report of the Asian Regional Workshop, Bangkok, Thailand, October 1983. Tokyo; United Nations University, 1988. 208p. (Food and Nutrition Bulletin, Supplement no. 13)	Third
Third	Aranda-Pastor, Jose, and Lenin Saenz, eds. The Process of Food and Nutrition Plannning; Proceedings of an International Conference, Antigua, Guatemala, April 1980. Guatemala; Division of Applied Nutrition, INCAP, 1981. 270p.	Second
Second	Arbuckle, W. S., and Julius H. Frandsen. Ice Cream. 4th ed. Westport, Conn.; Avi, 1986. 483p. (1st ed. as Ice Cream and Related Products, by J. H. Frandsen, 1961.)	Second
Second	Arnott, Margaret L., ed. Gastronomy: The Anthropology of Food and Food Habits. The Hague; Mouton, 1975. 354p.	Second
Third	Arora, S. K., ed. Chemistry and Biochemistry of Legumes. London; E. Arnold, 1983. 359p.	
First	Arroyave, Guillermo et al. Biochemical Methodology for the Assessment of Vitamin A Status; A Report of the International Vitamin A Consultative Group. Washington, D.C.; Nutrition Foundation, 1982. 92p.	First

Developed countries ranking		Third World ranking
Second	Arroyave, Guillermo et al. Evaluation of Sugar Fortification with Vitamin A at the National Level. Washington, D.C.; Pan American Health Organization, Regional Office of the World Health Organization, 1979. 82p. (PAHO Scientific Publication no. 384) (Available in Spanish.)	Second
Third	Arthur D. Little, Inc. Flavor: Its Chemical, Behavioral, and Commercial Aspects; Proceedings of a Symposium, Cambridge, Mass., April 1977 . . . edited by Charles M. Apt. Boulder, Colo.; Westview Press, 1978. 229p.	
	Ashworth, John C., ed. Proceedings of the 3d International Drying Symposium. Wolverhampton, U.K.; Drying Research, 1982. 2 vols.	Third
First	Aspinall, Gerald O., ed. The Polysaccharides. New York; Academic Press, 1982–1983. 2 vols.	Third
First	Association of Official Analytical Chemists. Official Methods of Analysis . . . Vol. II: Food Composition; Additives; Natural Contaminants. Edited by Kenneth Helrick. 15th ed. Washington, D.C.; Association of Official Analytical Chemists, 1990. pp. 685–1298. Vol. I about agricultural non-food chemistry. (1st ed., 1919. 1st-10th ed. published under earlier association name, Association of Official Agricultural Chemists.)	First
Second	Atkinson, Stephanie A., and Bo Lonnerdal, eds. Protein and Non-Protein Nitrogen in Human Milk. Boca Raton, Fla.; CRC Press, 1989. 249p.	Third
First	Augustin, Jorg, Barbara P. Klein, Deborah Becker and Paul B. Venugopal eds. Methods of Vitamin Assay, for the Association of Vitamin Chemists. 4th ed. New York; Wiley, 1985. 590p. (1st ed., New York and London; Interscience Publishers, 1947. 189p.)	First
Second	Austin, James E., ed. Global Malnutrition and Cereal Fortification. Cambridge, Mass.; Ballinger Pub. Co., 1979. 307p.	Second
Second	Austin, James E. Nutrition Programs in the Third World: Cases and Readings. Cambridge, Mass.; Oelgeschlager, Gunn & Hain, 1981. 456p.	First
First	Austin, James E., and Marian F. Zeitlin. Nutrition Intervention in Developing Countries: An Overview; Prepared by the Harvard Institute for International Development. Cambridge, Mass.; Oelgeschlager, Gunn & Hain, 1981. 227p.	First
Second	Aykroyd, Wallace R. The Conquest of Famine. London; Chatto & Windus, 1974. 216p.	Second
Second	Aykroyd, Wallace R. Wheat in Human Nutrition. Rome; Food and Agriculture Organization, 1970. 163p. (FAO Nutritional Studies no. 23)	Third
Second	Aykroyd, Wallace R., Joyce Doughty, and Ann Walker. Legumes in Human Nutrition. Rev. ed. Rome; Food and Agricul-	First

Developed countries ranking		Third World ranking
	ture Organization, 1982. 152p. (FAO Food and Nutrition Paper no. 20) (1964 ed., by W. R. Aykroyd and Joyce Doughty. 138p.)	
	Aylward, Francis, and Mogens Jul. Protein and Nutrition Policy in Low-Income Countries. New York; Wiley, 1975. 150p.	Third
Second	Ayres, John C., and John C. Kirschman, eds. Impact of Toxicology on Food Processing; Proceedings of a Symposium sponsored by the Institute of Food Technologists and the International Union of Food Science and Technology, June 1980. Westport, Conn.; Avi, 1981. 320p.	Second
Third	Ayres, John C., and John O. Mundt. Microbiology of Foods. San Francisco; W. H. Freeman, 1980. 708p.	Second

B

Developed countries ranking		Third World ranking
Third	Bailey, Allen J., ed. Recent Advances in the Chemistry of Meat; Proceedings of a Symposium . . . ARC Meat Research Institute, Langford, U.K., April 1983, Organized by the Food Chemistry Group of the Royal Society of Chemistry and the Food Group of the Society of Chemical Industry. London; Royal Society of Chemistry, 1984. 245p. (Royal Society of Chemistry Special Publication no. 47)	Second
First	Bailey, Alton E., and Daniel Swern, eds. Bailey's Industrial Oil and Fat Products . . . by Marvin W. Formo et al. 4th ed. New York; Wiley, 1979–1985. 3 vols. (1st ed., by A. E. Bailey, New York; Interscience Publishers, 1945. 735p.)	First
Third	Balderston, Judith B. et al. Malnourished Children of the Rural Poor: The Web of Food, Health, Education, Fertility, and Agricultural Production. Boston; Auburn House Pub. Co., 1981. 204p.	Second
First	Banks, W., and Charles T. Greenwood. Starch and Its Components. New York; Wiley, 1975. 342p.	Second
Second	Banwart, George J. Basic Food Microbiology. 2d ed. Westport, Conn.; Avi, 1989. 773p. (1st ed., 1979. 781p.)	Second
Second	Barker, Lewis M., ed. The Psychobiology of Human Food Selection. Westport, Conn.; Avi, 1982. 262p.	Second
Third	Barker, Randolph, and Robert W. Herdt. The Rice Economy of Asia. Washington, D.C.; Resources for the Future, 1985. 324p.	Second
Second	Barman, Thomas E. Enzyme Handbook. Berlin, etc.; Springer, 1969. 2 vols. (Accompanied by Supplement I, 1974. 517p.)	
First	Barnes, P. J., ed. Lipids in Cereal Technology. New York; Academic Press, 1983. 425p.	Second
Third	Basu, Tapan K., and C. J. Schorah. Vitamin C in Health and Disease. London; Croom Helm; Westport, Conn.; Avi, 1982. 152p.	

Developed countries ranking		Third World ranking
Second	Bauernfeind, J. Christopher, ed. Carotenoids as Colorants and Vitamin A Precursors: Technological and Nutritional Applications. New York; Academic Press, 1981. 938p.	
Second	Bauernfeind, J. Christopher. The Safe Use of Vitamin A: A Report of the International Vitamin A Consultative Group. New York; Nutrition Foundation, 1980. 44p.	First
Second	Bauernfeind, J. Christopher, ed. Vitamin A Deficiency and Its Control. Orlando, Fla.; Academic Press, 1986. 530p.	First
Second	Bauernfeind, J. Christopher, and Paul A. Lachance, eds. Nutrient Additions to Food: Nutritional, Technological and Regulatory Aspects. Trumbull, Conn.; Food & Nutrition Press, 1991. 622p.	
Third	Beal, Virginia A., and Mary Jane Laus, eds. Symposium on Dietary Data Collection, Analysis, and Significance; Proceedings . . . sponsored by the Dept. of Food Science and Nutrition, June 1981. Amherst; Massachusetts Agricultural Experiment Station, College of Food and Natural Resources, University of Massachusetts at Amherst, 1982. 164p. Massachusetts AES, College of Food and Natural Resources, Research Bulletin no. 675)	
Second	Beare-Rogers, Joyce, ed. Dietary Fat Requirements in Health and Development. Champaign, Ill.; American Oil Chemists Society, 1988. 206p.	Third
First	Beaton, George H., and J. M. Bengoa, eds. Nutrition in Preventive Medicine: The Major Deficiency Syndromes, Epidemiology, and Approaches to Control. Geneva; World Health Organization, 1976. 590p. (WHO Monograph Series no. 62)	First
Second	Beaton, George H., and Earle W. McHenry, eds. Nutrition: A Comprehensive Treatise. New York; Academic Press, 1964–1966. 3 vols.	
Second	Beaver, Paul C., Rodney C. Jung, and Eddie W. Cupp. Clinical Parasitology. 9th ed. Philadelphia; Lea & Febiger, 1984. 825p. (1st ed., by Charles F. Craig and Ernest C. Faust, 1937. 733p.)	Second
First	Becher, Paul, ed. Encyclopedia of Emulsion Technology. New York; M. Dekker, 1983. 3 vols.	
Second	Bechtel, Peter J. Muscle as Food. Orlando, Fla.; Academic Press, 1986. 459p.	Third
Second	Beghin, Ivan, Miriam Cap, and Bruno Dujardin. A Guide to Nutritional Assessment. Geneva; World Health Organization, 1988. 80p.	First
Third	Behrman, Richard E., and Robert Kliegman, eds. Nelson Textbook of Pediatrics. 14th ed. Philadelphia; W. B. Saunders, 1992. (5th ed. published as Mitchell-Nelson Textbook of Pediatrics, by Waldo E. Nelson, 1950. 1658p.) (Available in Span-	

Developed countries ranking		Third World ranking
	ish: Compendio de pediatría de Belson. Mexico; Neisa, 1991. 798p.)	
Third	Beitz, Donald C., and R. Gaurth Hansen, eds. Animal Products in Human Nutrition. New York; Academic Press, 1982. 545p.	
Second	Belitz, H. D., W. Grosch. Food Chemistry. Translated of 2d ed. of Lehrbuch der Lebensmittelchemie. Berlin, New York; Springer Verlag, 1987. 774p.	
First	Bender, Arnold E. Dictionary of Nutrition and Food Technology. 6th ed. London and Boston; Butterworths, 1990. 336p. (1st ed., New York; Academic Press, 1960. 143p.)	First
Second	Bender, Arnold E. Food Processing and Nutrition. London and New York; Academic Press, 1978. 243p.	
Second	Bender, Filmore E., Larry W. Douglass, and Amihud Kramer. Statistical Methods for Food and Agriculture. New York; Food Products Press, 1989. 345p. (1st ed., Westport, Conn.; Avi Pub. Co., 1982.)	First
	Bennion, Marion. Introductory Foods. 8th ed. New York and London; Macmillan Collier Macmillan, 1985. 632p. (1st ed., by Osee G. Hughes, 1940. 522p.)	Second
Third	Bennion, Marion. The Science of Food. San Francisco; Harper & Row, 1980. 598p.	
Second	Berg, Alan. Malnourished People: A Policy View. Washington, D.C.; World Bank, 1981. 108p.	First
First	Berg, Alan. The Nutrition Factor: Its Role in National Development. Washington, D.C.; Brookings Institution, 1973. 290p. (Available in Spanish: Estudios Sobre Nutricíon: su Importancia en el Desarrollo Socioeconómico. 1ed. México: Limusa-Noriega. 344p.)	First
Second	Berg, Alan, N. S. Scrimshaw, and D. L. Call, eds. Nutrition, National Development, and Planning; Proceedings of a National Conference. Cambridge, Mass.; MIT Press, 1973. 401p.	First
	Berger, Heribert, ed. Vitamins and Minerals in Pregnancy and Lactation; Proceedings of an International Symposium, Innsbruck, Austria, Sept. 1986. New York; Raven press, 1988. 450p.	Third
First	Bergmeyer, Hans U., Jurgen Bergmeyer, and Marianne Grassl, eds. Methods of Enzymatic Analysis. 3d ed., rev. and enl. Weinheim, Germany, and Deerfield Beach, Fla.; Verlag Chemie, 1983–1986. 12 vols. (1st English ed. trans. by Dermot H. Williamson. Weinheim/Bergstrasse; Verlag Chemie; New York; Academic Press, 1963. 1064p. 1st German ed. published, 1962, as Methoden der Enzymatischen Analyse.)	
Second	Beuchat, Larry R. Food and Beverage Mycology. 2d ed. New York; Van Nostrand Reinhold, 1987. 661p. (1st ed., Westport, Conn.; Avi Pub. Co., 1978. 527p.)	First

Developed countries ranking		Third World ranking
Second	Bingham, Sheila. Dictionary of Nutrition: A Consumer's Guide to the Facts of Food. London; Barrie & Jenkins, 1977. 319p.	
Second	Binkley, Roger W. Modern Carbohydrate Chemistry. New York; M. Dekker, 1988. 343p.	
Third	Biochemical Identification of Meat Species: A Seminar in the EEC Programme of Coordination of Livestock Productivity Management, Brussels, November 1984. London and New York; Elsevier Applied Science, 1985. 213p.	
Second	Birch, Gordon G. Analysis of Food Carbohydrate. London and New York; Elsevier Applied Science, 1985. 311p.	
Second	Birch, Gordon G. et al., eds. Developments in Food Carbohydrate. London; Applied Science Publishers, 1977. 3 vols. (Papers in vol. 1, edited by G. G. Birch and R. S. Shallenberger, were presented at an American Chemical Society Symposium organized by the Divisions of Carbohydrate Chemistry and Agricultural and Food Chemistry. Vol. 2, edited by C. K. Lee. Vol. 3, edited by C. K. Lee and M. G. Lindley.)	
First	Birch, Gordon G., N. Blakebrough, and K. J. Parker, eds. Enzymes and Food Processing; Papers from an Industry-University Cooperation Symposium organized under the auspices of the National College of Foods Technology, University of Reading, March-April 1980. London; Applied Science, 1981. 296p.	First
Second	Birch, Gordon G., J. G. Brennan, and K. J. Parker, eds. Sensory Properties of Foods: An Industry-University Cooperation Symposium organized under the auspices of the National College of Food Technology, University of Reading. London; Applied Science Publishers, 1977. 326p.	
Second	Birch, Gordon G., G. Campbell-Platt, and M. G. Lindley, eds. Foods for the '90s; Papers from a Symposium organized under the auspices of the Department of Food Science and Technology, University of Reading, April 1989. London and New York; Elsevier Applied Science, 1990. 250p.	Third
Third	Birch, Gordon G., and M. G. Lindley, eds. Developments in Food Flavours; Proceedings of an Industry-University Cooperation Symposium, National College of Food Technology, Dept. of Food Technology, University of Reading, March 1986. London and New York; Elsevier Applied Science, 1986. 287p.	
Second	Birch, Gordon G., and M. G. Lindley, eds. Interactions of Food Components; An Industry-University Cooperation Symposium organized under the auspices of the National College of Food Technology, University of Reading, April 1985. London and New York; Elsevier Applied Science Publishers, 1986. 343p.	
Second	Birch, Gordon G., and K. J. Parker, eds. Nutritive Sweeteners. London and Englewood, N.J.; Applied Science, 1982. 316p.	

Developed countries ranking		Third World ranking
Second	Birch, Gordon G., and K. J. Parker, eds. Control of Food Quality and Food Analysis; An Industry-University Cooperation Symposium organized under the auspices of the National College of Food Technology (Dept. of Food Technology), University of Reading, March 1983. London and New York; Elsevier Applied Science, 1984. 332p.	Third
Second	Birch, Gordon G., and K. J. Parker, eds. Dietary Fibre. London and New York; Applied Science, 1983. 304p.	Second
Second	Birch, Gordon G., and K. J. Parker, eds. Food and Health: Science and Technology; Proceedings of an Industry-University Cooperation Symposium organized under the auspices of the National College of Food Technology, University of Reading, April 1979. London; Applied Science, 1980. 532p.	
Second	Birch, Gordon G., Michael Spencer, and Allan G. Cameron. Food Science. 3d ed. Oxford and New York; Pergamon Press, 1986. 175p. (1st ed., 1972. 189p.)	Second
Second	Biswas, Margaret, and Per Pinstrup-Andersen, eds. Nutrition and Development. New York; United Nations University; Oxford and New York; Oxford University Press, 1985. 190p.	Second
Second	Blackburn, George L., John P. Grant, and Vernon R. Young, eds. Amino Acids: Metabolism and Medical Applications; Based on a Conference, March-April 1982, Raleigh, N.C. Boston; John Wright and PSG, 1983. 520p.	
Second	Blakley, Raymond L., and Stephen J. Benkovic, eds. Folates and Pterins. New York; Wiley, 1984–1986. 3 vols. (Vol. 3 edited by R. L. Blakley and V. Michael Whitehead.)	Third
Second	Blanshard, J. M. V., P. J. Frazier, and T. Galliard, eds. Chemistry and Physics of Baking: Materials, Processes, and Products; Proceedings of an International Symposium organized by the Food Chemistry Group, Royal Society of Chemistry and the School of Agriculture, University of Nottingham, the School of Agriculture, Sutton Bonington, April 1985. London; Royal Society of Chemistry, 1986. 276p. (Special Publication no. 56)	
Second	Blanshard, J. M. V., and P. Lillford. Food Structure and Behaviour. London; Academic Press, 1987. 291p.	Second
Second	Blaxter, Kenneth L., and J. C. Waterlow, eds. Nutritional Adaptation in Man; Proceedings of an International Symposium organized by the Rank Prize Funds, Royal Windsor, U.K., April 1984. London; J. Libbey, 1985. 244p.	
Third	Blaxter, Kenneth L., ed. Food Chains and Human Nutrition; Proceedings of an International Symposium organized by the Rank Prize Funds, Kenilworth, Warwickshire, U.K., April 1979. London; Applied Science Publishers, 1980. 470p.	Second
Third	Blaxter, Kenneth, and Leslie Fowden, eds. Food, Nutrition and Climate; Proceedings of an International Symposium organized	

Developed countries ranking		Third World ranking
	by the Rank Prize Funds, Dormy Hotel, Ferndown, Dorset, U.K., April 1981. London and Englewood, N.J.; Applied Science, 1982. 422p.	
Second	Block, Seymour S., ed. Disinfection, Sterilization, and Preservation. 3d ed. Philadelphia; Lea & Febiger, 1983. 1053p. (1st ed., edited by Carl A. Lawrence and S. S. Block, 1968. 808p.)	Third
Third	Bloom, Stephen R., and Julia M. Polak, eds. Gut Hormones. 2d ed. Edinburgh and New York; Churchill Livingstone, 1981. 605p. (1st ed., edited by S. R. Bloom, 1978. 664p.)	
Third	Board, R. G. A Modern Introduction to Food Microbiology. Oxford and Boston; Blackwell Scientific Publications, 1983. 236p. (Basic Microbiology no. 8) (Available in Spanish: Introduccíon Moderna a la Microbiología de los Aliementos. Zaragoza: Acribia, 1988. 284p.)	Third
	Bodwell, C. E., J. S. Adkins, and D. T. Hopkins, eds. Protein Quality in Humans: Assessment and in Vitro Estimation. Westport, Conn.; Avi, 1981. 435p.	Second
Second	Bodwell, C. E., and John W. Erdman, eds. Nutrient Interactions. New York; M. Dekker, 1988. 389p.	Third
Third	Bodwell, C. E., and L. Petit, eds. Plant Proteins for Human Food; Proceedings of a European Congress held in Nantes, France, Oct. 1981. The Hague and Boston; M. Nijhoff/W. Junk, 1983. 471p.	
Third	Bondy, Philip K., and Leon E. Rosenberg, eds. Metabolic Control and Disease. 8th ed. Philadelphia; Saunders, 1980. 1870p. (1st ed., edited by Garfield G. Duncan, 1942, as Diseases of Metabolism: Detailed Methods of Diagnosis and Treatment: A Text for the Practitioner. 985p.) (Avaliable in Spanish: Enfermedades del Metabolismo. Barcelon; Salvat. 1092p.)	Third
Second	Borgstrom, Bengt, and Howard L. Brockman, eds. Lipases. Amsterdam and New York; Elsevier, 1984. 527p.	
First	Borgstrom, Georg, ed. Fish as Food. New York; Academic Press, 1961–1965. 4 vols.	First
Third	Borgstrom, Georg. The Food and People Dilemma. Belmont, Calif.; Duxbury Press, 1973. 140p.	Third
	Boserup, Ester. Population and Technological Change: A Study of Long-Term Trends. Chicago; University of Chicago Press, 1981. 255p. (Available in Spanish: Poblacíon y Cambio Technológico: Estudio de las Tendencias a Largo Plazo. Barcelona; Crittica. 360p.	Third
Second	Bothwell, Thomas H. et al. Iron Metabolism in Man. Oxford; Blackwell Scientific Pub., 1979. 576p.	Third
Second	Bothwell, Thomas H., and Robert W. Charlton. Iron Deficiency in Women; Report for the International Nutritional Ane-	Third

Developed countries ranking		Third World ranking
	mia Consultative Group. New York; Nutrition Foundation, 1981. 68p.	
Third	Bouchard, Claude, and Francis E. Johnston, eds. Fat Distribution during Growth and Later Health Outcomes; Proceedings of a Symposium held at Manoir St.-Castin, Lac Beauport, Quebec, June 1987. New York; Liss, 1988. 363p. (Current Topics in Nutrition and Disease no. 17)	
Second	Bourne, Geoffrey H., ed. World Nutritional Determinants. Basel and New York; Karger, 1985. 225p.	Second
First	Bourne, Malcolm C. Food Texture and Viscosity: Concept and Measurement. New York; Academic Press, 1982. 325p.	
Second	Bourne, Malcolm C. Post Harvest Food Losses: The Neglected Dimension in Increasing the World Food Supply. Ithaca, N.Y.; New York State College of Agriculture and Life Sciences, Cornell University, 1977. 49p. (Cornell International Agriculture Mimeograph no. 53)	Second
Second	Bowes and Church's Food Values of Portions Commonly Used. 16th ed., rev. by Jean A. T. Pennington. Philadelphia, Pa.; J. B. Lippincott, 1993. 483p. (1st ed., 1937, as Food Values of Portions Commonly Served. Editors, 1963–1975, Charles F. Church and Helen N. Church.)	
Third	Boyd, Eldon M. Toxicity of Pure Foods . . . edited by Carl E. Boyd. Cleveland, Ohio; CRC Press, 1973. 260p.	
Second	Boyer, Paul D., ed. The Enzymes. 3d ed. New York; Academic Press, 1970–1990. 20 vols. (2d ed., edited by P. D. Boyer, Henry Lardy and Karl Myrback, 1959–1963. 8 vols.)	Second
Second	Branen, A. Larry, and P. Michael Davidson, eds. Antimicrobials in Foods. New York; M. Dekker, 1983. 465p.	
Second	Branen, A. Larry, P. Michael Davidson, and Seppo Salminen, eds. Food Additives. New York; M. Dekker, 1990. 736p.	Third
	Braverman, Joseph B. Braverman's Introduction to the Biochemistry of Foods. Completely new ed., by Z. Berk. Amsterdam and New York; Elsevier Scientific Pub. Co., 1976. 315p. (1st ed., 1963. 336p.)	Third
Third	Bray, R. C., P. C. Engel, and S. G. Mayhew, eds. Flavins and Flavoproteins; Proceedings of the 8th International Symposium, Brighton, England, July 1984. Berlin and New York; W. de Gruyter, 1984. 923p.	
	Brenndorfer, B. et al. Solar Dryers: Their Role in Post-Harvest Processing. London; Commonwealth Science Council, Commonwealth Secretariat, 1985. 337p.	Second
	Briend, André. Prevention et Traitement de la Malnutrition: Guide Pratique. Paris; Editions de l'Orstom, 1985. 146p. (Collection Initiations-Documentations Techniques; no. 62.)	Third

Developed countries ranking		Third World ranking
First	Briggs, D. E. et al. Malting and Brewing Science. 2d ed. London and New York; Chapman & Hall, 1981–1982. 2 vols. (Earlier ed., by J. S. Hough, D. E. Briggs and R. Stevens, 1971. 678p.)	Second
Second	Briggs, Michael H. Vitamins in Human Biology and Medicine. Boca Raton, Fla.; CRC Press, 1981. 255p.	Second
	Brisson, Germain J. Lipids in Human Nutrition: An Appraisal of Some Dietary Concepts. Englewood, N.J.; J. K. Burgess, 1981. 175p.	Third
Second	Brockerhoff, Hans, and Robert G. Jensen. Lipolytic Enzymes. New York; Academic Press, 1974. 330p.	
Second	Broderick, Harold M., ed. The Practical Brewer: A Manual for the Brewing Industry. 2d ed. Madison, Wis.; Master Brewers Association of the Americas, 1977. 475p. (1st ed., by Edward H. Vogel et al. New York; 1946. 228p.)	
Third	Bronner, Felix, and Jack W. Coburn, eds. Calcium Physiology. New York; Academic Press, 1982. 568p. (Disorders of Mineral Metabolism no. 2)	
Third	Brostoff, Jonathan, and Stephen J. Challacombe, eds. Food Allergy. London and Philadelphia; Saunders, 1982. 260p.	
	Brothwell, Don, and Patricia Brothwell. Food in Antiquity: A Survey of the Diet of Early Peoples. London; Thames & Hudson, 1969. 248p. (Available in German: Manna und Hirse: Eine Kulturgeschichte der Ernahrung, 1984)	Third
Third	Brouk, B. Plants Consumed by Man. London and New York; Academic Press, 1975. 479p.	
	Brown, E. Evan. World Fish Farming: Cultivation and Economics. 2d ed. Westport, Conn.; Avi, 1983. 516p. (1st ed., 1977. 397p.)	Second
Second	Brown, M. H., ed. Meat Microbiology. London and New York; Applied Science, 1982. 529p.	
First	Brown, Myrtle L., ed. Present Knowledge in Nutrition. 6th ed. Washington, D.C.; International Life Sciences Institute-Nutrition Foundation, 1990. 532p. (Rev. ed. of Nutrition Reviews' Present Knowledge in Nutrition. 1st ed., 1953. 1984 ed., edited by M. A. Eastwood.)	First
Third	Brownell, Kelly D., and John P. Foreyt, eds. Handbook of Eating Disorders: Physiology, Psychology, and Treatment of Obesity, Anorexia, and Bulimia. New York; Basic Books, 1986. 529p.	Third
Second	Brozek, Josef, and Beat Schurch, eds. Malnutrition and Behavior: Critical Assessment of Key Issues: An International Symposium at a Distance, 1982–1983. Lausanne, Switzerland; Nestle Foundation, 1984. 656p. (Nestle Foundation Publication Series no. 4)	First

Developed countries ranking		Third World ranking
Second	Brubacher, G., W. Muller-Mulot, and D. A. T. Southgate, eds. Methods for the Determination of Vitamins in Food, Recommended by COST 91. London and New York; Elsevier Applied Science, 1985. 166p.	
Third	Bruch, Hilde. Eating Disorders; Obesity, Anorexia Nervosa, and the Person Within. New York; Basic Books, 1973. 396p.	
Second	Brun, T. A., and M. C. Latham, eds. World Food Issues: Maldevelopment and Malnutrition. Ithaca, N.Y.; Cornell Program in International Agriculture, 1990. 126p. (World Food Issues no. 2)	Second
	Brunser, Oscar, ed. Clinical Nutrition of the Young Child. New York; Raven Press, 1991. 315p.	Third
Second	Burgess, Anne. Evaluation of Nutrition Interventions: An Annotated Bibiography and Review of Methodologies and Results. 2d ed. Rome; Food and Agriculture Organization, 1982. 194p. (FAO Food and Nutrition Paper no. 24)	Second
Third	Burkitt, Denis P. Don't Forget Fiber in Your Diet: To Help Avoid Many of Our Commonest Diseases. Completely rev. and updated ed. New York; Arco Pub., 1984. 128p. (Previously published, 1979, as Eat Right to Keep Healthy and Enjoy Life More.)	Third
First	Burkitt, Denis P., and H. C. Trowell. Refined Carbohydrate Foods and Disease: Some Implications of Dietary Fibre. London and New York; Academic Press, 1975. 356p.	Third
Third	Burt, J. R., ed. Fish Smoking and Drying. The Effect of Smoking and Drying on the Nutritional Properties of Fish. Barking, U.K.; Elsevier Science Publishers, 1988. 166p.	Second
Third	Bushuk, Walter, ed. Rye: Production, Chemistry, and Technology. St. Paul, Minn.; American Association of Cereal Chemists, 1976. 181p. (AACC Monograph Series no. 5)	

C

Developed countries ranking		Third World ranking
Second	Cagan, Robert H., and Morley R. Kare, eds. Biochemistry of Taste and Olfaction; Proceedings of a Symposium . . . April 1980, Monell Chemical Senses Center. New York; Academic Press, 1981. 539p.	
Third	Caliendo, Mary Alice. Nutrition and the World Food Crisis. New York; Macmillan, 1979. 368p.	
Third	Cameron, Allan G. The Science of Food and Cooking. 3d ed. London; E. Arnold, 1985. 252p.	Third
Second	Cameron, Margaret, and Yngve Hofvander. Manual on Feeding Infants and Young Children; Sponsored by the UN/ACC Subcommittee on Nutrition. 3d ed. Oxford; Oxford University	First

Developed countries ranking		Third World ranking
	Press, 1983. 214p. (1st ed., New York; Protein Advisory Group of the United Nations System, 1971. 239p.)	
Second	Cameron, Margaret, and Wija A. van Staveren. Manual on Methodology for Food Consumption Studies. Oxford and New York; Oxford University Press, 1988. 259p.	Second
Second	Campbell-Platt, Geoffrey. Fermented Foods of the World: A Dictionary and Guide. London and Boston; Butterworths, 1987. 291p.	Second
Second	Canada. Bureau of Nutritional Sciences. Recommended Nutrient Intakes for Canadians. Ottawa; Health and Welfare Canada, 1983. 181p. (Revision of Dietary Standard for Canada.)	
Second	Canned Foods: Principles of Thermal Process Control, Acidification and Container Closure Evaluation . . . edited and illustrated by staff members of The Food Processors Institute. 5th ed. Washington, D.C.; The Institute, 1988. 231p. (3d ed., rev., 1980. 224p.)	
Third	Carpenter, Kenneth J. The History of Scurvy and Vitamin C. Cambridge and New York; Cambridge University Press, 1986. 288p.	
Third	Carpenter, Kenneth J., ed. Pellagra. Stroudsburg, Pa.; Hutchinson Ross Pub. Co., 1981. 391p.	
Second	Carter, M. W. et al., eds. Radionuclides in the Food Chain. Berlin and New York; Springer-Verlag, 1988. 518p.	
Second	Carterette, Edward C., and Morton P. Friedman, eds. Tasting and Smelling. New York; Academic Press, 1978. 321p. (Handbook of Perception no. 6A)	
	Casley, D. J., and D. A. Lury. Data Collection in Developing Countries. 2d ed. Oxford; Clarendon Press; New York; Oxford University Press, 1987. 244p. (1st ed., 1981. 244p.)	Second
	Castro, Josue de. The Geography of Hunger. Boston; Little, Brown, 1952. 337p. (Translation of Geopolitica da Fome.)	Third
	Cathie, John. The Political Economy of Food Aid. New York; St. Martin's Press, 1981. 190p.	Third
Third	Chambers, Robert. Rural Development: Putting the Last First. London and New York; Longman, 1983. 246p.	Second
Second	Chan, H. W.-S. Autoxidation of Unsaturated Lipids. London; Academic Press, 1987. 296p.	
Second	Chan, H. W.-S., ed. Biophysical Methods in Food Research. Oxford and Boston; Published for the Society of Chemical Industry by Blackwell Scientific Publications, 1984. 204p.	
Second	Chan, Harvey T., ed. Handbook of Tropical Foods. New York; M. Dekker, 1983. 639p.	Second
Second	Chanarin, Israel. The Megaloblastic Anaemias. Oxford; Blackwell Scientific, 1969. 1000p.	
Third	Chandra, Ranjit K., ed. Food Allergy; Proceedings of a Satel-	

Developed countries ranking		Third World ranking
	lite Symposium of the 6th International Congress of Immunology, St. John's, Newfoundland, July 1986, under the auspices of the International Union of Nutritional Sciences and the Memorial University of Newfoundland. St. John's, Newfoundland, Canada; Nutrition Research Education Foundation, 1987. 387p.	
	Chandra, Ranjit K., ed. Food Intolerance. New York; Elsevier, 1984. 260p.	Third
Second	Chandra, Ranjit K., ed. Nutrition and Immunology. New York; Liss, 1988. 342p.	Third
Third	Chandra, Ranjit K., ed. Trace Elements in Nutrition of Children, II; Proceedings . . . Nestle Nutrition Workshop, 23rd, Marrakech, Morocco, May 1989. Vevey; Nestle Nutrition; New York; Raven Press, 1991. 232p.	Third
Second	Chandra, Ranjit K., ed. Trace Elements in Nutrition of Children; Proceedings . . . Nestle Nutrition Workshop, 8th, Munich, January 1984. Vevey; Nestle Nutrition; New York; Raven Press, 1985. 306p. (Nestle Foundation Nutrition Series no. 8)	Second
Second	Chandra, Ranjit K., and P. M. Newberne. Nutrition, Immunity, and Infection: Mechanisms of Interactions. New York; Plenum Press, 1977. 246p.	First
Third	Chapman, Dennis, ed. Biological Membranes; Physical Fact and Function. London and New York; Academic Press, 1968–1984. 5 vols. (Vols. 2–5 lack subtitle. Vols. 2–3 edited by D. Chapman and D. F. H. Wallach.)	
Second	Charalambous, George, ed. Analysis of Foods and Beverages: Modern Techniques. Orlando, Fla.; Academic Press, 1984. 652p.	
Third	Charalambous, George, ed. Handbook of Food and Beverage Stability: Chemical, Biochemical, Microbiological, and Nutritional Aspects. Orlando, Fla.; Academic Press, 1986. 840p.	Third
Second	Charalambous, George, and George Inglett, eds. Chemistry of Foods and Beverages: Recent Developments; Proceedings of the 2d International Flavor Conference, Athens, July 1981 and Formulated Foods and Their Ingredients: Recent Progress in Chemistry, Nutrition, and Technology, Anaheim, Calif., Nov. 1981. New York; Academic Press, 1982. 348p.	
Second	Charalambous, George, and George Inglett, eds. Instrumental Analysis of Foods: Recent Progress; Proceedings . . . International Flavor Conference, 3rd, Corfu, Greece, July 1983. New York; Academic Press, 1983. 2 vols.	
Second	Charalambous, George, and George Inglett, eds. The Quality of Foods and Beverages: Chemistry and Technology; Proceedings of the 2d International Flavor Conference, Athens, Greece, July 1981. New York; Academic Press, 1981. 2 vols.	

Developed countries ranking		Third World ranking
Second	Charley, Helen. Food Science. 2d ed. New York; Wiley, 1982. 564p. (1st ed., New York; Ronald Press Co., 1970. 520p.)	Third
Third	Charm, Stanley E. The Fundamentals of Food Engineering. 3d ed. Westport, Conn.; Avi, 1978. 646p. (1st ed., 1963. 592p.)	
Third	Chavez, Adolfo, and Celia Martinez. Growing up in a Developing Community: A Bio-Ecologic Study of the Development of Children from Poor Peasant Families in Mexico. Mexico City; Instituto Nacional de la Nutricion, 1982. 155p.	Second
Second	Chen, Lincoln C., and Nevin S. Scrimshaw, eds. Diarrhea and Malnutrition: Interactions, Mechanisms, and Interventions. New York; Plenum Press, 1983. 318p. (Sponsored by the United Nations University, Tokyo.)	First
Second	Chen, Linda H., ed. Nutritional Aspects of Aging. Boca Raton, Fla.; CRC Press, 1986. 2 vols.	
Third	Chichester, Clinton O., ed. The Chemistry of Plant Pigments. New York; Academic Press, 1972. 218p. (Advances in Food Research, Supplement no. 3)	
Second	Christensen, Clyde M., ed. Storage of Cereal Grains and Their Products. 3d ed. St. Paul, Minn.; American Association of Cereal Chemists, 1982. 544p. (1st ed., edited by J. A. Anderson.)	First
Third	Christiansen, C., J. S. Johansen, and B. J. Riis, eds. Osteoporosis 1987; Proceedings of an International Symposium . . . Denmark, Sept.-Oct. 1987. Copenhagen; Osteopress, 1987. 2 vols.	
	Christie, Andrew B., and Mary C. Christie. Food Hygiene and Food Hazards for All Who Handle Food. 2d ed. London; Faber, 1977. 232p. (1st ed., 1971. 216p.)	Third
First	Christie, William W. Lipid Analysis: Isolation, Separation, Identification, and Structural Analysis of Lipids. 2d ed. Oxford and New York; Pergamon Press, 1982. 207p. (1st ed., 1973. 338p.)	
	Cleland, John, and John Hobcraft, eds. Reproductive Change in Developing Countries; Insights from the World Fertility Survey. London and New York; Oxford University Press, 1985. 301p.	Second
	Clugston, Graeme A., and Kalyan Bagchi. Iodine-Deficiency Disorders in South-East Asia. New Delhi; WHO Regional Office for South-East Asia, 1985. 96p. (SEARO Regional Health Papers no. 10)	Second
Second	Clydesdale, Fergus M., ed. Food Science and Nutrition: Current Issues and Answers. Englewood Cliffs, N.J.; Prentice-Hall, 1979. 226p.	
Second	Clydesdale, Fergus M., and Kathryn L. Wiemer. Iron Fortification of Foods. Orlando, Fla.; Academic Press, 1985. 176p.	
Third	Concon, Jose M. Food Toxicology. New York; M. Dekker, 1988. 2 vols.	

Developed countries ranking		Third World ranking
Third	Conning, D. V., and A. B. G. Lansdown. Toxic Hazards in Food. New York; Raven Press, 1983. 297p.	
Third	Conover, W. J.. Practical Nonparamatic Statistics. 2d ed. New York; Wiley, 1980. 493p. (1st ed., 1971. 462p.)	Third
Second	Considine, Douglas M., and Glenn D. Considine, eds. Foods and Food Production Encyclopedia. New York; Van Nostrand Reinhold, 1982. 2305p.	Second
Second	Consolazio, C. Frank, Robert E. Johnson, and Louis J. Pecora. Physiological Measurements of Metabolic Functions in Man. New York; Blakiston Division, McGraw-Hill, 1963. 505p.	
Third	Cook, Arthur H. Barley and Malt: Biology, Biochemistry, Technology. New York; Academic Press, 1962. 740p.	
Second	Copson, David A. Microwave Heating. 2d ed. Westport, Conn.; Avi, 1975. 615p. (1st ed., 1962. 433 p.)	
Second	Coultate, Tom P. Food: The Chemistry of Its Components. 2d ed. London; Royal Society of Chemistry, 1989. 325p. (1st ed., 1984. 197p.)	
Third	Counsell, J. N., ed. Natural Colours for Food and Other Uses; Proceedings of an International Symposium, London, October 1979. London; Applied Science Publishers, 1981. 167p.	
	Coursey, Donald G. Yams: An Account of the Nature, Origins, Cultivation and Utilisation of the Useful Members of the Dioscoreaceae. London; Longmans, 1967. 230p.	Third
Second	Cravioto, Joaquin, Leif Hambraeus, and Bo Vahlquist, eds. Early Malnutrition and Mental Development; Proceedings of a Symposium . . . Saltsjobaden, Sweden, 1973. Stockholm; Almqvist & Wiksel, 1974. 244p. (Jointly sponsored by the National Institute of Child Health and Human Development, Swedish International Development Authority, Swedish Nutrition Foundation, and World Health Organization.)	Second
Second	Crompton, D. W. T., M. C. Nesheim, and Z. S. Pawlowski, eds. Ascariasis and Its Public Health Significance: A Volume based on the Agenda and Discussions of the 1984 Banff Conference, Organized by WHO Parasitic Diseases Programme and Division of Nutritional Sciences, Cornell University, Ithaca, N.Y. London and Philadelphia; Taylor & Francis, 1985. 289p.	Third
Third	Crueger, Wulf, and Anneliese Crueger. Biotechnology: A Textbook of Industrial Microbiology . . . English ed. edited by Thomas D. Brock. 2d ed. Sunderland, Mass.; Sinauer Associates; Madison, Wis.; Science Tech., 1990. 357p. (Translation of Lehrbuch der Angewandten Mikrobiologie. 1st English ed., 1984. 308p.)	
Third	Cunningham, Frank E., and N. A. Cox. The Microbiology of Poultry Meat Products. Orlando, Fla.; Academic Press, 1987. 359p.	Third

Developed countries ranking		Third World ranking
	D	
Second	D'Appolonia, Bert L., and Wallace H. Kunerth, eds. The Farinograph Handbook. 3d ed., rev. and expanded. St. Paul, Minn.; American Association of Cereal Chemists, 1984. 64p. (1st ed., 1960. 105p.)	
Second	Daussant, J., J. Mosse, and J. Vaughan, eds. Seed Proteins. London and New York; Academic Press, 1983. 335p. (Annual Proceedings of the Phytochemical Society of Europe no. 20)	Third
Third	Davidek, Jiri, Jan Velisek, and Jan Pokorny, eds. Chemical Changes during Food Processing. Amsterdam and New York; Elsevier, 1990. 448p.	Third
Third	Davidsohn, A., and B. M. Milwidsky. Synthetic Detergents. 7th ed. Burnt Mill, Harlow, Essex, U.K.; Longman Scientific & Technical; New York; Wiley, 1987. 315p. (1st ed. titled, Shoe Creams and Polishing Waxes by J. Davidsohn and A. Davidsohn. London; Leonard Hill, 1938. 141p.)	
Second	Davidson and Passmore's Human Nutrition and Dietetics. Edited by R. Passmore and M. A. Eastwood, et al. 8th ed. Edinburgh and New York; Churchill Livingstone, 1986. 666p. (1st ed., by Stanley Davidson, A. P. Meiklejohn and R. Passmore. Edinburgh; Livingstone, 1959. 844p.)	First
Second	Davidson, Robert L. Handbook of Water-Soluble Gums and Resins. New York; McGraw-Hill, 1980. 700p.	Third
Second	Davies, R., Gordon G. Birch, and K. J. Parker, eds. Intermediate Moisture Foods; Proceedings of a Symposium . . . National College of Food Technology, Weybridge, England. London; Applied Science Publishers, 1976. 306p.	
Second	Dawber, Thomas R. The Framingham Study: The Epidemiology of Atherosclerotic Disease. Cambridge, Mass.; Harvard University Press, 1980. 257p.	
First	De Leenheer, Andre P., Willy E. Lambert, and Marcel G. M. De Ruyter, eds. Modern Chromatographic Analysis of the Vitamins. New York; M. Dekker, 1985. 556p.	
Second	De Luca, Luigi M., and Stanley S. Shapire, eds. Modulation of Cellular Interactions by Vitamin A and Derivatives (Retinoids); Proceedings of a Conference . . . March 1980, New York. New York; New York Academy of Sciences, 1981. 430p. (Annals of the New York Academy of Science no. 359)	
Second	Decareau, Robert V. Microwaves in the Food Processing Industry. Orlando, Fla.; Academic Press, 1985. 234p.	
Second	DeGroot, Leslie J. et al., eds. Endocrinology. 2d ed. Philadelphia; Saunders, 1989. 3 vols. (1st ed., New York; Grune & Stratton, 1979. 3 vols.)	
	Delange, F., and R. Ahluwalia, eds. Cassava Toxicity and Thyroid: Research and Public Health Issues; Proceedings of a	Second

Developed countries ranking		Third World ranking
	Workshop, Ottawa, May-June 1982. Ottawa; International Development Research Centre, 1983. 148p. (IDRC no. 207e)	
Second	DeLuca, Hector F., ed. The Fat-Soluble Vitamins. New York; Plenum Press, 1978. 287p. (Handbook of Lipid Research no. 2)	
First	DeMan, John M. Principles of Food Chemistry. 2d ed. New York; Van Nostrand Reinhold, 1990. 469p. (1st ed., Westport, Conn.; Avi Pub. Co., 1976. 426p.)	Second
First	DeMan, John M. et al., eds. Rheology and Texture in Food Quality. Westport, Conn.; Avi, 1976. 588p.	First
Third	Dennis, Colin, ed. Post-Harvest Pathology of Fruits and Vegetables. London and New York; Academic Press, 1983. 264p.	Second
First	Desrosier, Norman W., and James N. Desrosier. The Technology of Food Preservation. 4th ed. Westport, Conn.; Avi, 1977. 558p. (1st ed., 1959. 418p.)	First
Third	Desrosier, Norman W., and Donald K. Tressler. Fundamentals of Food Freezing. Westport, Conn.; Avi, 1977. 629p.	Third
	Dey, Jennie. Women in Rice-Farming Systems: Focus, Sub-Saharan Africa. Rome; Food and Agriculture Organization, 1984. 106p. (Women in Agriculture no. 2)	Third
Third	Dickens, Frank, P. J. Randle, and W. J. Whelan, eds. Carbohydrate Metabolism and Its Disorders. London and New York; Academic Press, 1968–1981. 3 vols.	
Second	Dickes, G. J., and P. V. Nicholas. Gas Chromatography in Food Analysis. London and Boston; Butterworths, 1976. 393p.	
First	Dickinson, Eric, ed. Food Emulsions and Foams; Proceedings of an International Symposium organized by the Food Chemistry Group, Royal Society of Chemistry, Leeds, March 1986. London; The Society, 1987. 290p. (Special Publication no. 58)	
First	Dickinson, Eric, and George Stainsby. Colloids in Food. London and New York; Applied Science, 1982. 533p.	
Third	Diehl, Joery M., and Claus Leitzmann, eds. Measurement and Determinants of Food Habits and Food Preferences; Report of an EC Workshop, Giessen, Germany, May 1985. Wageningen; EURO NUT, 1986. 303p. (EURO-NUT Report no. 7)	Third
Second	Diehl, Johannes F. Safety of Irradiated Foods. New York; M. Dekker, 1990. 345p.	
Third	DiLiello, Leo R. Methods in Food and Dairy Microbiology. Westport, Conn.; Avi, 1982. 142p.	Third
	Diseases of Children in the Subtropics and Tropics . . . edited by J. Paget Stanfield 4th ed. London; E. Arnold, 1990. 1008p. (1st ed., edited by H. C. Trowell and D. B. Jelliffe, 1958. 919p.)	Third
Second	Dixon, Malcolm, and Edwin C. Webb. Enzymes. 3d ed., completely rev. New York; Academic Press, 1979. 1116p. (1st ed., 1958. 782p.)	

Developed countries ranking		Third World ranking
Third	Dixon, Wilfrid, and Frank J. Massey. Introduction to Statistical Analysis. 4th ed. New York; McGraw-Hill, 1983. 678p. (1st ed., published in Eugene, Or., 1949. 220p.)	
	Dobbing, John, ed. Maternal Nutrition and Fetal Growth: Eating for Two?; Based on a Workshop sponsored by Nestle Nutrition, held at the Chateau de Rochegude, Vaucluse, France, June 1980. London and New York; Academic Press, 1981. 197p.	Third
Third	Dobbing, John, ed. Maternal Nutrition and Lactational Infertility . . . based on papers discussed at the 9th Nestle Nutrition Workshop, England, 1984. Vevey, Switzerland; Nestle Nutrition; New York; Raven Press, 1985. 149p.	Third
First	Dobbing, John, ed. Sweetness; Proceedings of a Symposium . . . Geneva, May 1986, Sponsored by the International Life Sciences Institute. London and New York; Springer-Verlag, 1987. 282p.	
Second	Doberenz, A. R., J. A. Milner, and B. S. Schweigert, eds. Food and Agricultural Research Opportunities to Improve Human Nutrition; Proceedings of the USDA Diet and Health Symposia Workshop, University of California, Davis, September 1985; University of Delaware, September 1985; and University of Illinois, October 1985. Newark, Del.; College of Human Resources, University of Delaware, 1986. 136, 59, 220p.	
Third	Dorland, Wayne E., and James A. Rogers. The Fragrance and Flavor Industry. Mendham, N.J.; W. E. Dorland Co., 1977. 443p.	
	Douglass, Gordon K., ed. Agricultural Sustainability in a Changing World Order. Boulder, Colo.; Westview Press, 1984. 282p.	Third
	Dowdy, Shirley M., and Stanley Wearden. Statistics for Research. 2d ed. New York; Wiley, 1991. (1st ed., 1983. 537p.)	Second
Second	Doyle, Michael P., ed. Foodborne Bacterial Pathogens. New York; M. Dekker, 1989. 796p.	Second
Second	Dravnieks, Andrew. Atlas of Odor Character Profiles. Philadelphia; American Society for Testing Materials, 1985. 354p.	
Second	Dreher, Mark L. Handbook of Dietary Fiber: An Applied Approach. New York; Dekker, 1987. 468p.	
Second	Dreosti, Ivor E., and Richard M. Smith, eds. Neurobiology of the Trace Elements. Clifton, N.J.; Humana Press, 1983. 2 vols.	
	Duckham, A. N., J. G. W. Jone, and E. H. Roberts, eds. Food Production and Consumption: The Efficiency of Human Food Chains and Nutrient Cycles. Amsterdam; North-Holland; New York; American Elsevier, 1976. 541p.	Third
First	Duckworth, Ronald B., ed. Water Relations of Foods; Proceedings of an International Symposium, Glasgow, September 1974,	

Developed countries ranking		Third World ranking
	International Union of Food Science and Technology. London and New York; Academic Press, 1975. 716p.	
First	Dunn, John T. et al., compilers and eds. Towards the Eradication of Endemic Goiter, Cretinism, and Iodine Deficiency; Proceedings of the 5th Meeting of the PAHO/WHO Technical Group . . . Washington, D.C.; PAHO, Pan American Sanitary Bureau, Regional Office of the World Health Organization, 1986. 419p.	Second
First	Durnin, John V. G. A., and R. Passmore. Energy, Work and Leisure. London; Heinemann, 1967. 166p.	
	Dwyer, Daisy, and Judith Bruce, eds. A Home Divided: Women and Income in the Third World. Stanford, Calif.; Stanford University Press, 1988. 289p.	Second
Third	Dziedzic, S. Z., and M. W. Kearsley, eds. Glucose Syrups: Science and Technology. London; Elsevier Applied Science, 1984. 276p.	

E

Developed countries ranking		Third World ranking
First	Earle, R. L. Unit Operations in Food Processing. 2d ed. Oxford and New York; Pergamon Press, 1983. 207p. (1st ed., 1966. 342 p.) (Available in Spanish: Ingeniería de los Alimentos. 2ed. Zaragoza; Acribia, 1987. 213p.)	
	Eckholm, Erik P. Losing Ground: Environmental Stress and World Food Prospects. 1st ed. New York; Norton, 1976. 223p.	Third
Second	Edmondson, D. E., and D. V. McCormick, eds. Flavins and Flavoproteins, 1987; Proceedings of the 9th International Symposium, Atlanta, Ga., June 1987. Berlin and New York; W. de Gruyter, 1987. 775p.	
Second	Engen, Trygg. The Perception of Odors. New York; Academic Press, 1982. 202p.	
Second	Erickson, David R., ed. Edible Fats and Oils Processing: Basic Principles and Modern Practices. World Conference Proceedings . . . Maastricht, Netherlands, 1989. Champaign, Ill.; American Oil Chemists' Society, 1990. 442p.	Second
Second	Erickson, David R. et al., eds. Handbook of Soy Oil Processing and Utilization. St. Louis, Mo.; American Soybean Association; Champaign, Ill.; American Oil Chemists' Society, 1980. 598p.	First
First	Eskin, N. A. M. Biochemistry of Foods. 2d ed. San Diego; Academic Press, 1990. 557p. (1971 ed. with Harold M. Henderson and Ronald J. Townsend. 240p.)	Second
Second	Eskin, N. A. M. Plant Pigments, Flavors and Textures; The Chemistry and Biochemistry of Selected Compounds. New York; Academic Press, 1979. 211p.	

Developed countries ranking		Third World ranking
First	Eveleth, Phyllis B., and J. M. Tanner. Worldwide Variation in Human Growth. 2d ed. Cambridge and New York; Cambridge University Press, 1990. 397p. (1st ed., 1976. 497p.)	Second

F

Developed countries ranking		Third World ranking
First	Fabriani, Giuseppe, and Claudia Litnas, eds. Durum Wheat: Chemistry and Technology. St. Paul, Minn.; American Association of Cereal Chemists, 1988. 332p.	
First	Falkner, Frank, and J. M. Tanner, eds. Human Growth: A Comprehensive Treatise. 2d ed. New York; Plenum Press, 1986–1988. 3 vols. (1st ed., 1978–1980. 3 vols.)	First
Second	Faridi, Hamed, ed. Rheology of Wheat Products. St. Paul, Minn.; American Association of Cereal Chemists, 1985. 273p.	
Third	Farkas, Jozsef. Irradiation of Dry Food Ingredients. Boca Raton, Fla.; CRC Press, 1988. 153p.	
Second	Fazzalari, F. A., ed. Compilation of Odor and Taste Threshold Values Data; Sponsored by Committee E-18 on Sensory Evaluation of Materials and Products, American Society for Testing and Materials. Philadelphia; ASTM, 1978. 497p. (ASTM Data Series no. DS 48A)	
First	Feeney, Robert E., and John R. Whitaker, eds. Food Proteins: Improvement Through Chemical and Enzymatic Modification; Proceedings of a Symposium . . . 1st Chemical Congress of the North American Continent, Mexico City, December 1975, Sponsored by the Division of Agricultural and Food Chemistry. Washington, D.C.; American Chemical Society, 1977. 312p.	
Second	Feeney, Robert E., and John R. Whitaker, eds. Modification of Proteins: Food, Nutritional, and Pharmacological Aspects; Proceedings of a Symposium jointly sponsored by the Divisions of Agricultural and Food Chemistry and Biological Chemistry, 180th Meeting of the American Chemical Society, Las Vegas, Aug. 1980. Washington, D.C.; ACS, 1982. 402p. (Advances in Chemistry Series no. 198)	
Second	Fellows, Peter. Food Processing Technology; Principles and Practice. Chichester, U.K.; E. Horwood; New York; VCH, 1988. 505p.	Second
First	Fenaroli, Giovanni. Handbook of Flavor Ingredients . . . adapted from the Italian . . . edited, trans. and rev. by Thomas E. Furia and Nicolo Bellanca. 2d ed. Cleveland; CRC Press, 1975. (1st ed., 1971. 803p.)	
First	Fennema, Owen R., ed. Food Chemistry. 2d ed., rev. and expanded. New York; M. Dekker, 1985. 991p. (1st ed., 1976.	First

Developed countries ranking		Third World ranking
	792p.) (Available in Spanish: Introduccíon a la Ciencia de los Alimentos. Barcelona: Revertè, 1992. 918.)	
Third	Fennema, Owen R., ed. Proteins at Low Temperatures; Based on a Symposium sponsored by the Division of Agriculture and Food Chemistry, 175th Meeting of the American Chemical Society, Anaheim, Calif., March 1978. Washington, D.C.; ACS, 1979. 233p. (Advances in Chemistry Series no. 180)	
Second	Fennema, Owen R., and Wei-hsien Chang. Role of Chemistry in the Quality of Processed Food. Westport, Conn.; Food & Nutrition Press, 1986. 336p.	Third
Second	Fennema, Owen R., William D. Powrie, and Elmer H. Marth. Low-Temperature Preservation of Foods and Living Matter. New York; M. Dekker, 1973. 598p.	
Second	Ferrando, R. Traditional and Non-Traditional Foods. Rome; Food and Agriculture Organization, 1981. 156p. (FAO Food and Nutrition Series no. 2)	Second
Second	Fildes, Valerie A. Breasts, Bottles and Babies: A History of Infant Feeding. Edinburgh; Edinburgh University Press, 1986. 462p.	
Second	Filer, L. J. et al., eds. Glutamic Acid: Advances in Biochemistry and Physiology; Proceedings of an International Symposium . . . Milan, May 1978. New York; Raven Press, 1979. 400p.	
Third	Finley, John W., and Daniel E. Schwass, eds. Xenobiotic Metabolism: Nutritional Effects; Proceedings of a Symposium sponsored by the Division of Agricultural and Food Chemistry at the 187th Meeting of the American Chemical Society, St. Louis, Mo., April 1984. Washington, D.C.; ACS, 1985. 382p. (ACS Symposium Series no. 277)	
Second	Fishbein, Martin, and Icek Ajzen. Belief, Attitude, Intention, and Behavior: An Introduction to Theory and Research. Reading, Mass.; Addison-Wesley Pub. Co., 1975. 578p.	
Third	Fisher, Patty, and Arnold E. Bender. The Value of Food. 3d ed. Oxford and New York; Oxford University Press, 1979. 208p. (1st ed., 1970. 174p.) (Available in Spanish: Valor Nutritivo de los Alimentos. 1ed. México: Limusa-Noriega, 1987. 205p.)	
First	Fogarty, William M., and Catherine T. Kelly, eds. Microbial Enzymes and Biotechnology. 2d ed. London and New York; Elsevier Applied Science, 1990. 472p. (1st ed., 1983. 382p.)	
Second	Fomon, Samuel J., and Thomas A. Anderson. Infant Nutrition. 2d ed. Philadelphia; Saunders, 1974. 575p. (1st ed., 1967. 299p.) (Available in Spanish: Nutrición Infantil. 2ed. Bogotà; Interamericana, 1976.)	Second
Second	Fomon, Samuel J., and William C. Heird, eds. Energy and Protein Needs during Infancy; Based on a Meeting, Washington,	Second

Developed countries ranking		Third World ranking
	D.C., December 1984. Orlando, Fla.; Academic Press, 1986. 248p.	
Second	Food Additives Tables . . . compiled by Food Law Research Centre, Institute of European Studies, University of Brussels, M. Fondu editors, and Updated ed. Amsterdam; Elsevier Scientific, 1980–1984. 4 vols.	
Third	Food and Agriculture Organization. Food Balance Sheets, 1975–77 Average, and per Capita Food Supplies, 1961–65 Average, 1967 to 1977. Rome; FAO, 1980. 1012p.	Second
	Food and Agriculture Organization. Food Balance Sheets = Bilana Alimentaires = Hojas de blance de Alimentos, 1984–1986 Average. Rome; FAO, 1991. 384p.	Third
	Food and Agriculture Organization. Food, Nutrition and Agriculture: Guidelines for Agricultural Training Curricula in Africa. Rome; FAO, 1982. 205p. (FAO Food and Nutrition Paper no. 22)	Second
	Food and Agriculture Organization. The Technology of Traditional Milk Products in Developing Countries. Rome; FAO, 1990. 333p. (FAO Animal Production and Health Paper no. 85)	Third
	Food and Agriculture Organization. Utilization of Tropical Foods. Rome; FAO, 1989. 8 vols. (FAO Food and Nutrition Paper no. 47/1–8) (Contents: 47/1, Cereals; 47/2, Roots and Tubers; 47/3, Trees; 47/4, Tropical Beans; 47/5, Tropical Oil-Seeds; 47/6, Sugars, Spices and Stimulants; 47/7, Fruits and Leaves; 47/8, Animal Products. Vols. average 60p.)	Second
Second	Food and Agriculture Organization and World Health Organization. Dietary Fats and Oils in Human Nutrition; Report of an Expert Consultation . . . September 1977. Rev. and augmented ed. Rome; FAO, 1980. 102p. (FAO Food and Nutrition Series no. 30) (Supersedes FAO Food and Nutrition Paper no. 3, 1977. 94p.)	First
	Food and Agriculture Organization. Food Policy and Nutrition Division. Food, Nutrition and Agriculture: Guidelines for Curriculum Content for Agricultural Training in Southeast Asia . . . prepared by Nutrition Programmes Service. Rome; FAO, 1981? 141p. (University of the Philippines, Los Banos, FAO, and the U.S. Agency for International Development participating.)	Third
	Food and Agriculture Organization. Nutrition Planning, Assessment, and Evaluation Service, Food Policy and Nutrition Division. Integrating Nutrition into Agricultural and Rural Development Projects: Six Case Studies. Rome; FAO, 1984. 132p. (Nutrition in Agriculture no. 2)	Second
	Forbes, Gilbert B. Human Body Composition: Growth, Aging, Nutrition, and Activity. New York; Springer-Verlag, 1987. 350p.	Second

Developed countries ranking		Third World ranking
Third	Forsberg, Robert A., ed. Triticale; Proceedings of a Symposium sponsored by Divisions C-1 and C-6 of the Crop Science Society of America, Fort Collins, Colo., August 1979. Madison, Wis.; CSSA and American Society of Agronomy, 1985. 82p. (CSSA Special Publication no. 9)	
Second	Fox, Brian A., and Allan G. Cameron. Food Science: A Chemical Approach. 4th ed. London; Hodder and Stoughton, 1982. 370p. (First published as Chemical Approach to Food and Nutrition, 1961.)	
Second	Fox, P. F., ed. Cheese: Chemistry, Physics, and Microbiology. London and New York; Elsevier Applied Science, 1987. 2 vols.	
First	Fox, P. F., ed. Developments in Dairy Chemistry. London and New York; Applied Science; New York; Elsevier Science, 1982. 4 vols.	
Third	Fox, P. F., and J. J. Condon, eds. Food Proteins; Proceedings of the Kellogg Foundation International Symposium, University College, Cork, Republic of Ireland, Sept. 1981. London and New York; Applied Science, 1982. 361p.	
Second	Francis, Dorothy E. M. Nutrition for Children. Oxford and Boston; Blackwell Scientific; St. Louis; Blackwell Mosby Book Distributors, 1986. 164p.	
Second	Francis, F. J., and F. M. Clydesdale. Food Colorimetry: Theory and Applications. Westport, Conn.; Avi, 1975. 477p.	
Second	Frankle, Reva T., and Anita Yanochik Owen. Nutrition in the Community: The Art of Delivering Services. 2d ed. St. Louis, Mo.; Times Mirror/Mosby College Pub., 1986. 427p. (1st ed., 1978. 395p.)	Third
Third	Frazier, William C., and Dennis C. Westhoff. Food Microbiology. 4th ed. New York; McGraw-Hill, 1988. 539p. (1st ed., 1958. 471p.) (Available in Spanish: Microbiología de los Alimentos. 3rd. Zaragoza: Acribia, 1985. 538p.)	First
Second	Frey, Kenneth J., and R. A. Olson, eds. Nutritional Quality of Cereal Grains. Madison, Wis.; American Society of Agronomy, 1987. 511p.	Third
First	Friberg, Stig. Food Emulsions. New York; M. Dekker, 1976. 480p.	
Second	Frieden, Earl, ed. Biochemistry of the Essential Ultratrace Elements. New York; Plenum, 1984. 426p.	
Third	Friedman, Mendel, ed. Nutritional and Toxicological Aspects of Food Safety; Proceedings of a Symposium on Food Safety: Metabolism and Nutrition, sponsored by the Pacific Conference on Chemistry and Spectroscopy, San Francisco, Oct. 1982. New York; Plenum, 1984. 584p.	
Second	Friedman, Mendel, ed. Nutritional and Toxicological Significance of Enzyme Inhibitors in Foods; Proceedings of an Ameri-	

Developed countries ranking		Third World ranking
	can Institute of Nutrition/FASEB Symposium . . . Anaheim, Calif., 1985. New York; Plenum Press, 1986. 572p.	
Third	Friedman, Mendel, ed. Nutritional Improvement of Food and Feed Proteins; Proceedings of a Symposium sponsored by the Protein Subdivision of the Division of Agricultural and Food Chemistry of the American Chemical Society, Chicago, 1977. New York; Plenum Press, 1978. 882p. (Advances in Experimental Medicine and Biology no. 105)	Third
Second	Friedman, Mendel, ed. Protein Crosslinking; Proceedings of a Symposium . . . San Francisco, Aug.-Sept. 1976. New York; Plenum Press, 1977. 2 vols.	
Third	Friedrich, W. Vitamins. Berlin and New York; W. de Gruyter, 1988. 1058p.	
Second	Friend, J., and M. J. C. Rhodes, eds. Recent Advances in the Biochemistry of Fruits and Vegetables. London and New York; Academic Press, 1981. 275p. (Annual Proceedings of the Phytochemical Society of Europe no. 19)	
First	Furia, Thomas E., ed. CRC Handbook of Food Additives. 2d ed. Cleveland; CRC Press, 1972–1981. 2 vols. (Vol. 2 published in Boca Raton, Fla.; 1st ed., 1968. 771p.)	Third
	G	
First	Galler, Janina R., ed. Nutrition and Behavior. New York; Plenum Press, 1984. 514p. (Human Nutrition: A Comprehensive Treatise, Vol. 5)	
First	Gaman, P. M., and K. B. Sherrington. The Science of Food: An Introduction to Food Science, Nutrition, and Microbiology. 3d ed. Oxford and New York; Pergamon Press, 1990. (1st ed., 1977. 300p.)	Second
Second	Garrow, J. S. Energy Balance and Obesity in Man. 2d ed., rev. Amsterdam and New York; Elsevier/North Holland, 1978. 243p. (1st ed., 1974. 335p.)	Second
Second	Garrow, J. S. Treat Obesity Seriously: A Clinical Manual. Edinburgh and New York; Churchill Livingstone, 1981. 246p.	
Third	Garti, Nissim, and Kiyotaka Sato, eds. Crystallization and Polymorphism of Fats and Fatty Acids. New York; M. Dekker, 1988. 450p.	
Third	Gastineau, Clifford F. et al., eds. Fermented Food Beverages in Nutrition; Proceedings of an International Symposium . . . Rochester, Minn., Mayo Clinic, June 1977. New York; Academic Press, 1979. 537p.	
Second	Geigy Scientific Tables . . . edited by C. Lentner. 8th ed., rev. and enl. West Caldwell, N.J.; Ciba-Geigy, 1981. 4 vols. (Translation of Wissenschaftliche Tabellen.) (5th ed. by J. R. Geigy. Basle and New York: S. Karger, 1959. 547p.)	

Developed countries ranking		Third World ranking
Second	Geissman, Theodore A. The Chemistry of Flavonoid Compounds. Oxford and New York; Pergamon Press, 1962. 666p.	
First	Geldard, Frank A. The Human Senses. 2d ed. New York; Wiley, 1972. 584p. (1st ed., 1953. 365p.)	
Second	George, Susan. How the Other Half Dies: The Real Reasons for World Hunger. Montclair, N.J.; Allanheld, Osmun, 1977. 308p. (Available in Spanish: Cómo Muerre la Otra Mitad del Mundo. 1ed. México; Siglo, 1980. 328p.)	Second
Third	Gershwin, M. Eric, Richard S. Beach, and Lucille S. Hurley. Nutrition and Immunity. Orlando, Fla.; Academic Press, 1985. 417p.	Third
	Ghosh, Pradip K., ed. Health, Food and Nutrition in Third World Development. Westport, Conn.; Greenwood Press, 1984. 617p.	Second
Third	Gibson, Rosalind S. Principles of Nutritional Assessment. New York; Oxford University Press, 1990. 691p.	Second
Third	Gifft, Helen H., Marjorie B. Washbon, and Gail G. Harrison. Nutrition, Behavior, and Change. Englewood Cliffs, N.J.; Prentice-Hall, 1972. 392p.	
Second	Gittinger, J. Price, Joanne Leslie, and Caroline Hoisington, eds. Food Policy: Integrating Supply, Distribution, and Consumption. Baltimore, Md.; Published for the World Bank by Johns Hopkins University Press, 1987. 567p.	Second
	Glantz, Michael H., ed. Drought and Hunger in Africa: Denying Famine a Future; Based on presentations at a Colloquium, Boulder, Colo., Aug. 1985. Cambridge and New York; Cambridge University Press, 1987. 457p.	Second
First	Glicksman, Martin, ed. Food Hydrocolloids. Boca Raton, Fla.; CRC Press, 1982–1983. 3 vols.	Third
Second	Glicksman, Martin. Gum Technology in the Food Industry. New York; Academic Press, 1969. 590p.	
	Goldberger, Joseph. Goldberger on Pellagra . . . edited by Milton Terris. Baton Rouge; Louisiana State University Press, 1964. 395p.	Third
Second	Goldblith, Samuel A., and Maynard A. Joslyn. Milestones in Nutrition. Westport, Conn.; Avi, 1964. 797p. (Anthology of Food Sciences no. 2)	Second
Second	Goldman, Armond S., Stephanie A. Atkinson, and Lars A. Hanson, eds. Human Lactation 3: The Effects of Human Milk on the Recipient Infant; Proceedings of an International Conference . . . 1986, Konstanz, Germany. New York; Plenum Press, 1987. 400p.	Second
Second	Goodman and Gilman's The Pharmacological Basis of Therapeutics . . . edited by Alfred G. Gilman, and 8th ed. New York; Pergamon Press, 1990. 1811p. (1st ed., by Louis S. Goodman	

Developed countries ranking		Third World ranking
	and Alfred Gilman, New York; Macmillan, 1941. 1387p.) (Available in Spanish: Bases Farmacológicas de la Terapéutica. 7ed. Buenos AIres: Mèdica Panamericana, 1986. 216p.)	
	Gopalan, C., ed. Combating Undernutrition: Basic Issues and Practical Approaches. New Delhi?; Nutrition Foundation of India, 1987. 439p. (Papers originally published in the Bulletin of the Nutrition Foundation of India.)	Second
	Gopalan, C., and Meera Chatterjee. Use of Growth Charts for Promoting Child Nutrition: A Review of Global Experience. New Delhi; Nutrition Foundation of India, 1985. 120p. (Special Publications Series no. 2)	Third
Second	Gormley, T. R., G. Downey, and D. O'Beirne. Food, Health and the Consumer. London and New York; Elsevier Applied Science, 1987. 317p.	
Third	Gosney, W. B. Principles of Refrigeration. Cambridge; Cambridge University Press, 1982. 666p.	
Second	Gottschalk, Werner, and Hermann P. Muller, eds. Seed Proteins: Biochemistry, Genetics, Nutritive Value. The Hague and Boston; M. Nijhoff/W. Junk, 1983. 531p.	
Second	Gould, Wilbur A and Ronald W. Gould. Total Quality Assurance for the Industries. 3d ed. Baltimore, Md.; CTI Publications. 1993. (1st ed., 1988.)	
Second	Gould, Wilbur A. Tomato Production, Processing and Quality Evaluation. 2d ed. Westport, Conn.; Avi, 1983. 445p. (1st ed., 1974.)	
Third	Gorham, J. Richard, ed. Ecology and Management of Food-Industry Pests. Arlington, Va.; Association of Official Analytical Chemists, 1991. 595p. (FDA Technical Bulletin no. 4)	
	Grace, M. R. Cassava Processing. Rome; Food and Agrculture Organization, 1977. 155p. (FAO Plant Production and Protection Series no. 3) (Issued in 1956 under title: Processing of Cassava and Cassava Products in Rural Industries; in 1971 under title: Processing of Cassava.)	Third
	Gracey, Michael, ed. Diarrhoeal Disease and Malnutrition: A Clinical Update. Edinburgh and New York; Churchill Livingstone, 1985. 230p.	Third
Second	Gracey, Michael, and Frank Falkner, eds. Nutritional Needs and Assessment of Normal Growth; Presented at the 7th Nestle Nutrition Workshop, Rome, May-June 1983. Vevey, Switzerland; Nestle Nutrition; New York; Raven Press, 1985. 226p.	Third
Second	Graham, Horace D., ed. The Safety of Foods. 2d ed. Westport, Conn.; Avi, 1980.	
	Grant, John P. Handbook of Total Parenteral Nutrition. Philadelphia; Saunders, 1980. 197p.	Third
	Gray, Cheryl W. Food Consumption Parameters for Brazil and	Third

Developed countries ranking		Third World ranking
	Their Application to Food Policy. Washington, D.C.; International Food Policy Research Institute, 1982. 78p. (IFPRI Research Report no. 32)	
Second	Great Britain. Ministry of Agriculture, Fisheries, and Food. Manual of Nutrition. 9th ed. London; H.M.S.O., 1985. 131p. (1st ed., prepared by Magnus Pyke, 1945. 64p.)	
Third	Great Britain. Working Party on the Composition of Foods for Infants and Young Children. The Composition of Mature Human Milk: Report of a Working Party . . . London; H.M.S.O., 1977. 47p.	Third
Third	Green, John H., and Amihud Kramer. Food Processing Waste Management. Westport, Conn.; Avi, 1979. 629p.	
Third	Green, L. F., ed. Development in Soft Drinks Technology. London; Applied Science Publishers, 1978. 3 vols. (Vol. 3 edited by H. W. Houghton.)	
Third	Greenberg, David M., ed. Metabolic Pathways. 3d ed. New York; Academic Press, 1967–1975. 7 vols. (1st ed., 1954, as Chemical Pathways of Metabolism.)	
	Greene, Lawrence S., and Francis E. Johnston, eds. Social and Biological Predictors of Nutritional Status, Physical Growth, and Neurological Development. New York; Academic Press, 1980. 344p.	Second
Second	Grenby, Trevor H., ed. Progress in Sweeteners. London and New York; Elsevier Applied Science, 1989. 394p.	
Second	Grob, Robert L., ed. Modern Practice of Gas Chromatography. 2d ed. New York; Wiley, 1985. 897p. (1st ed., 1977. 654p.)	
Second	Gross, Jeana. Pigments in Fruits. London and Orlando, Fla.; Academic Press, 1987. 303p.	
Second	Gruenwedel, Dieter W., and John R. Whitaker, eds. Food Analysis: Principles and Techniques. New York; M. Dekker, 1984–1987. 4 vols. (Vol. 1, Physical Characterization; vol. 2, Physicochemical Techniques; vol. 3, Biological Techniques; vol. 4, Separation Techniques; vol. 5, Proximate Analysis; vol. 6, Physical Techniques; vol. 7, Spectroscopy; vol. 8, Electroanalytical Techniques.)	
Third	Guggenheim, Yechiel K. Nutrition and Nutritional Diseases: The Evolution of Concepts. Lexington, Mass.; Collamore Press, 1981. 378p.	Third
Second	Guilbault, George G. Analytical Uses of Immobilized Enzymes. New York; M. Dekker, 1984. 453p.	
Second	Guilbault, George G. Handbook of Enzymatic Methods of Analysis. New York; M. Dekker, 1976. 738p. (Clinical and Biochemical Analysis no. 4)	
Third	Gunstone, Frank D. Palm Oil. Chichester, England and New York; Wiley, 1987. 100p.	Third

Developed countries ranking		Third World ranking
Second	Gunstone, Frank D., John L. Harwood, and Fred B. Padley, eds. The Lipid Handbook. London and New York; Chapman & Hall, 1986. 314p.	
Second	Gunstone, Frank D., and Frank A. Norris. Lipids in Foods: Chemistry, Biochemistry, and Technology. 1st ed. Oxford and New York; Pergamon Press, 1983. 170p.	
Third	Gurr, Michael I. Role of Fats in Food and Nutrition. London and New York; Elsevier Applied Science Publishers, 1984. 170p.	
Second	Gurr, Michael I., and J. L. Harwood. Lipid Biochemistry: An Introduction. 4th ed. London and New York; Chapman & Hall, 1991. 406p. (1st ed., Ithaca, N.Y.; Cornell University Press, 1971. 231p.)	
Third	Gutcho, Marcia H. Edible Oils and Fats: Recent Developments. Park Ridge, N.J.; Noyes Data, 1979. 402p. (Food Technology Review no. 49)	
Second	Guthrie, Helen A., and Robin S. Bagby. Introductory Nutrition. 7th ed., rev. St. Louis, Mo.; Times Mirror/Mosby College Pub., 1989. 656p. (1st ed., 1967. 464p.)	Second
Third	Guthrie, Rufus K. Food Sanitation. 3d ed. New York; Van Nostrand Reinhold, 1988. 330p. (1st ed., Westport, Conn.; Avi, 1972. 247p.)	
Third	Gwatkin, Davidson R., Janet R. Wilcox, and Joe D. Wray. Can Health and Nutrition Interventions Make a Difference? Washington, D.C.; Overseas Development Council, 1980. 76p. (ODC Monograph no. 13)	Second
	H	
	Hall, David W. Handling and Storage of Food Grains in Tropical and Subtropical Areas. Rome; Food and Agriculture Organization, 1970. 350p. (FAO Development Paper no. 90)	Second
	Hall, R., and J. Kobberling, eds. Thyroid Disorders Associated with Iodine Deficiency and Excess; Papers presented at a Symposium, Freiburg, Germany, April 1984. New York; Raven Press, 1985. 453p. (Serono Symposia Publications no. 22)	Third
Third	Hallgren, Bo et al., eds. Diet and Prevention of Coronary Heart Disease and Cancer; Proceedings of the 4th International Berzelius Symposium sponsored by the Swedish Society of Medicine. New York; Raven Press, 1986. 213p.	
Second	Hallowell, E. R. Cold Freezer Storage Manual. 2d ed. Westport, Conn.; Avi, 1980. 356p. (Earlier ed., by W. R. Woolrich and E. R. Hallowell, 1970. 338p.)	
Second	Hambraeus, Leif, and Stig Sjolin, eds. The Mother/Child Dyad: Nutritional Aspects; Proceedings of a Symposium . . . Uppsala, Sweden, June 1977, Jointly sponsored by Uppsala University	

Developed countries ranking		Third World ranking
	and the Swedish Nutrition Foundation. Stockholm; Almqvist & Wiksell, 1979. 155p. (Symposia of the Swedish Nutrition Foundation no. 14)	
Second	Hamilton, Eva May N., Eleanor N. Whitney, and Frances S. Sizer. Nutrition: Concepts and Controversies. 5th ed. St. Paul, Minn.; West Pub. Co., 1990. 736p. (1st ed., by E. M. Hamilton and E. N. Whitney, 1979. 627p.)	
Third	Hamilton, R. J., and A. Bhati, eds. Fats and Oils: Chemistry and Technology; Based on the Symposium of Recent Advances in Chemistry and Technology of Fats and Oils, December 1979. London; Applied Science, 1980. 255p.	
Third	Hamilton, R. J., and J. B. Rossell. Analysis of Oils and Fats. London and New York; Elsevier Applied Science Publishers, 1986. 441p.	
Third	Hamilton, Sahni, Barry Popkin, and Deborah Spicer. Women and Nutrition in Third World Countries. New York; Praeger, 1984. 147p.	Third
Third	Hampe, Edward C., and Merle Wittenberg. The Food Industry: Lifeline of America. 2d ed., rev. by Lillian E. Edds. Ithaca, N.Y.; Cornell University, 1980. 383p. (1st ed. entitled: The Lifeline of America: Development of the Food Industry. New York: McGraw-Hill, 1964. 390p.)	
Second	Hansen, R. Gaurth, Bonita W. Wyse, and Ann W. Sorenson. Nutritional Quality Index of Foods. Westport, Conn.; Avi, 1979. 636p.	
Second	Harborne, Jeffrey B., ed. The Flavonoids: Advances in Research Since 1980. London and New York; Chapman & Hall, 1988. 621p.	
Second	Harborne, Jeffrey B. Phytochemical Methods: A Guide to Modern Techniques of Plant Analysis. 2d ed. London and New York; Chapman & Hall, 1984. 288p. (1st ed., 1973. 278p.)	
First	Harborne, Jeffrey B., and Tom J. Mabry, eds. The Flavonoids, Advances in Research. London and New York; Chapman & Hall, 1982. 744p. (Updates an earlier work, The Flavonoids, 1975.)	
Third	Harler, Campbell R. Tea Manufacture. London and New York; Oxford University Press, 1963. 126p.	
Third	Harper, W. James, and Carl W. Hall. Dairy Technology and Engineering. Westport, Conn.; Avi, 1976. 631p.	
Second	Harris, James R., ed. Electron Microscopy of Proteins. London and New York; Academic Press, 1981–1982. 6 vols. (Vols. 5–6 edited by James R. Harris and Robert W. Horne.)	
Third	Harris, Kenton L., and Carl J. Lindblad, compilers. Postharvest Grain Loss Assessment Methods: A Manual of Methods for the Evaluation of Postharvest Losses. American Association of Ce-	

Developed countries ranking		Third World ranking
	real Chemists, 1978. 193p. (Based on two conferences: The Postharvest Grain Losses Methods Workshop, Harpers Ferry, W.Va., September 1976; and The Workshop on Postharvest Grain Loss Methodology, Slough, U.K., June 1977.)	
Third	Hartog, Adel P. den, and Wija A. van Staveren. Manual for Social Surveys on Food Habits and Consumption in Developing Countries. Wageningen; Pudoc, 1983. 114p. (Rev. ed. of Field Guide on Food Habits and Food Consumption.)	Third
Second	Hathcock, John N., ed. Nutritional Toxicology. New York; Academic Press, 1982. 2 vols.	
Second	Hathcock, John N., and Julius Coon, eds. Nutrition and Drug Interrelations; Proceedings of an International Symposium . . . Iowa State University, August 1976. New York; Academic Press, 1978. 927p.	
Third	Hautvast, Joseph G. A., and Wijnand Klaver, eds. The Diet Factor in Epidemiological Research. Wageningen; J. G. A. Hautvast, 1982. 154p.	
Third	Hayes, P. R. Food Microbiology and Hygiene. London and New York; Elsevier Applied Science Publishers, 1985. 403p.	Second
Second	Heath, Henry B., and Gary Reineccius. Flavor Chemistry and Technology. Westport, Conn.; Avi, 1986. 442p.	
Third	Heddle, John A. Mutagenicity; New Horizons in Genetic Toxicology. New York; Academic Press, 1982. 471p.	
Second	Heimann, Werner. Fundamentals of Food Chemistry. Chichester; E. Horwood; Westport, Conn.; Avi, 1980. 344p. (Translation of Grundzuge der Lebensmittelchemie.)	Second
Second	Heiser, Charles B., Jr. Seed to Civilization: The Story of Food. New ed. Cambridge; Harvard University Press, 1990. 228p. (1st ed., San Francisco; W. H. Freeman, 1973. 243p.)	
	Hendrickse, R. G. et al. Paediatrics in the Tropics. Oxford and Boston; Blackwell Scientific, 1991. 960p.	Third
Third	Henrickson, Robert L. Meat, Poultry, and Seafood Technology. Englewood Cliffs, N.J.; Prentice-Hall, 1978. 276p.	
	Herbert, Victor. Nutrition Cultism: Facts and Fictions. Philadelphia; George F. Stickley Co., 1980. 234p.	Second
Second	Herschdoerfer, S. M., ed. Quality Control in the Food Industry. 2d ed. London and Orlando, Fla.; Academic Press, 1984–1987. 4 vols. (1st ed., 1967–1972.)	
Second	Hersom, A. C., and E. D. Hulland. Canned Foods: Thermal Processing and Microbiology. 7th ed. Edinburgh and New York; Churchill Livingstone, 1980. 380p. (1st ed., by John G. Baumgartner, as Canned Foods; An Introduction to Their Microbiology. London; Churchill, 1943. 157p.)	
Second	Hetzel, Basil S. The Story of Iodine Deficiency: An Interna-	Third

Developed countries ranking		Third World ranking
	tional Challenge in Nutrition. Oxford and New York; Oxford University Press, 1989. 236p.	
First	Hetzel, Basil S., John T. Dunn, and John B. Stanbury, eds. The Prevention and Control of Iodine Deficiency Disorders; Based on the Inaugural Meeting of the ICCIDD, Kathmandu, Nepal, March 1986. Amsterdam and New York; Elsevier, 1987. 354p. (Major Health Issues no. 2)	First
Second	Himes, John H., ed. Anthropometric Assessment of Nutritional Status. New York; Wiley-Liss, 1991. 431p.	Third
Second	Hobbs, Betty C., and J. H. B. Christian, eds. The Microbiological Safety of Food; Proceedings of the 8th International Symposium on Food Microbiology, Reading, U.K. London and New York; Academic Press, 1973. 487p.	
Third	Holland, B., I. D. Unwin, D. H. Buss, and R. A. McCance. Cereals and Cereal Products: Third Supplement to McCance and Widdowson's The Composition of Foods. Nottingham, U.K.; Royal Society of Chemistry, 1988. 147p.	
Third	Holmes, Frederic L. Lavoisier and the Chemistry of Life: An Exploration of Scientific Creativity. Madison, Wis.; University of Wisconsin Press, 1985. 565p. (Wisconsin Publications in the History of Science and Medicine no. 4)	
Third	Holten, Carl H. Lactic Acid; Properties and Chemistry of Lactic Acid and Derivates. Weinheim; Verlag Chemie, 1971. 566p.	
Third	Horan, Michael J. et al., eds. NIH Workshop on Nutrition and Hypertension; Proceedings of a Symposium . . . New York; Biomedical Information, 1985. 385p.	
Second	Horisberger, Marc, and Umberto Bracco, eds. Lipids in Modern Nutrition; Papers from the 2d Nestle Nutrition Research Symposium, Vevey, Switzerland, Sept. 1985. New York; Raven Press, 1987. 248p. (Nestle Nutrition Workshop Series no. 13)	
Second	Hoseney, R. Carl. Principles of Cereal Science and Technology. St. Paul, Minn.; American Association of Cereal Chemists, 1986. 327p.	Second
First	Hough, C. A. M., K. J. Parker, and A. J. Vlitos, eds. Developments in Sweeteners. London; Applied Science, 1979–1983. 2 vols.	
Second	Houston, D. F., ed. Rice: Chemistry and Technology. St. Paul, Minn.; American Association of Cereal Chemists, 1972. 517p. (AACC Monograph Series no. 4)	Second
Second	Hudson, B. J. F., ed. Developments in Food Proteins. London and Englewood, N.J.; Applied Science Publishers, 1982. 4 vols.	
First	Hulme, Alfred C. The Biochemistry of Fruits and Their Products. London and New York; Academic Press, 1970. 2 vols.	

Developed countries ranking		Third World ranking
Second	Hulse, Joseph H., Evangeline M. Laing, and Odette E. Pearson. Sorghum and the Millets: Their Composition and Nutritive Value. London and New York; Academic Press, 1980. 997p.	Second
Third	Hultin, Herbert, and Max Milner, eds. Postharvest Biology and Biotechnology; Proceedings of a Symposium . . . Philadelphia, June 1977, sponsored by the Institute of Food Technologists and International Union of Food Science and Technology. Westport, Conn.; Food & Nutrition Press, 1978. 462p.	
Third	Hummel, Charles. Macaroni Products: Manufacture, Processing and Packing. 2d ed., rev. London; Food Trade Press, 1966. 287p. (1st ed., 1950. 223p.)	
Third	Hurley, Lucille S. Developmental Nutrition. Englewood Cliffs, N.J.; Prentice-Hall, 1980. 335p.	Third
Third	Hurley, Lucille S. et al., eds. Trace Elements in Man and Animals; Proceedings . . . Sixth International Symposium, May-June 1987, Pacific Grove, Calif. New York; Plenum Press, 1988. 724p.	
Second	Hytten, Frank, and Geoffrey Chamberlain, eds. Clinical Physiology in Obstetrics. Oxford and Boston; Blackwell Scientific Publications, 1980. 506p. (Successor to The Physiology of Human Pregnancy, by F. Hytten and Isabella Leitch, 1st-2d eds.)	
	I	
Second	Iglesias, Hector A., and Jorge Chirife. Handbook of Food Isotherms: Water Sorption Parameters for Food and Food Components. New York; Academic Press, 1982. 347p.	
Second	Igoe, Robert S. Dictionary of Food Ingredients. 2d ed. New York; Van Nostrand Reinhold, 1989. 225p. (1st ed., 1983. 173p.)	
Second	Inglett, George E., ed. Maize; Recent Progress in Chemistry and Technology; Proceedings . . . 7th World Cereal and Bread Congress, Prague, Czechoslovakia, June-July 1982. New York; Academic Press, 1982. 251p.	
Third	Inglett, George E., and George Charalambous, eds. Tropical Foods: Chemistry and Nutrition; Proceedings of an International Conference . . . Honolulu, March 1979. New York; Academic Press, 1979. 2 vols.	Third
Second	Inglett, George E., and Lars Munch, eds. Cereals for Food and Beverages: Recent Progress in Cereal Chemistry and Technology; Proceedings of an International Conference . . . Carlsberg Research Center, 1979. London and New York; Academic Press, 1980. 557p.	
Third	Institute of Food Science and Technology (U.K.). Food Additives: The Professional and Scientific Approach. London; Institute of Food Science and Technology, 1986. 20p.	

Developed countries ranking		Third World ranking
Second	Institute of Food Science and Technology (U.K.). Food and Drink Manufacture: Good Manufacturing Practice: A Guide to Its Responsible Management. (1st ed. London; IFST, 1987. 55p.)	
Second	Institute of Food Science and Technology (U.K.). Guidelines for the Handling of Chilled Foods. 2d ed. London; IFST, 1990. (1st ed., 1982.)	
Third	Institute of Medicine (U.S.). The Impact of Diet and Physical Activity on Pregnancy and Lactation: Women's Work in the Developing World. Washington, D.C.; National Academy Press, 1990. 129p.	Second
Second	Institute of Medicine (U.S.). Nutrition during Pregnancy: Part 1, Weight Gain; Part 2, Nutrient Supplements. Washington, D.C.; National Academy Press, 1990. 450p.	Third
Second	Institute of Medicine (U.S.). Subcommittee on Lactation. Nutrition during Lactation. Subcommittee on Lactation, Committee on Nutritional Status during Pregnancy and Lactation, Food and Nutrition Board, Institute of Medicine, National Academy of Sciences. Washington, D.C.; National Academy Press, 1991. 309p.	Third
	Instituto de Nutricion de Centro America y Panama. Evaluacion Nutricional de la Poblacion de Centro America y Panama: El Salvador. Guatemala; INCAP, 1969. 1 vol. (INCAP no. 25)	Second
First	International Congress of Nutrition, 11th, August-September 1978, Rio de Janeiro, Brazil. Nutrition and Food Science: Present Knowledge and Utilization; Proceedings . . . organized by the Brazilian Nutrition Sociey, edited by Walter Santos et al. New York; Plenum Press, 1980. 3 vols.	Second
Second	International Congress of Nutrition, 12th, 1981, San Diego, Calif. Nutrition in Health and Disease and International Development; Proceedings . . . edited by Alfred E. Harper and George K. Davis. New York; A. R. Liss, 1981. 1034p.	
First	International Congress of Nutrition, 13th, August 1985, Brighton, England; Proceedings . . . edited by T. G. Taylor and N. K. Jenkins, held under the auspices of the International Union of Nutritional Science. London; J. Libbey, 1986. 977p.	
Third	International Nutritional Anemia Consultative Group. The Effects of Cereals and Legumes on Iron Availability. Washington, D.C.; Nutrition Foundation, 1982. 44p.	Third
	International Rice Research Institute. Women in Rice Farming; Proceedings of a Conference . . . International Rice Research Institute, P.O. Box 933, Manila, Philippines, Sept. 1983. Aldershot, Hants, U.K. and Brookfield, Vt.; Gower; Manila; IRRI, 1985. 531p.	Third
Third	International Union of Biochemistry. Nomenclature Committee. Enzyme Nomenclature 1984: Recommendations . . . on the No-	

Developed countries ranking		Third World ranking
	menclature and Classification of Enzyme-Catalysed Reactions. Orlando, Fla.; Published for the International Union of Biochemistry by Academic Press, 1984. 646p. (Earlier ed., 1978.)	
	Irwin, M. Isabel. Nutritional Requirements of Man: A Conspectus of Research. New York; Nutrition Foundation, 1980. 592p.	Third
	Iyengar, Govindaraja V., W. E. Kollmer, and H. J. M Bowen. The Elemental Composition of Human Tissues and Body Fluids: A Compilation of Values for Adults . . . trans. into English. Weinheim and New York; Verlag Chemie, 1978. 151p. (Rev. and extended version of Normale Konzentrationen Verschiedener Elemente in Organen und Korperflussigkeiten.)	Third
	J	
Third	Jackson, A. T. Process Engineering in Biotechnology. Englewood Cliffs, N.J.; Prentice-Hall, 1991. 147p.	Third
Third	Jackson, A. T., and J. Lamb. Calculations in Food and Chemical Engineering: Theory, Worked Examples and Problems. London; Macmillan, 1981. 209p.	
Third	Jackson, John M., and Byron M. Shinn. Fundamentals of Food Canning Technology. Westport, Conn.; Avi, 1979. 406p.	Second
First	James, W. P. T., and Olof Theander, eds. The Analysis of Dietary Fiber in Food. New York; M. Dekker, 1981. 276p. (Basic and Clinical Nutrition no. 3)	
Third	Jeejeebhoy, Khursheed N., ed. Total Parenteral Nutrition in the Hospital and at Home. Boca Raton, Fla.; CRC Press, 1983. 255p.	
	Jelliffe, Derrick B. Infant Nutrition in the Sub-Tropics and Tropics. 2d ed. Geneva; World Health Organization, 1968. 335p. (WHO Monograph Series no. 29) (1st ed., 1955. 237p.) (Available in Spanish: Nutrición Infantil en Países en Desarrollo. México; LImusa-Noriega. 246p.	First
First	Jelliffe, Derrick B., and E. F. Patrice Jelliffe. The Assessment of the Nutritional Status of the Community. 2d ed. Oxford; Oxford University Press, 1979. 271p. (1st ed. Gcneva; World Health Organization, 1966.)	Third
Second	Jelliffe, Derrick B., and E. F. Patrice Jelliffe. Community Nutritional Assessment: With Special Reference to Less Technically Developed Countries. Oxford and New York; Oxford University Press, 1989. 633p.	First
Second	Jelliffe, Derrick B., and E. F. Patrice Jelliffe. Growth Monitoring and Promotion in Young Children: Guidelines for the Selection of Methods and Training Techniques. New York; Oxford University Press, 1990. 134p.	First
First	Jelliffe, Derrick B., and E. F. Patrice Jelliffe. Human Milk in	First

Developed countries ranking		Third World ranking
	the Modern World: Psychosocial, Nutritional, and Ecomonic Significance. Oxford and New York; Oxford University Press, 1978. 500p.	
Second	Jelliffe, Derrick B., and E. F. Patrice Jelliffe, eds. Nutrition and Growth. New York; Plenum Press, 1979. 452p. (Human Nutrition: A Comprehensive Treatise, Vol. 2.)	First
Second	Jelliffe, Derrick B., and E. F. Patrice Jelliffe, eds. Programmes to Promote Breastfeeding. Oxford and New York; Oxford University Press, 1988. 490p.	Second
Third	Jelliffe, E. F. Patrice, and Derrick B. Jelliffe, eds. Adverse Effects of Foods. New York; Plenum, 1982. 614p.	
Second	Jellinek, Gisela. Sensory Evaluation of Food: Theory and Practice. Chichester, England; E. Horwood, 1985. 429p. (Translation of Sensorische Lebensmittel-Prufung.)	
	Jenkins, G. H. Introduction to Cane Sugar Technology. Amsterdam and New York; Elsevier Pub. Co., 1966. 478p.	Third
Third	Jensen, Robert G., and Margaret C. Neville, eds. Human Lactation: Milk Components and Methodologies; Proceeding of a Symposium on Methods in Human Lactation, 1984, Winter Park, Colorado. New York; Plenum Press, 1985. 307p.	Second
Second	Jerome, Norge W., Randy F. Kandel, and Gretel H. Pelto, eds. Nutritional Anthropology: Contemporary Approaches to Diet and Culture. Pleasantville, N.Y.; Redgrave Pub. Co., 1980. 433p. (Papers originally presented at three Symposia . . . at the annual Meetings of the American Anthropological Association, 1973 and 1974.)	Second
Second	Johnson, Arnold H., and Martin S. Peterson, eds. Encyclopedia of Food Technology. Westport, Conn.; Avi, 1974. 993p.	
First	Johnson, Leonard R. et al., eds. Physiology of the Gastrointestinal Tract. 2d ed. New York; Raven Press, 1987. 1780p. 2 vols. (1st ed., 1981.)	
Second	Johnston, Francis E. Nutritional Anthropology. New York; A. R. Liss, 1987. 304p.	
Second	Joint FAO/IAEA/WHO Expert Committee. Wholesomeness of Irradiated Food; Report . . . Geneva; World Health Organization, 1981. 34p. (WHO Technical Report Series no. 659)	
Second	Joint FAO/UNICEF/WHO Expert Committee. Methodology of Nutritional Surveillance: Report. Geneva; World Health Organization, 1976. 66p. (WHO Technical Report Series no. 593)	First
Third	Joint FAO/WHO Codex Alimentarius Commission. Recommended International General Standard for Irradiated Foods and Recommended International Code of Practice for the Operation of Radiation Facilities for the Treatment of Foods. Rome; Joint FAO/WHO Food Standards Programme, FAO; New York; UNIPUB, 1980. 19p.	

Developed countries ranking		Third World ranking
Third	Joint FAO/WHO Expert Committee on Nutrition. Food and Nutrition Strategies in National Development. Rome; Food and Agriculture Organization, 1976. 64p.	Second
Third	Joint FAO/WHO Expert Consultation. Requirements of Vitamin A, Iron, Folate and Vitamin B12; Report . . . Rome; Food and Agriculture Organization, 1988. 107p. (FAO Food and Nutrition Series no. 23)	Second
Third	Joint FAO/WHO Expert Group on Requirements of Ascorbic Acid, Vitamin D, Vitamin B12, Folate, and Iron. Report . . . Geneva; World Health Organization, 1970. 75p. (WHO Technical Report Series No. 452; FAO Nutrition Meetings Report Series no. 47)	Second
Second	Joint FAO/WHO Expert Group, Rome, Sept. 1965. Requirements of Vitamin A, Thiamine, Riboflavine and Niacin. Rome; Food and Agriculture Organization, 1967. 86p. (FAO Nutrition Meetings Report Series No. 41; WHO Technical Report Series no. 362)	Second
First	Joint FAO/WHO/UNU Expert Consultation. Energy and Protein Requirements II: Report . . . Geneva; World Health Organization, 1985. 206p. (WHO Technical Report Series no. 724) (Earlier ed., 1973. 118p.)	
Third	Joint UNICEF/WHO Committee on Health Policy. National Decision-Making for Primary Health Care; A Study. Geneva; World Health Organization, 1981. 69p.	
First	Joint WHO/UNICEF/USAID/Helen Keller International/IVACG Meeting. Control of Vitamin A Deficiency and Xerophthalmia; Report . . . Geneva; World Health Organization, 1982. 70p. (WHO Technical Report Series no. 672)	First
First	Josephson, Edward S. Preservation of Food by Ionizing Radiation. Boca Raton, Fla.; CRC Press, 1983. 3 vols.	
Third	Jukes, D. J. Food Legislation of the UK: A Concise Guide. 2d ed. London and Boston; Butterworths, 1987. 151p.	
Second	Jul, Mogens. The Quality of Frozen Foods. London and Orlando, Fla.; Academic Press, 1984. 292p.	
Second	Juliano, Bienvenido O., ed. Rice: Chemistry and Technology. 2d ed., rev. St. Paul, Minn.; American Association of Cereal Chemists, 1985. 774p. (1st ed., edited by D. F. Houston, 1972. 517p.	
Second	Junshi, Chen, and T. Colin Campbell et al. Diet, Life-Style, and Mortality in China: A Study of the Characteristics of 65 Chinese Counties = Chung-kuo ti shan shih, sheng huo fang shih ho ssu wang lu: liu shih wu ko hsien ti tiao cha yen chiu. Oxford; Oxford University Press; Ithaca, N.Y.; Cornell University Press; People's Republic of China; People's Medical Pub. House, 1990. 894p.	Third

Developed countries ranking		Third World ranking
	K	
Third	Kadoya, Takashi, ed. Food Packaging. San Diego; Academic Press, 1990. 424p.	
Second	Kapsalis, John G. Objective Methods in Food Quality Assessment. Boca Raton, Fla.; CRC Press, 1987. 275p.	
Second	Kare, Morley R., and Joseph G. Brand, eds. Interaction of the Chemical Senses with Nutrition; Proceedings of the 3d International Conference . . . Monell Chemical Senses Center, October 1984. Orlando, Fla.; Academic Press, 1986. 477p.	
First	Kare, Morley R., and Bruce P. Halpern, eds. Physiological and Behavioral Aspects of Taste; Proceedings of a Conference, Cornell University, June 1960. Chicago; University of Chicago Press, 1961. 149p.	
First	Karel, Marcus. Physical Principles of Food Preservation. New York; M. Dekker, 1975. 474p. (Part 2 of: Principles of Food Science.)	
First	Karmas, Endel, and Robert S. Harris, eds. Nutritional Evaluation of Food Processing. 3d ed. New York; Van Nostrand Reinhold, 1988. 786p. (1st ed., edited by R. S. Harris and Harry von Loesecke. New York; Wiley, 1960. 612p.)	
Third	Karrer, Walter. Konstitution und Vorkommen der Organischen Pflanzenstoffe (Exclusive Alkaloide). 2d ed. Basel; Birkhauser, 1976. 1205p. (1st ed., 1958. 1207p.)	
Second	Katch, Frank I. Nutrition, Weight Control, and Exercise. 3d ed. Philadelphia; Lea & Febiger, 1988. 342p. (1st ed. Boston; Houghton Mifflin, 1977. 365p.)	
First	Kawamura, Yojiro, and Morley R. Kare, eds. Umami: A Basic Taste: Physiology, Biochemistry, Nutrition, Food Science; Proceedings of the 1st International Symposium on Umami, Lihue, Hawaii, October 1985. New York; M. Dekker, 1987. 649p.	
Second	Kay, Daisy E. Food Legumes. London; Tropical Products Institute, Ministry of Overseas Development, 1979. 435p. (TPI Crop and Product Digests no. 3)	Second
Second	Kefford, J. F., and B. V. Chandler. The Chemical Constituents of Citrus Fruits. New York; Academic Press, 1970. 246p.	
Third	Kelsey, Jennifer L., W. Douglas Thompson, and Alfred S. Evans. Methods in Observational Epidemiology. New York; Oxford University Press, 1986. 366p. (Monographs in Epidemiology and Biostatistics no. 10)	
Second	Kennedy, John F., and Charles A. White. Bioactive Carbohydrates in Chemistry, Biochemistry and Biology. Chichester, U.K.; E. Horwood; New York; Halsted Press, 1983. 331p.	
Second	Kent, Norman L. Technology of Cereals: An Introduction for Students of Food Science and Agriculture. 3d ed. Oxford and New York; Pergamon, 1983. 221p. (Rev. ed. of Technology of	Second

Developed countries ranking		Third World ranking
	Cereals with Special Reference to Wheat. 2d ed., 1975.) (Available in Spanish: Tecnología de los Cereales. 2ed. Zaragoza; Acribia, 1987. 220p.)	
Second	Keys, Ancel B. Seven Countries: A Multivariate Analysis of Death and Coronary Heart Disease. Cambridge, Mass.; Harvard University Press, 1980. 381p.	
Second	Kies, Constance, ed. Nutritional Bioavailability of Iron; Proceedings of a Symposium held at the American Chemical Society Meeting, Atlanta, Ga., March 1981. Washington, D.C.; American Chemical Society, 1982. 204p. (ACS Symposium Series no. 203)	
Third	King, Maurice H. et al. Nutrition for Developing Countries, With Special Reference to the Maize, Cassava, and Millet Areas of Africa. Nairobi, Kenya; Oxford University Press, 1972. 1 vol.	Second
Third	King, Richard D., ed. Developments in Food Analysis Techniques. London; Applied Science Publishers, 1978–1980. 3 vols.	
Second	Kinsella, John E. Seafoods and Fish Oils in Human Health and Disease. New York; M. Dekker, 1987. 317p.	
Second	Kinsella, John E., and William G. Soucie, eds. Food Proteins; Proceedings of the Protein and Co-Products Symposium . . . 1988. Champaign, Ill.; American Oil Chemists' Society, 1989. 431p.	
Second	Kleiber, Max. The Fire of Life: An Introduction to Animal Energetics. Rev. ed. Huntington, N.Y.; R. E. Krieger Pub. Co., 1975. 453p. (1st ed., New York; Wiley, 1961. 454p.)	
Third	Klein, Robert E. et al., eds. Evaluating the Impact of Nutrition and Health Programs; Proceedings of the Pan American Health Organization International Conference . . . 1977, Panama. New York; Plenum Press, 1979. 462p.	Second
Second	Knorr, Dietrich, ed. Food Biotechnology. New York; M. Dekker, 1987. 613p.	
Second	Kon, Stanislaw K. Milk and Milk Products in Human Nutrition. 2d ed., rev. Rome; Food and Agriculture Organization, 1972. 80p. (FAO Nutritional Studies no. 27) (1st ed., 1959. 75p.)	Third
Second	Kosikowski, Frank. Cheese and Fermented Milk Foods. 2d ed., 3d printing with revisions. Brooktondale, N.Y.; F. V. Kosikowski and Associates, 1982. 711p. (1st ed., Ithaca, N.Y.; Distributed by Edwards Bros., Ann Arbor, Mich., 1966. 429p.)	
Second	Kraft, Allen A. Psychrotrophic Bacteria in Foods: Disease and Spoilage. Boca Raton, Fla.; CRC Press, Inc., 1992. 274p.	
First	Kramer, Amihud, and Bernard A. Twigg. Quality Control for the Food Industry. 3d ed. Westport, Conn.; Avi, 1970–1973. 2	Second

Developed countries ranking		Third World ranking
	vols. (1st-2d ed. published as Fundamentals of Quality Control for the Food Industry.)	
Second	Kramer, Donald E., and John Liston, eds. Seafood Quality Determination; Proceedings of the International Symposium . . . coordinated by the University of Alaska Sea Grant College Program, Anchorage, November 1986. Amsterdam and New York; Elsevier, 1987. 677p.	
Third	Kramer, John K. G., Frank D. Sauer, and Wallace J. Pigden, eds. High and Low Erucic Acid Rapeseed Oils: Production, Usage, Chemistry, and Toxicological Evaluation. New York; Academic Press, 1983. 582p.	
Second	Krause, Marie V. Food, Nutrition, and Diet Therapy. 8th ed. Philadelphia; Saunders, 1992. 933p. (3d ed., 1961. 716p.)	Third
Second	Kritchevsky, David, Charles Bonfield, and James W. Anderson, eds. Dietary Fiber: Chemistry, Physiology, and Health Effects; Proceedings of the George Vahouny Fiber Conference, held April 1988, Washington, D.C. New York; Plenum Press, 1990. 499p.	
Third	Kruger, James E., David Lineback, and Clyde E. Stauffer, eds. Enzymes and Their Role in Cereal Technology. St. Paul, Minn; American Association of Cereal Chemists, 1987. 403p.	
Third	Kumar, Rajiv, ed. Vitamin D: Basic and Clinical Aspects. Boston; M. Nijhoff, 1984. 786p.	
Second	Kunau, Wolf-H., and Ralph T. Holman, eds. Polyunsaturated Fatty Acids. Champaign, Ill.; American Oil Chemists' Society, 1977. 258p. (AOCS Monograph no. 4)	
Third	Kurtz, Robert C., ed. Nutrition in Gastrointestinal Disease. New York; Churchill Livingstone, 1981. 146p. (Contemporary Issues in Clinical Nutrition no. 1)	
	L	
Second	LaBuza, Theodore P. Shelf-Life Dating of Foods. Westport, Conn.; Food & Nutrition Press, 1982. 500p.	
First	LaBuza, Theodore P., and John W. Erdman. Food Science and Nutritional Health: An Introduction. St. Paul, Minn.; West Pub. Co., 1984. 558p. (Rev. ed. of: Food and Your Well-Being, 1977.)	Second
Third	Lampert, Lincoln M. Modern Dairy Products: Composition, Food Value, Processing, Chemistry, Bacteriology, Testing, Imitation Dairy Products. 3d ed. New York; Chemical Pub. Co., 1975. 437p. (First published, 1947, as Milk and Dairy Products.)	
Second	Lappe, Frances Moore, and Joseph Collins. Food First: Beyond the Myth of Scarcity. Rev. and updated ed. New York; Ballan-	Third

Developed countries ranking		Third World ranking
	tine Books, 1979. 619p. (Available in Spanish: Comer es Primero; Más Allá De La Escasez. Mexico; Siglo XXI, 1982. 416p.)	
Second	Larson, Bruce L., and Vearl R. Smith. Lactation: A Comprehensive Treatise. New York; Academic Press, 1974. 3 vols.	
Second	Larsson, Kare, and Stig E. Friberg, eds. Food Emulsions. 2d ed., rev. and expanded. New York; M. Dekker, 1990. 510p. (1st ed., edited by Stig Friberg, 1976. 480p.)	
Second	Lasztity, Radomir. The Chemistry of Cereal Proteins. Boca Raton, Fla.; CRC Press, 1984. 203p.	Second
Third	Lasztity, Radomir, and Mate Hidvegi, eds. Amino Acid Composition and Biological Value of Cereal Proteins; Proceedings of the International Association for Cereal Chemistry Symposium, Budapest, Hungary, May-June 1983. Dordrecht and Boston; D. Reidel, 1985. 662p.	
First	Latham, Michael C. Human Nutrition in Tropical Africa; A Textbook for Health Workers with Special Reference to Community Health Problems in East Africa. Rome; Food and Agriculture Organization, 1979. 286p. (FAO Food and Nutrition Series no. 11, Rev. 1)	Second
Third	Latham, Michael C., and Marjorie S. van Veen, eds. International Conference on Dietary Guidelines; Proceedings . . . Ryerson Polytechnical Institute, Toronto, June 1988. Ithaca, N.Y.; Cornell University Program in International Nutrition, 1989. 207p. (Cornell International Nutrition Monograph Series no. 21)	Third
Third	Lawrence, Andrew A. Natural Gums for Edible Purposes. Park Ridge, N.J.; Noyes Data, 1976. 338p. (Food Technology Review no. 36)	Third
Third	Lawrence, Felicity, ed. Additives: Your Complete Survival Guide. London; Century, 1986. 288p.	
Third	Lawrence, James F., ed. Food Constituents and Food Residues: Their Chromatographic Determination. New York; M. Dekker, 1984. 617p.	
First	Lawrie, Ralston A., ed. Developments in Meat Science. London; Elsevier Applied Science Publishers, 1980. 4 vols.	
First	Lawrie, Ralston A. Meat Science. 4th ed. Oxford and New York; Pergamon Press, 1985. 267p. (1st ed., 1966. 368p.)	Third
Second	Lebenthal, Emanuel. Textbook of Gastroenterology and Nutrition in Infancy. 2d ed. New York; Raven Press, 1989. 2 vols. (1st ed., 1981.) (Available in Spanish: Gastroenterologiá y Nutrición en Pediatría. Barcelona; Salvat, 1984.)	Second
Second	Lebenthal, Emanuel, ed. Total Parenteral Nutrition: Indications, Utilization, Complications, and Pathophysiological Considerations. New York; Raven Press, 1986. 514p.	

Developed countries ranking		Third World ranking
Second	Lee, Frank A. Basic Food Chemistry. 2d ed. Westport, Conn.; Avi, 1983. 564p. (1st ed., 1975. 430p.)	Second
Second	Lee, Richard B., and Irven DeVore, eds. Man the Hunter; Proceedings of a Symposium . . . University of Chicago, 1966. Chicago; Aldine Pub. Co., 1969. 415p.	
Second	Lees, Robert S., and Marcus Karel, eds. Omega-3 Fatty Acids in Health and Disease. New York; M. Dekker, 1990. 240p.	
Second	Lehninger, Albert L. Biochemistry; The Molecular Basis of Cell Structure and Function. 2d ed. New York; Worth Publishers, 1975. 1104p. (1st ed., 1970. 833p.) (Available in Spanish: Bioquímica. Barcelona: Omega. 1144p.)	
Second	Leniger, Hendrik A., and W. A. Beverloo. Food Process Engineering. Dordrecht, Holland and Boston; D. Reidel Pub. Co., 1975. 552p.	
Third	Lennarz, William J., ed. The Biochemistry of Glycoproteins and Proteoglycans. New York; Plenum Press, 1980. 381p.	
Second	Lessof, M. H., ed. Clinical Reactions to Food. Chichester, England and New York; Wiley, 1983. 662p.	
	Leung, Woot-Tsuen Wu. Food Composition Table for Use in Africa. Bethesda, Md.; Food and Agriculture Organization, 1968. 306p.	Third
Second	Leung, Woot-Tsuen Wu. Food Composition Table for Use in East Asia. Washington, D.C.; U.S. Govt. Print. Off., 1973. 334p.	Third
	Leung, Woot-Tsuen Wu. Food Composition Table for Use in Latin America. Washington, D.C.; U.S. Govt. Print. Off., 1961. 145p.	Third
Third	Leveille, Gilbert A., Mary Ellen Zabik, and Karen J. Morgan. Nutrients in Foods. Cambridge, Mass.; Nutrition Guild, 1983. 291p.	
Third	Lewis, Alvin E., Biostatistics. 2d ed. New York; van Nostrand Reinhold, 1984. 198p. (1st ed., 1966. 227p.) (Available in Spanish: Bioestadística. México; Cecsa, 1969. 288p.)	Third
Second	Lewis, Michael J. Physical Properties of Foods and Food Processing Systems. Weinheim; VCH; Chichester, England; E. Horwood, 1987. 465p.	
First	Liener, Irvin E., ed. Toxic Constituents of Plant Foodstuffs. 2d ed. New York; Academic Press, 1980. 502p. (1st ed., 1969. 500p.)	First
	Lifshitz, Fima, ed. Carbohydrate Intolerance in Infancy. New York; M. Dekker, 1982. 255p. (Clinical Disorders in Pediatric Nutrition no. 1)	Third
	Lifshitz, Fima, ed. Pediatric Nutrition: Infant Feedings, Deficiencies, Diseases. New York; M. Dekker, 1982. 621p. (Clinical Disorders in Pediatric Nutrition no. 2)	Third

Developed countries ranking		Third World ranking
Third	Lindblad, B. S., ed. Perinatal Nutrition; Proceedings . . . 6th Annual Bristol-Myers Symposium on Nutrition Research, Saltsjobaden, Sweden, August 1986. San Diego; Academic Press, 1988. 394p. (Bristol-Meyers Nutrition Symposium no. 6)	Third
Second	Linder, Maria C., ed. Nutritional Biochemistry and Metabolism: With Clinical Applications. 2d ed. New York; Elsevier, 1991. 436p. (1st ed., 1985.) (Available in Spanish: Nutrición: Aspectos Bioquímicos, Metabólicos y Clínicos. Pamplona; Eunas, 1988. 480p.)	Third
Second	Lineback, David R., and George E. Inglett, eds. Food Carbohydrates; Proceedings of a Symposium sponsored by the Institute of Food Technologists and the International Union of Food Science and Technology, June 1981. Westport, Conn.; Avi, 1982. 494p.	
Second	Linko, P. et al., eds. Food Process Engineering; Proceedings of the 2d International Congress on Engineering and Food and the 8th European Food Symposium, Helsinki University of Technology, Espoo, Finland, Aug. 1979. London; Applied Science, 1980. 2 vols.	
Third	Linskens, H. F., and J. F. Jackson, eds. Plant Fibers. Berlin and New York; Springer-Verlag, 1989. 377p.	
	Livingston, G. E., ed. Nutritional Status Assessment of the Individual; Proceedings of a National Conference . . . New York, October 1987. Trumbull, Conn.; Food & Nutrition Press, 1989. 479p.	Third
Third	Livingston, G. E., Raymond J. Moshy, and Charlotte M. Chang, eds. The Role of Food Product Development in Implementing Dietary Guidelines: Proceedings of an International Conference, sponsored by the American Health Foundation, May 1980, New York. Westport, Conn.; Food & Nutrition Press, 1982. 212p.	Third
Third	Lloyd-Still, John D., ed. Malnutrition and Intellectual Development. Littleton, Mass.; Publishing Sciences Group, 1976. 194p.	
Third	Lock, Arthur. Practical Canning. 3d ed, rev. and enlarged. London; Food Trade Press, 1969. 415p. (1st ed., 1949. 246p.)	
Third	Lohman, Timothy G., Alex F. Roche, and Reynaldo Martorell. Anthropometric Standardization Reference Manual. Champaign, Ill.; Human Kinetics Books, 1988. 177p.	Third
Second	Loncin, Marcel, and Richard L. Merson. Food Engineering, Principles and Selected Applications. New York; Academic Press, 1979. 494p.	
	Longree, Karla, and Gertrude Armbruster. Quantity Food Sanitation. 4th ed. New York; Wiley, 1987. 452p. (1st ed., New York; Interscience Publishers, 1967. 397p.)	Third
Second	Lopez, Anthony. A Complete Course in Canning and Related	Second

Developed countries ranking		Third World ranking
	Processes. 12th ed., rev. and enl. Baltimore; Canning Trade, 1987. 3 vols.	
Second	Lorenz, Klaus J., and Karel Kulp, eds. Handbook of Cereal Science and Technology. New York; M. Dekker, 1991. 882p.	Second
Second	Lowenberg, Miriam E. et al. Food and People. 3d ed. New York; Wiley, 1979. 382p. (1st ed., 1968, as Food and Man.) (Available in Spanish: Alimentos y el Hombre. México; Limusa-Noriega. 348p.)	
Third	Lueck, Erich. Antimicrobial Food Additives; Characteristics, Uses, Effects . . . trans. from the German by Grant F. Edwards. Berlin and New York; Springer-Verlag, 1980. 280p.	
Second	Luh, Bor S., and Jasper G. Woodroof, eds. Commercial Vegetable Processing. 2d ed. New York; Van Nostrand Reinhold, 1988. 784p. (1st ed., 1975. 755 p.)	Second

M

Developed countries ranking		Third World ranking
First	Maarse, Henk, ed. Volative Compounds in Foods and Beverages. 1st ed. New York; M. Dekker, 1991. 764p.	
First	Maarse, Henk, and R. Belz. Isolation, Separation, and Identification of Volatile Compounds in Aroma Research. Berlin; Akademie-Verlag; Hingham, Mass.; Kluwer Boston, 1985. 290p. (Earlier ed., 1981. 290p.)	
Third	MacCarthy, Diarmuid, ed. Concentration and Drying of Foods; Proceedings of the Kellogg Foundation 2d International Food Research Symposium, held at University College, Cork, Republic of Ireland, September 1985. London and New York; Elsevier Applied Science Publishers, 1986. 303p.	Third
Third	Macdonald, I., and A. Vrana, eds. Metabolic Effects of Dietary Carbohydrates. Basel and New York; Karger, 1986. 271p.	
First	Machlin, Lawrence J., ed. Handbook of Vitamins: Nutritional, Biochemical, and Clinical Aspects. 2d ed. New York; M. Dekker, 1991. 595p. (1st ed., 1984. 614p.)	First
Second	Machlin, Lawrence J., ed. Vitamin E: A Comprehensive Treatise. New York; M. Dekker, 1980. 660p.	
Third	Mackinney, Gordon, and Angela C. Little. Color of Foods. Westport, Conn.; Avi, 1962. 308p.	Third
Second	Macrae, R., ed. HPLC in Food Analysis. London and New York; Academic Press, 1982. 340p.	
Second	Le Magnen, Jacques. Hunger. Cambridge and New York; Cambridge University Press, 1985. 157p.	
Third	Mahan, L. Kathleen, and Jane M. Rees. Nutrition in Adolescence. St. Louis; Times Mirror/Mosby College Pub., 1984. 331p.	
Second	Manley, Duncan. Technology of Biscuits, Crackers and	

Developed countries ranking		Third World ranking
	Cookies. 2d ed. Chichester, England; Ellis Horwood, 1991. 500p. (1st ed., 1983. 446p.)	
Second	Mann, Charles K., and Barbara Huddleston, eds. Food Policy; Frameworks for Analysis and Action. Bloomington, Ind.; Indiana University Press, 1986. 243p.	Third
Second	Manoff, Richard K. Social Marketing: New Imperative for Public Health. New York; Praeger, 1985. 293p.	Second
Second	Manske, R. H. F., and H. L. Holmes, eds. The Alkaloids: Chemistry and Physiology. New York; Academic Press, 1950+. (Editors vary. Vols. 21–38 have subtitle Chemistry and Pharmacology. 39 vols. in 1991.)	
	Manson-Bahr, Philip E. C., and D. R. Bell. Manson's Tropical Diseases. 19th ed. London; Bailliere Tindall, 1987. 1557p. (1st-6th eds. by Patrick Manson, 7th-16th eds. by Philip Manson-Bahr.)	Third
Third	Marinetti, Guido V., ed. Lipid Chromatographic Analysis. 2d ed., rev. and expanded. New York; M. Dekker, 1976. 3 vols. (1st ed., London; E. Arnold; New York; M. Dekker, 1967–1969. 2 vols.)	
Second	Markakis, Pericles, ed. Anthocyanins as Food Colors. New York; Academic Press, 1982. 263p.	
Second	Martin, Roy E. et al., eds. Chemistry and Biochemistry of Marine Food Products. Westport, Conn.; Avi, 1982. 474p.	First
Third	Martorell, Reynaldo. Nutrition and Health Status Indicators: Suggestions for Surveys of the Standard of Living in Developing Countries. Washington, D.C.; World Bank, Development Research Center, 1981. 97p.	Second
First	Mason, John B. et al. Nutritional Surveillance. Geneva; World Health Organization, 1984. 194p.	First
Second	Masters, Keith. Spray Drying Handbook. 4th ed. New York; J. Wiley, 1985. 696p. (1st ed., Cleveland, Ohio; CRC Press, 1972. 668p.)	
Second	Mata, Leonardo J. The Children of Santa Maria Cauque: A Prospective Field Study of Health and Growth. Cambridge, Mass.; MIT Press, 1978. 395p.	Second
Second	Mathlouthi, M., ed. Food Packaging and Preservation: Theory and Practice. London and New York; Elsevier Applied Science, 1986. 402p.	
Second	Matthews, Ruth H., ed. Legumes: Chemistry, Technology, and Human Nutrition. New York; M. Dekker, 1989. 389p.	
Third	Matz, Samuel A., ed. Bakery Technology and Engineering. 3d ed. New York; Van Nostrand Reinhold, 1992. 853p. (1st ed., Westport, Conn.; Avi, 1960. 669p.)	
First	Matz, Samuel A., ed. The Chemistry and Technology of Ce-	First

Developed countries ranking		Third World ranking
	reals as Food and Feed. 2d ed. McAllen, Tex.; Pan-Tech International; New York; Van Nostrand Reinhold, 1991. 751p. (1st ed., Westport, Conn.; Avi Pub. Co., 1959. 732p.)	
Third	Matz, Samuel A. Food Texture. Westport, Conn.; Avi, 1962. 286p.	
Second	Matz, Samuel A. Snack Food Technology. 3d ed. Westport, Conn.; Avi Pub. Co., 1992. 450p. (1st ed., 1976. 349p.)	
Third	Matz, Samuel A. Technology of the Materials of Baking. McAllen, Tex.; Pan-Tech International, 1989. 296p.	
Third	Mauron, J., ed. Nutritional Adequacy, Nutrient Availability and Needs; Proceedings of the Nestle Nutrition Research Symposium, Vevey, Switzerland, September 1982. Basel and Boston; Birkhauser Verlag, 1983. 382p.	Third
Third	Maxwell, Morton H., Charles R. Kleeman, and Robert G. Narins, eds. Clinical Disorders of Fluid and Electrolyte Metabolism. 4th ed. New York; McGraw-Hill, 1987. 1268p. (1st ed., 1962. 512p.)	Second
Second	Mayer, Jean. U.S. Nutrition Policies in the Seventies. San Francisco; W. H. Freeman, 1973. 256p.	
Second	McArdle, William D. Exercise Physiology: Energy, Nutrition, and Human Performance. 3d ed. Philadelphia; Lea & Febiger, 1991. (1st ed., by W. D. McArdle, Frank I. Katch and Victor L. Katch, 1981. 508p.)	
First	McCance, R. A. and E. M. Widdowson. The Composition of Foods; McCance and Widdowson's The Composition of Foods. 5th ed., rev. and extended, by B. Holland et al. London; Royal Society of Chemistry and Ministry of Agriculture, Fisheries and Food, 1991. 462p. (1st Suppl., by A. A. Paul; 2d Suppl., by S. P. Tan; listed separately; 3d Suppl., B. Holland; listed separately.)	First
First	McCance, R. A., and Elsie M. Widdowson, eds. Calorie Deficiencies and Protein Deficiencies; Proceedings of a Colloquium, Cambridge, April 1967. London; Churchill, 1968. 386p.	Second
Second	McCormick, Donald B., and Lemuel D. Wright, eds. Vitamins and Coenzymes. New York; Academic Press, 1970–1980. 6 vols. (Methods in Enzymology no. 18, 62, 66–67)	Third
Third	McGilvery, Robert W. Biochemistry, a Functional Approach. 3d ed. Philadelphia; Saunders, 1983. 909p. (1st ed., 1970. 769p.)	
Second	McKenzie, Hugh A., ed. Milk Proteins; Chemistry and Molecular Biology. New York; Academic Press, 1970–1971. 2 vols.	Second
First	McLaren, Donald S. A Colour Atlas of Nutritional Disorders. London and Chicago; Wolfe Medical Publications, 1981. 109p.	Second
First	McLaren, Donald S., ed. Nutrition in the Community: A Criti-	Second

Developed countries ranking		Third World ranking
	cal Look at Nutrition Policy, Planning, and Programmes. 2d ed. Chichester and New York; Wiley, 1983. 472p. (1st ed., Wiley, 1976. 393p.)	
Second	McLaren, Donald S. Nutritional Opthalmology. 2d ed. of Malnutrition and the Eye. London and New York; Academic Press, 1980. 438p.	Second
Second	McLaren, Donald S., and David Burman, eds. Textbook of Paediatric Nutrition. 2d ed. Edinburgh and New York; Churchill Livingstone, 1982. 464p. (1st ed., 1976. 416p.)	Second
Second	McLaren, Donald S., and Michael M. Meguid. Nutrition and Its Disorders. 4th ed., rev. and enl. Edinburgh and New York; Churchill Livingstone, 1988. 293p. (1st ed., 1972. 280p.) (Available in Spanish: Nutrición y sus Trastornos. México; Manual Moderno, 1983. 313p.)	Second
Third	McLean, J. A., and G. Tobin. Animal and Human Calorimetry. Cambridge, Mass. and New York; Cambridge University Press, 1987. 338p.	
Third	McLoughlin, Peter F. M., ed. African Food Production Systems, Cases and Theory. Baltimore; Johns Hopkins Press, 1970. 318p.	Third
Third	McWilliams, Margaret. Food Fundamentals. 4th ed. New York and London; Macmillan Collier Macmillan, 1986. 600p. (1st ed. New York; Wiley, 1966. 379p.)	Second
Second	McWilliams, Margaret. Foods: Experimental Perspectives. New York; Macmillan, 1989. 584p.	
Third	McWilliams, Margaret, and Harriett Paine. Modern Food Preservation. Fullerton, Calif.; Plycon Press, 1977. 198p.	Third
Second	Means, Gary E., and Robert E. Feeney. Chemical Modification of Proteins. San Francisco; Holden-Day, 1971. 254p.	
Third	Meilgaard, Morten, and Gail V. Civille. Sensory Evaluation Techniques. Boca Raton, Fla.; CRC Press, 1987. 2 vols.	
Third	Mellor, J. D. Fundamentals of Freeze-Drying. London and New York; Academic Press, 1978. 386p.	Third
Second	Merrill, Annabel L. Energy Value of Foods: Basis and Derivation. Rev. ed. Washington, D.C.; U.S. Dept. of Agriculture, Human Nutrition Research Branch, Agricultural Research Service, 1973. 105p. (Earlier ed., 1955.)	
Third	Merrill, Richard A., and Peter B. Hutt, eds. Food and Drug Law: Cases and Materials. Mineola, N.Y.; Foundation Press, 1980. 959p.	
Third	Middlekauff, Roger D., and Philippe Shubik, eds. International Food Regulation Handbook: Policy, Science, Law. New York; M. Dekker, 1989. 562p.	
Second	Mills, Colin F., ed. Zinc in Human Biology. London and New York; Springer-Verlag, 1989. 388p.	

Developed countries ranking		Third World ranking
	Mills, Colin F., I. Bremner, and J. K. Chesters, eds. Trace Elements in Man and Animals; Proceedings of the 5th International Symposium . . . (TEMA-5), Aberdeen, Scotland, June-July 1984. Farnham Royal, Slough, U.K.; Commonwealth Agricultural Bureaux, 1985. 977p.	Third
Second	Milner, Max, Nevin Scrimshaw, and Daniel I. C. Wang, eds. Protein Resources and Technology: Status and Research Needs. Westport, Conn.; Avi, 1978. 629p. (Sect. I, by N. S. Scrimshaw and D. I. Wang, published by the National Science Foundation, 1975.)	
Second	Min, David B., and Thomas H. Smouse, eds. Flavor Chemistry of Fats and Oils. Champaign, Ill.; American Oil Chemists' Society, 1985. 309p. (AOCS Monograph no. 15)	
Second	Minifie, Bernard W. Chocolate, Cocoa, and Confectionery: Science and Technology. 3d ed. New York; Van Nostrand Reinhold, 1989. 904p. (1st U.S. ed., Westport, Conn.; Avi Pub. Co., 1970. 624p.)	
Third	Minor, Lewis J. Nutritional Standards. Westport, Conn.; Avi, 1983. 281p.	Third
Second	Mintz, Sidney W. Sweetness and Power: The Place of Sugar in Modern History. New York; Viking, 1985. 274p.	
First	Mitchell, J. R., and D. A. Ledward, eds. Functional Properties of Food Macromolecules. London and New York; Elsevier Applied Science Publishers, 1986. 433p.	
Second	Mitzner, Karen, Nevin Scrimshaw, and Robert Morgan, eds. Improving the Nutritional Status of Children during the Weaning Period: A Manual for Policymakers, Program Planners, and Fieldworkers. Cambridge, Mass.; 1984. 258p.	Second
Second	Mohsenin, Nuri N. Thermal Properties of Foods and Other Agricultural Materials. New York; Gordon and Breach, 1980. 407p.	
Third	Moment, Gairdner B., ed. Nutritional Approaches to Aging Research. Boca Raton, Fla.; CRC Press, 1982. 266p.	Third
	Morley, David. Paediatric Priorities in the Developing World. London; Butterworth, 1973. 470p.	First
Third	Morley, David, Jon E. Rohde, and Glen Williams, eds. Practicing Health for All. Oxford and New York; Oxford University Press, 1983. 333p.	Second
	Morris, Morris David. Measuring the Condition of the World's Poor: The Physical Quality of Life Index. New York; Published for the Overseas Development Council by Pergamon Press, 1979. 176p.	Third
First	Morton, E. D., and A. J. MacLeod, eds. Food Flavours. Amsterdam and New York; Elsevier Scientific, 1982–1983. 1 vol. in 3 pts.	

Developed countries ranking		Third World ranking
Second	Morton, I. D., ed. Cereals in a European Context; Proceedings of the 1st European Conference on Food Science and Technology, Bournemouth, U.K., 1986. New York; VCH; Chichester, Eng.; E. Horwood, 1987. 523p.	
Second	Moskowitz, Howard R., ed. Applied Sensory Analysis of Foods. Boca Raton, Fla.; CRC Press, 1988. 2 vols.	
Second	Moskowitz, Howard R., ed. Food Texture: Instrumental and Sensory Measurement. New York; M. Dekker, 1987. 335p.	
Third	Mosley, W. Henry, ed. Nutrition and Human Reproduction; Papers presented at a Conference . . . Bethesda, Maryland, February 1977, organized by the National Institute of Child Health and Human Development and the Subcommittee on Nutrition and Fertility of the Committee on International Nutrition Programs of the National Research Council. New York; Plenum Press, 1978. 515p.	
Third	Mountney, George J. Poultry Products Technology. 2d ed. Westport, Conn.; Avi Pub. Co., 1976. 369p. (1st ed., 1966. 264p.)	
Second	Mountney, George J., and Wilbur A. Gould. Practical Food Microbiology and Technology. 3d ed. New York; Van Nostrand Reinhold, 1988. 351p. (2d ed., by Harry H. Weiser, 1971. 345p.)	Second
Second	Muller, Hans G. An Introduction to Tropical Food Science. Cambridge and New York; Cambridge University Press, 1988. 316p. (Available in Spanish: Nutrición y Ciencia de los Alimentos. Zaragoza; Acribia, 1986. 325p.)	Second
Second	Muller, Hans G., and G. Tobin. Nutrition and Food Processing. 1st American ed. London; Croom Helm; Westport, Conn.; American ed. by Avi, 1980. 302p.	Third
First	Munro, Hamish N., and J. B. Allison. Mammalian Protein Metabolism. New York; Academic Press, 1964–1970. 4 vols.	First
Third	Munro, Hamish N., and Darla E. Danford, eds. Nutrition, Aging, and the Elderly. New York; Plenum Press, 1989. 395p. (Human Nutrition: A Comprehensive Treatise, Vol. 6	Third
	Murdoch, William W. The Poverty of Nations: The Political Economy of Hunger and Population. Baltimore; Johns Hopkins University Press, 1980. 382p.	Third

N

Developed countries ranking		Third World ranking
Second	Nabors, Lyn O., and Robert C. Gelardi. Alternative Sweeteners. New York; M. Dekker, 1986. 355p.	
Third	Nagy, Steven, and John A. Attaway, eds. Citrus Nutrition and Quality; Proceedings of a Symposium . . . Division of Agricultural and Food Chemistry, 179th Meeting of the American	

Developed countries ranking		Third World ranking
	Chemical Society, Houston, March 1980. Washington, D.C.; ACS, 1980. 456p. (ACS Symposium Series no. 143)	
First	Nagy, Steven, and Philip E. Shaw. Tropical and Subtropical Fruits: Composition, Properties and Uses. Westport, Conn.; Avi, 1980. 570p.	Second
Second	Nagy, Steven, Phillip E. Shaw, and Matthew K. Veldhuis, eds. Citrus Science and Technology. Westport, Conn.; Avi, 1977. 2 vols.	Second
Second	National Canners Association. Research Laboratories. Laboratory Manual for Food Canners and Processors. 3d ed. Westport, Conn.; Avi, 1968. 2 vols. (Previous eds. published as A Laboratory Manual for the Canning Industry.)	
Second	National Research Council (U.S.). Population Growth and Economic Development: Policy Questions. Washington, D.C.; National Academy Press, 1986. 108p.	
First	National Research Council (U.S.). Recommended Dietary Allowances. 10th ed. Washington, D.C.; National Academy Press, 1989. 284p. (1st rev. ed., 1958. 36p.)	First
Second	National Research Council (U.S.). World Food and Nutrition Study; Supporting Papers . . . Washington, D.C.; National Academy of Sciences, 1977. 5 vols.	
	National Research Council (U.S.). Assembly of Life Sciences. Committee on Nutrition of the Mother and Preschool Child. Laboratory Indices of Nutritional Status in Pregnancy. Washington, D.C.; National Academy of Sciences, 1978. 195p.	Third
	National Research Council (U.S.). Board on Science and Technology for International Development. Postharvest Food Losses in Developing Countries. Washington, D.C.; National Academy of Sciences, 1978. 206p. (Text in English with summaries in French and Spanish.)	Third
Third	National Reseearch Council (U.S.). Board on Science and Technology for International Development. Applications of Biotechnology to Traditional Fermented Foods. Washington, D.C.; National Academy Press, 1992. 199p.	Third
First	National Research Council (U.S.). Committee on Codex Specifications. Food Chemicals Codex. 3d ed. Washington, D.C.; National Academy Press, 1981. 735p., and Supplement, 1983. 34p; 2d Suppl., 1986. 58p.; Third Suppl. 1992. 90p.	
First	National Research Council (U.S.). Committee on Diet and Health. Diet and Health: Implications for Reducing Chronic Disease Risk. Washington, D.C.; National Academy Press, 1989. 749p.	
First	National Research Council (U.S.). Committee on Diet, Nutrition, and Cancer. Diet, Nutrition, and Cancer. Washington, D.C.; National Academy Press, 1982. 496p.	Second

Developed countries ranking		Third World ranking
Second	National Research Council (U.S.). Committee on Food Consumption Patterns. Assessing Changing Food Consumption Patterns. Washington, D.C.; National Academy Press, 1981. 284p.	
Second	National Research Council (U.S.). Committee on Nutrition of the Mother and Preschool Child. Alternative Dietary Practices and Nutritional Abuses in Pregnancy; Proceedings of a Workshop. Washington, D.C.; National Academy Press, 1982. 211p.	
Second	National Research Council (U.S.). Committee on Nutrition of the Mother and Preschool Child. Nutrition Services in Perinatal Care. Washington, D.C.; National Academy press, 1981. 72p.	
First	National Research Council (U.S.). Coordinating Committee on Evaluation of Food Consumption Surveys. National Survey Data on Food Consumption: Uses and Recommendations. Washington, D.C.; National Academy Press, 1984. 133p.	
First	National Research Council (U.S.). Coordinating Committee on Evaluation of Food Consumption Surveys. Subcommittee on Criteria for Dietary Evaluation. Nutrient Adequacy: Assessment Using Food Consumption Surveys. Washington, D.C.; National Academy Press, 1986. 146p.	Third
Third	National Research Council (U.S.). Food Protection Committee. Food Colors. Washington, D.C.; National Academy of Sciences, 1971. 46p.	
Second	National Research Council (U.S.). Food Protection Committee of the Food and Nutrition Board. Toxicants Occurring Naturally in Foods. 2d ed. Washington, D.C.; National Academy of Sciences, 1973. 624p. (1st ed., 1966. 301p.)	Third
Third	NATO Advanced Study Institute. Post-Harvest Physiology and Crop Preservation . . . edited by Morris Lieberman. New York; Published with NATO Scientific Affairs Division by Plenum Press, 1983. 572p. (NATO Advanced Study Institutes Series. Series A, Life Sciences no. 4)	Second
Second	Nelson, Philip E., James V. Chambers, and Judy H. Rodriguez, eds. Principles of Aseptic Processing and Packaging. Washington, D.C.; Food Processors Institute, 1987. 120p.	Third
Second	Nelson, Philip E., and Donald K. Tressler, eds. Fruit and Vegetable Juice Processing Technology. 3d ed. Westport, Conn.; Avi, 1980. 603p. (1st ed., by D. K. Tressler and Maynard A. Joslyn, 1961. 1028p.)	First
	Nettleton, Joyce A. Seafood Nutrition: Facts, Issues, and Marketing of Nutrition in Fish and Shellfish. Huntington, N.Y.; Osprey Books, 1985. 280p.	Third
Third	Neuberger, A., and T. H. Jukes, eds. Biochemistry of Nutrition I. Baltimore, Md.; University Park Press, 1979. 331p.	Third
First	Neurath, Hans, and Robert L. Hill, eds. The Proteins. 3d ed. New York; Academic Press, 1975–1982. 5 vols. (1st ed., as	Second

Developed countries ranking		Third World ranking
	The Proteins; Chemistry, Biological Activity, and Methods, by H. Neurath and Kenneth Bailey, 1953–1954. 2 vols.)	
Third	Newell, Guy R. Nutrition and Cancer: Etiology and Treatment. New York; Raven Press, 1981. 445p.	
Second	Nizel, Abraham E. Nutrition in Preventive Dentistry: Science and Practice. 2d ed. Philadelphia; Saunders, 1981. 611p. (1st ed., 1972. 506p.)	
	Nobel Conference, 3rd, Saltsjobaden, Sweden, 1981. Acute Enteric Infections in Children: New Prospects for Treatment and Prevention; Proceedings . . . edited by Tord Holme et al. Amsterdam and New York; Elsevier/North-Holland Biomedical Press, 1981. 549p.	Third
Third	Nordin, B. E. C., ed. Calcium, Phosphate, and Magnesium Metabolism: Clinical Physiology and Diagnostic Procedures. Edinburgh and New York; Churchill Livingstone, 1976. 683p.	Third
Second	Novin, Donald, Wanda Wyrwicka, and George A. Bray, eds. Hunger: Basic Mechanisms and Clinical Implications. New York; Raven Press, 1976. 494p.	Second
	Nutrition Canada. Nutrition: A National Priority; A Report to the Department of National Health and Welfare. Ottawa; Information Canada, 1973. 136p.	Third
Third	Nutrition Intervention in Developing Countries: An Overview . . . prepared by the Harvard Institute for International Development, and James E. Austin and Marian F. Zeitlin. Project directors. Cambridge, Mass.; Oelgeschlager, Gunn & Hain, 1981. 227p.	Second
	O	
Second	O'Mahony, Michael. Sensory Evaluation of Food: Statistical Methods and Procedures. New York; M. Dekker, 1986. 487p.	
Second	Ockerman, Herbert W. Food Science Sourcebook. 2d ed. New York; Van Nostrand Reinhold, 1991. 2 vols. (1st ed. published as Source Book for Food Scientists. Westport, Conn.; Avi Pub. Co., 1978. 962p.)	
Second	Okos, Martin R., ed. Physical and Chemical Properties of Food. St. Joseph, Mich.; American Society of Agricultural Engineers, 1986. 407p. (ASAE Publication no. 9–86)	
Second	Olson, R. A., and K. J. Frey, eds. Nutritional Quality of Cereal Grains: Genetic and Agronomic Improvement. Madison, Wis.; American Society of Agronomy, 1987. 511p.	
First	Olson, Robert E., ed. Protein-Calorie Malnutrition; Proceedings of a Symposium . . . Faculties of Medicine of Chiang Mai and St. Louis Universities and the International Union of Nutritional Sciences, January 1973, Chiang Mai. New York; Academic Press, 1975. 467p.	Second

Developed countries ranking		Third World ranking
Third	Oomen, H. A., and G. J. Grubben. Tropical Leaf Vegetables in Human Nutrition. 2d ed. Amsterdam; Koninklijk Instituut voor de Tropen, 1978. 140p. (Connumication - Department of Agricultural Research, Koninklijk Instituut voor de Tropen no. 69) (1st ed., 1977. 133p.)	Second
Second	Ory, Robert L., and Allen J. St. Angelo, eds. Enzymes in Food and Beverage Processing; Proceedings . . . 172d Meeting of the American Chemical Society, San Francisco, August 1976. Washington, D.C.; American Chemical Society, 1977. 325p. (ACS Symposium Series no. 47)	

P

Developed countries ranking		Third World ranking
Third	Packaging Institute International. Glossary of Packaging Terms: Standard Definitions of Trade Terms Commonly Used in Packaging. 6th ed. Stamford, Conn.; PII, 1988. 287p. (2d ed., New York; 1955. 322p.)	
Third	Packard, Vernal S. Processed Foods and the Consumer: Additives, Labeling, Standards, and Nutrition. Minneapolis; University of Minnesota Press, 1976. 359p.	
Second	Padley, F. B., and J. Podmore, eds. The Role of Fats in Human Nutrition. Weinheim, Germany, and Deerfield Beech, Fla.; VCH; Chichester, England; Published for the Society of Chemical Industry, London, by Ellis Horwood, 1985. 210p.	Third
Second	Paige, David M., ed. Clinical Nutrition. 2d ed. St. Louis; Mosby, 1988. 937p. (Rev. ed. of Manual of Clinical Nutrition, 1983.)	Second
Second	Palling, S. J., ed. Developments in Food Packaging. London; Applied Science, 1980. 1 vol.	
	Pan American Health Organization. Health of Adolescents and Youths in the Americas. Washington, D.C.; PAHO, Pan American Sanitary Bureau, Regional Office of the World Health Organization, 1985. 329p. (Scientific Publication no. 489)	Third
Second	Pancoast, Harry M., and W. Ray Junk. Handbook of Sugars. 2d ed. Westport, Conn.; Avi, 1980. 598p. (1st ed., 1973, by W. R. Junk, published as Handbook of Sugars for Processors, Chemists, and Technologists. 327p.)	
Second	Pantastico, E. B., ed. Postharvest Physiology, Handling and Utilization of Tropical and Subtropical Fruits and Vegetables. Westport, Conn.; Avi, 1975. 560p.	Third
Second	Paquot, C., and A. Hautfenne, preparers. Standard Methods for the Analysis of Oils, Fats, and Derivatives; International Union of Pure and Applied Chemistry. 7th ed., rev. and enlarged. Oxford and Boston; Blackwell Scientific, 1987. 1 vol. (Earlier ed. as Standard Methods of the Oils and Fats Division of the IUPAC.)	

Developed countries ranking		Third World ranking
Second	Passmore, R. et al. Handbook on Human Nutritional Requirements. Rome; Food and Agriculture Organization, 1974. 66p. (FAO Nutritional Studies No. 28; WHO Monograph Series no. 61)	Second
	Patwardhan, Vinayak N. The State of Nutrition in the Arab Middle East. Nashville, Tenn.; Vanderbilt University Press, 1972. 308p.	Third
	Paulino, Leonardo A. Food in the Third World: Past Trends and Projections to 2000. Washington, D.C.; International Food Policy Research Institute, 1986. 76p. (IFPRI Research Report no. 52)	Third
Third	Pearson, Albert M., and Thayne R. Dutson. Meat and Poultry Microbiology. Westport, Conn.; Avi, 1986. 436p.	Third
Second	Pearson, Albert M., and F. W. Tauber. Processed Meats. 2d ed. Westport, Conn.; Avi, 1984. 427p. (1st ed., by W. E. Kramlich, A. M. Pearson and F. W. Tauber, 1973.)	Second
Second	Pearson's Composition and Analysis of Foods . . . edited by R. S. Kirk and Ronald Sawyer. 9th ed. New York; John Wiley and Sons, 1991. 708p. (1st ed., by Morris B. Jacobs, as The Chemical Analysis of Foods and Food Products. New York; Van Nostrand Co., 1938. 537p.)	
Second	Pederson, Carl S. Microbiology of Food Fermentations. 2d ed. Westport, Conn.; Avi, 1979. 384p. (1st ed., 1971. 283p.)	Second
Second	Peleg, Micha, and Edward B. Bagley, eds. Physical Properties of Foods; Papers of the IFT-IUFOST Basic Symposium, Las Vegas, Nevada, 1982. Westport, Conn.; Avi, 1983. 532p.	
Third	Pellett, Peter L., and Vernon R. Young, eds. Nutritional Evaluation of Protein Foods; Report of a Working Group sponsored by the International Union of Nutritional Sciences and the United Nations University World Hunger Programme. Tokyo; United Nations University, 1980. 154p. (Food and Nutrition Bulletin. Supplement no. 4) (WHTR-3/UNUP-129.)	Second
Second	Pelto, Gretel H., Pertti J. Pelto, and Ellen Messer, eds. Research Methods in Nutritional Anthropology. Tokyo; United Nations University, 1989. 201p. (Food and Nutrition Bulletin. Supplement no. 11)	Second
Second	Pennington, Jean A. T. Dietary Nutrient Guide. Westport, Conn.; Avi, 1976. 276p.	
Second	Peterson, Martin S., and Arnold H. Johnson. Encyclopedia of Food Science. Westport, Conn.; Avi, 1978. 1005p.	
Second	Phillips, Glyn O., David J. Wedlock, and Peter A. Williams, eds. Gums and Stabilisers for the Food Industry 2: Applications of Hydrocolloids; Proceedings of the 2d International Conference . . . Wrexham, England, July 1983. (1st ed. Oxford and New York; Pergamon Press, 1984. 569p.)	

Developed countries ranking		Third World ranking
Second	Phillips, Glyn O., David J. Wedlock, and Peter A. Williams, eds. Gums and Stabilisers for the Food Industry 3; Proceedings of the 3d International Conference . . . Wrexham, England, July 1985. London and New York; Elsevier Applied Science Publishers, 1986. 675p.	
Second	Piggott, J. R., ed. Statistical Procedures in Food Research. London and New York; Elsevier Applied Science, 1986. 415p.	
First	Pigman, Ward, and Derek Horton, eds. The Carbohydrates: Chemistry and Biochemistry. 2d ed. New York; Academic Press, 1970–1980. 4 parts in 2 vols. (1957 ed., by W. Pigman, as The Carbohydrates; Chemistry, Biochemistry, Physiology. 902p.)	
Second	Pike, Ruth L., and Myrtle L. Brown, eds. Nutrition, An Integrated Approach. 3d ed. New York; Wiley, 1984. 1068p. (1st ed., 1967. 542p.)	
Second	Pilch, Susan M., ed. Physiological Effects and Health Consequences of Dietary Fiber. Bethesda, Md.; Life Sciences Research Office, FASEB, 1987. 234p.	
Third	Pinstrup-Andersen, Per, Alan Berg, and Martin Forman, eds. International Agricultural Research and Human Nutrition; Proceedings of a Workshop sponsored by the U.N. Administrative Committee on Coordination, Subcommittee on Nutrition, held at the International Livestock Centre for Africa, Feb.-March 1984. Washington, D.C.; International Food Policy Research Institute, 1984. 326p.	Third
Second	Pinstrup-Anderson, Per, ed. Food Subsidies in Developing Countries: Costs, Benefits, and Policy Options. Baltimore; Johns Hopkins University Press for International Food Policy Research Institute, 1988. 374p.	Second
Third	Pipes, Peggy L. Nutrition in Infancy and Childhood. 4th ed. St. Louis; Times Mirror/Mosby College Pub., 1989. 425p. (1st ed., 1977. 205p.)	Third
Third	Pirie, Norman W., ed. Food Protein Sources. Cambridge and New York; Cambridge University Press, 1975. 260p.	Third
Second	Pitcher, Wayne H., ed. Immobilized Enzymes for Food Processing. Boca Raton, Fla.; CRC Press, 1980. 219p.	
	Pitt, John I., and Ailsa D. Hocking. Fungi and Food Spoilage. Sydney and Orlando; Academic Press, 1985. 413p.	Third
Second	Pollitt, Ernesto, and Peggy Amante, eds. Energy Intake and Activity. New York; Published by A. R. Liss for the United Nations University, 1984. 418p.	Third
First	Pollitt, Ernesto, and Rudolph L. Leibel, eds. Iron Deficiency, Brain Biochemistry, and Behavior. New York; Raven Press, 1982. 214p.	Second

Developed countries ranking		Third World ranking
Third	Pollock, James R. Brewing Science. London and New York; Academic Press, 1979. 2 vols.	
Second	Pomeranz, Yeshajahu. Functional Properties of Food Components. Orlando, Fla.; Academic Press, 1985. 536p.	Second
First	Pomeranz, Yeshajahu, ed. Wheat: Chemistry and Technology. 3d ed. St. Paul, Minn.; American Association of Cereal Chemists, 1988. 2 vols. (2d ed., 1971. 821p.)	First
Second	Pomeranz, Yeshajahu, and Clifton E. Meloan. Food Analysis: Theory and Practice. 2d ed. New York; Van Nostrand Reinhold, 1987. 797p. (Rev. ed. Westport, Conn.; Avi Pub. Co., 1978. 710p.)	Second
First	Potter, Norman N. Food Science. 4th ed. Westport, Conn.; Avi, 1986. 735p. (Also available in Japanese and Spanish. 1st ed., 1968. 653p.) (Available in Spanish: Ciencia de los Alimentos. México; Harla, 1978. 680p.)	Second
Second	Prasad, Ananda S., ed. Clinical, Biochemical, and Nutritional Aspects of Trace Elements. New York; A. R. Liss, 1982. 577p. (Current Topics in Nutrition and Disease no. 6)	Second
Second	Prasad, Ananda S., ed. Trace Elements in Human Health and Disease; Proceedings of an International Symposium . . . Detroit, July 1974. New York; Academic Press, 1976. 2 vols.	
Third	Prasad, Ananda S. et al., eds. Zinc Deficiency in Human Subjects; Proceedings of an International Symposium, Ankara, Turkey, April 1982. New York; A. R. Liss, 1983. 268p.	
	Prescott, Samuel C. Prescott & Dunn's Industrial Microbiology. 4th ed., edited by Gerald Reed. Westport, Conn.; Avi, 1982. 883p. (1st ed., New York and London; McGraw-Hill, 1940. 541p.)	Third
First	Price, J. F. The Science of Meat and Meat Products. 3d ed. Westport, Conn.; Food & Nutrition Press, 1987. 639p. (Previous eds. issued by the American Meat Institute Foundation.)	First
Second	Priestly, R. J., ed. Effects of Heating on Foodstuffs. London; Applied Science, 1979. 417p.	
	Pruthi, J. S. Spices and Condiments: Chemistry, Microbiology, Technology. New York; Academic Press, 1980. 449p. (Earlier ed., New Delhi; National Book Trust, India, 1976. 269p.)	Second
First	Pryde, Everett H., ed. Fatty Acids. Champaign, Ill.; American Oil Chemists' Society, 1979. 644p. (AOCS Monograph no. 7/7)	
Second	Puffer, Ruth R., and Carlos V. Serrano. Patterns of Mortality in Childhood: Report of the Inter-American Investigation of Mortality in Childhood. Washington, D.C.; Pan American Health Organization, 1973. 470p. (PAHO Scientific Publication no. 262)	Second

Developed countries ranking		Third World ranking
	Purchase, I. F. H., ed. Mycotoxins. Amsterdam and New York; Elsevier Scientific Pub. Co., 1974. 443p.	Second
	Puri, Subbhash C., and Denneth Mullen. Applied Statistics for Food and Agricultural Scientists. Boston; G. K. Hall, 1980. 311p.	Third
Second	Pyke, Magnus. Food and Society. London; Murray, 1968. 178p.	
Second	Pyke, Magnus. Food Science and Technology. 4th ed., rev. and enl. by Lelio Parducci. London; J. Murray, 1981. 304p. (1st ed., 1964. 211p.)	Second

R

Developed countries ranking		Third World ranking
Second	Radley, J. A., ed. Examination and Analysis of Starch and Starch Products. London; Applied Science, 1976. 220p.	
Third	Ramachandran, G. N., and A. H. Reddi, eds. Biochemistry of Collagen. New York; Plenum Press, 1976. 536p.	
Second	Rao, M. A., and S. S. H. Rizvi, eds. Engineering Properties of Foods. New York; M. Dekker, 1986. 398p.	
Third	Rasper, Vladimir F., ed. Cereal Polysaccharides in Technology and Nutrition; Proceedings of a Symposium held in conjunction with the Annual Meeting of the American Association of Cereal Chemists, October 1983, Kansas City, Missouri. St. Paul, Minn.; American Association of Cereal Chemists, 1984. 184p.	
Second	Rayner, Leslie. Dictionary of Foods and Food Processes (English-German-French-Spanish- Italian). England; Food Science Publishers, 1990. 290p.	Third
Third	Rechcigl, Miloslav, ed. CRC Handbook of Naturally Occurring Food Toxicants. Boca Raton, Fla.; CRC Press, 1983. 339p.	
Second	Rechcigl, Miloslav, ed. Diets, Culture Media, and Food Supplements. Cleveland, Ohio; CRC Press, 1977. 4 vols. (CRC Handbook Series in Nutrition and Food, Section G)	
Third	Rechcigl, Miloslav. Effect of Nutrient Deficiencies in Man. West Palm Beach, Fla.; CRC Press, 1978. 388p. (CRC Handbook Series in Nutrition and Food, Section E—Nutrional Disorders no. 3)	
First	Rechcigl, Miloslav, ed. Handbook of Nutritive Value of Processed Food. Boca Raton, Fla.; CRC Press, 1982. 2 vols.	First
Second	Rechcigl, Miloslav, ed. Nutrition and the World Food Problem. Basel, Switzerland; S. Karger, 1979. 374p.	Third
Second	Rechcigl, Miloslav, ed. Nutritional Requirements. Cleveland, Ohio; CRC Press, 1977. 1 vol. (CRC Handbook Series in Nutrition and Food, Section D	Third
Third	Reddy, Bandaru S., and Leonard A. Cohen, eds. Diet, Nutri-	

Developed countries ranking		Third World ranking
	tion, and Cancer: A Critical Evaluation. Boca Raton, Fla.; CRC Press, 1986. 2 vols.	
First	Reed, Gerald. Enzymes in Food Processing. 2d ed. New York; Academic Press, 1975. 573p. (1st ed., 1966. 483p.)	First
Third	Reed, Gerald, and Tilak W. Nagodawithana. Yeast Technology. 2d ed. New York; Van Nostrand Reinhold, 1991. 454p. (1st ed., by G. Reed and Henry J. Peppler, 1973. 378p.)	Second
	Reh, Emma. Manual on Househood Food Consumption Surveys. Rome; Food and Agriculture Organization, 1962. 96p. (FAO Nutritional Studies no. 18)	Third
Second	Renner, Edmund. Milk and Dairy Products in Human Nutrition . . . trans. by M. Wotzilka. 4th ed. Munich; Volkswirtschaftlicher Verlag, 1983. 450p. (Translation of Milch und Milshprodukte in der Ernahrung des Menschen, 4th ed.) (1st ed., 1974. 454p.)	Second
Second	Reutlinger, Shlomo, and Marcelo Selowski. Malnutrition and Poverty: Magnitude and Policy Options. Baltimore; Johns Hopkins University Press, 1976. 82p. (World Bank Occ. Paper no. 23)	Second
Third	Reynolds, Robert D., and James E. Leklem, eds. Vitamin B-6: Its Role in Health and Disease. Proceedings . . . Conference on Vitamin B-6 Nutrition and Metabolism, 1984, Banff, Alberta. New York; Liss, 1985. 510p.	
Third	Rha, ChoKyun, ed. Theory, Determination and Control of Physical Properties of Food Materials. Dordrecht, Holland, and Boston; Reidel Pub. Co., 1975. 415p. (Series in Food Material Science no. 1)	
Third	Richardson, Treva M. Sanitation for Foodservice Workers. 3d ed. Boston; CBI Pub. Co., 1981. 275p. (2d ed. Boston; Cahners Books, 1974. 148 p.)	
Second	Riemann, Hans, and Frank L. Bryan, eds. Food-Borne Infections and Intoxications. 2d ed. New York; Academic Press, 1979. 748p. (1st ed., 1969. 698p.)	
Third	Ritchie, Jean A. S. Nutrition and Families. London; Macmillan, 1983. 171p.	
Second	Roberts, Howard R., ed. Food Safety. New York; Wiley, 1981. 339p.	Second
Second	Roberts, T. A. Food Microbiology: Advances and Prospects. London and New York; Academic Press, 1983. 394p.	
Third	Robertson, Gordon L. Food Packaging; Principles and Practice. New York; Marcel Dekker, Inc., 1993. 676p.	
Second	Robinson, Corinne H. et al. Normal and Therapeutic Nutrition. 17th ed., rev. New York; Macmillan, 1990. 759p. (11th ed., by Fairfax T. Proudfit and C. H. Robinson, 1960. 859p.) (Avail-	Third

Developed countries ranking		Third World ranking
	able in Spanish: Fundamentos de Nutrición Normal. México; Cesa, 1979. 606p.)	
Second	Robinson, David S. Food: Biochemistry and Nutritional Value. Harlow, U.K.; Longman; New York; Wiley, 1987. 554p.	
Third	Robinson, R. K. The Vanishing Harvest: A Study of Food and Its Conservation. Oxford; Oxford University Press, 1983. 273p.	
Second	Robinson, Richard K., ed. Dairy Microbiology. 2d ed. London and New York; Elsevier Applied Science, 1990. 2 vols. (1st ed. London and Englewood, N.J.; Applied Science, 1981.) (Available in Spanish: Microbiología Lactológica. Zaragoza; Acribia, 1987. 298p.)	Third
Third	Robinson, Richard K., ed. Modern Dairy Technology. London and New York; Elsevier Applied Science Publishers, 1986. 2 vols.	Third
	Robson, John R. K. et al. Malnutrition: Its Causation and Control (With Special Reference to Protein Calorie Malnutrition). New York; Gordon & Breach, 1972. 2 vols.	Third
Second	Roche, Alexander F., and Frank Falkner, eds. Nutrition and Malnutrition; Identification and Measurement; Proceedings . . . Burg Wartenstein Conference on Physical Anthropology and Nutritional Status, Austria, 1973. New York and London; Plenum Press, 1974. 367p. (Advances in Experimental Medicine and Biology no. 49)	
First	Rockland, Louis B., George F. Stewart, and R. B. Duckworth, eds. Water Activity: Influences on Food Quality; Proceedings . . . International Symposium on Properties of Water, 2d, 1978, Osaka, Japan; sponsored by Internation Union of Food Science and Technology. New York; Academic Press, 1981. 921p.	
Second	Roe, Daphne A. Drug-Induced Nutritional Deficiencies. 2d ed. Westport, Conn.; Avi, 1985. 336p. (1st ed., 1976. 272p.)	Second
Second	Roe, Daphne A. Geriatric Nutrition. 2d ed. Englewood Cliffs, N.J.; Prentice-Hall, 1987. 267p. (1st ed., 1983. 271p.)	Second
Third	Roe, Daphne A. Handbook on Drug and Nutrient Interactions: A Problem-Oriented Reference Guide. 4th ed. Chicago; American Dietetic Association, 1989. 134p. (1st ed., 1976, by Donna C. March, as Handbook: Interactions of Selected Drugs with Nutritional Status in Man, 1976. 119p.)	
Third	Roe, Daphne A., ed. Nutrition and the Skin. New York; Liss, 1986. 199p.	
First	Roe, Daphne A. A Plague of Corn: The Social History of Pellagra. Ithaca, N.Y.; Cornell University Press, 1973. 217p.	Third
Third	Romans, John R., and P. Thomas Ziegler. The Meat We Eat. 11th ed. Danville, Ill.; Interstate Printers, 1977. 780p. (1st ed., by P. Thomas Ziegler, 1944. 377p.)	

Developed countries ranking		Third World ranking
First	Rose, A. H., ed. Fermented Foods. London and New York; Academic Press, 1982. 337p.	
Third	Rose, A. H., and J. S. Harrison, eds. The Yeasts. New York; Academic Press, 1969–1970. 3 vols.	Third
Third	Rosner, Bernard A., Fundamentals of Biostatistics. 3d ed. Boston; PWS-Kent Pub. Co., 1990. 655p. (Earlier ed., 1986. Boston; Duxbury Press, 1986. 584p.)	Third
Second	Rotberg, Robert I., and Theodore K. Rabb, eds. Hunger and History: The Impact of Changing Food Production and Consumption Patterns on Society. Cambridge and New York; Cambridge University Press, 1985. 336p. (Originally published as The Journal of Interdisciplinary History, XIV, no. 2, Autumn 1983.)	Third
	Rowe, John W. and Richard W. Besdine, eds. Geriatric Medicine. 2d ed. Boston; Little, Brown, 1988. 534p. (Rev. and updated ed. of Health and Disease in Old Age. 1st ed., 1982.)	Third
Second	Rubner, Max. A Nutrition Foundation's reprint of The Laws of Energy Consumption in Nutrition . . . trans. by Allan Markoff, Alex Sandri-White; edited by Robert J.T. Joy. New York; Academic Press, 1982. 371p. (Translation of: Die Gesetze des Energieverbrauchs bie der Ernahrung. This translation was originally published as paperbound technical report by the U.S. Army Research Institute of Environmental Medicine, 1968.)	
Third	Rush, David, Zena Stein, and Mervyn Susser. Diet in Pregnancy: A Randomized Controlled Trial of Nutritional Supplements. New York; A. R. Liss, 1980. 200p. (Birth Defects Original Article Series Vol. 16 no. 3)	Third
First	Ryall, A. Lloyd, and Werner J. Lipton. Handling, Transportation, and Storage of Fruits and Vegetables. 2d ed. Westport, Conn.; Avi, 1979. 2 vols. (1st ed., 1972.)	First

S

Developed countries ranking		Third World ranking
Second	Sahn, David E., ed. Seasonal Variability in Third World Agriculture: The Consequences for Food Security. Baltimore; Johns Hopkins University Press, 1989. 366p.	Second
Second	Sahn, David E., Richard Lockwood, and Nevin S. Scrimshaw, eds. Methods for the Evaluation of the Impact of Food and Nutrition Programmes; Report of a Workshop . . . Tokyo; United Nations University, 1984. 291p. (Food and Nutrition Bulletin. Supplement no. 8)	Second
Third	Salunkhe, D. K., J. K. Chavan, and S. S. Kadam. Postharvest Biotechnology of Cereals. Boca Raton, Fla.; CRC Press, 1985. 208p.	Third

Developed countries ranking		Third World ranking
First	Salunkhe, D. K., and B. B. Desai. Postharvest Biotechnology of Oilseeds. Boca Raton, Fla.; CRC Press, 1986. 264p.	First
Third	Salunkhe, D. K., and S. S. Kadam, eds. CRC Handbook of World Food Legumes: Nutritional Chemistry, Processing Technology, and Utilization. Boca Raton, Fla.; CRC Press, 1989. 3 vols.	Third
Second	Sanjur, Diva. Social and Cultural Perspectives in Nutrition. Englewood Cliffs, N.J.; Prentice-Hall, 1982. 336p.	
First	Sauberlich, Howerde E., J. H. Skala, and R. P. Dowdy. Laboratory Tests for the Assessment of Nutritional Status. Cleveland, Ohio; CRC Press, 1974. 136p. (Originally appeared in CRC Critical Reviews in Clinical Laboratory Sciences, v. 4, issue 3.)	Second
Second	Schneider, Howard A., Carl E. Anderson, and David B. Coursin, eds. Nutritional Support of Medical Practice. 2d ed. Hagerstown, Md.; Harper & Row, 1983. 702p. (1st ed., 1977. 555 p.)	
	Schofield, Sue. Development and the Problems of Village Nutrition. Montclair, N.J.; Allanheld, Osmun, 1979. 145p.	Third
Third	Schultz, H. W. Food Law Handbook. Westport, Conn.; Avi, 1981. 662p.	
Third	Schultz, H. W., E. A. Day, and R. O. Sinnhuber, eds. Lipids and Their Oxidation; Proceedings of the second in a series of Symposia on Foods, Oregon State University, 1961. Westport, Conn.; Avi, 1962. 442p.	
Third	Schulz, G. E., and R. H. Schirmer. Principles of Protein Structure. New York; Springer-Verlag, 1979. 314p.	
Third	Schurch, Beat, ed. Evaluation of Nutrition Education in Third World Communities; A Nestle Foundation Workshop, Lutry/Lausanne, September 1982. Bern; Hans Huber, 1983. 235p. (Nestle Foundation Publication Series no. 3)	Second
Second	Schurch, Beat, and Ann-Marie Favre, compilers. Urbanization and Nutrition in the Third World: An Annotated Bibliography. Lausanne, Switzerland; Nestle Foundation, 1985. 160p.	Second
Second	Schurch, Beat, and Nevin S. Scrimshaw, eds. Activity, Energy Expenditure and Energy Requirements of Infants and Children; Proceedings of an I/D/E/C/G Workshop, Cambridge, Mass., November 1989. Lausanne, Switzerland; I/D/E/C/G, 1990. 411p.	Second
Second	Schurch, Beat, and Nevin S. Scrimshaw, eds. Chronic Energy Deficiency: Consequences and Related Issues; Proceedings . . . International Dietary Energy Consultancy Group, Scientific Meeting, 1987, Guatemala City. Lausanne, Switzerland; The Group, 1988. 201p.	Second
Third	Schuster, Gregor, and W. F. Adams, eds. Emulgatoren fur	

Developed countries ranking		Third World ranking
	Lebensmittel (Emulsions for Foodstuff). Berlin and New York; Springer, 1985. 474p. (In German.)	
First	Schwimmer, Sigmund. Source Book of Food Enzymology. Westport, Conn.; Avi, 1981. 967p.	First
Second	Scott, R. Cheesemaking Practice. 2d ed. London and New York; Elsevier Applied Science Publishers, 1986. 529p. (1st ed., 1981. 475p.)	
Second	Scrimshaw, Nevin S., and Aaron M. Altschul, eds. Amino Acid Fortification of Protein Foods; Report of an International Conference, Massachusetts Institute of Technology, September 1969. Cambridge Mass.; MIT Press, 1971. 664p.	Second
	Scrimshaw, Nevin S., and Moises Behar, eds. Nutrition and Agricultural Development: Significance and Potential for the Tropics; Proceedings of the 14th International Biological Symposium, Guatemala City, Guatemala, December 1974, Held in celebration of the 25th Anniversary of the Institute of Nutrition of Central America and Panama. New York; Plenum Press, 1976. 500p.	Second
	Scrimshaw, Nevin S., and John E. Gordon, eds. Malnutrition, Learning, and Behavior; Proceedings of an International Conference . . . Massachusetts Institute of Technology, 1967. Cambridge Mass.; MIT Press, 1968. 566p.	Second
First	Scrimshaw, Nevin S., Carl E. Taylor, and John E. Gordon. Interactions of Nutrition and Infection. Geneva; World Health Organization, 1968. 329p. (WHO Monograph Series no. 57)	First
First	Scrimshaw, Nevin S., and Mitchel B. Wallerstein, eds. Nutrition Policy Implementation: Issues and Experience. New York; Plenum Press, 1982. 558p. (Sponsored by the United Nations University.)	First
Second	Scrimshaw, Susan, and Elena Hurtado. Rapid Assessment Procedures for Nutrition and Primary Health Care: Anthropological Approaches to Improving Programme Effectiveness. Tokyo; United Nations University; Los Angeles; UCLA Latin American Center Pub., 1987. 70p.	Second
First	Scriver, Charles R. et al., eds. The Metabolic Basis of Inherited Disease. 6th ed. New York; McGraw-Hill, 1989. 2 vols. (1st ed., 1960, edited by John B. Stanbury, James B. Wyngaarden and Donald S. Fredrickson. 1477p.)	First
First	Sebrell, W. H., and Robert S. Harris, eds. The Vitamins; Chemistry, Physiology, Pathology, Methods. 2d ed. New York; Academic Press, 1967. 7 vols. (Vols. 1–5 edited by W. H. Sebrell and R. S. Harris; v. 6–7 edited by P. Gyorgy and W. N. Pearson. Vols. 6–7 are rev. ed. of Vitamin Methods, by P. Gyorgy, 1950–51.)	First
Second	Seib, Paul A., and Bert M. Tolbert, eds. Ascorbic Acid: Chem-	

Developed countries ranking		Third World ranking
	istry, Metabolism, and Uses; Proceedings of the 2d Chemical Congress of the North American Continent (180th ACS National Meeting), Las Vegas, Nevada, August 1980. Washington, D.C.; American Chemical Society, 1982. 604p.	
Second	Sen, Amartya. Poverty and Famines: An Essay on Entitlement and Deprivation. Oxford; Clarendon Press, New York; Oxford University Press, 1981. 257p.	
	Shack, Kathryn W., ed. Teaching Nutrition in Developing Countries: Or, The Joys of Eating Dark Green Leaves; Report from an International Workshop . . . Santa Barbara, Calif., June 1977. Santa Monica, Calif.; Meals for Millions Foundation, 1977. 193p.	Third
Second	Shallenberger, R. S. Advanced Sugar Chemistry: Principles of Sugar Stereochemistry. Westport, Conn.; Avi, 1982. 323p.	
Second	Shallenberger, R. S., and G. G. Birch. Sugar Chemistry. Westport, Conn.; Avi, 1975. 221p.	
First	Shils, Maurice E., James A. Olson, and Moshe Shike, eds. Modern Nutrition in Health and Disease. 8th ed. Philadelphia; Lea & Febiger, 1994. 2 vols. (Early eds., edited by Michael G. Wohl and Robert S. Goodhart, as Modern Nutrition in Health and Disease; Dietotherapy.)	First
Third	Sikorski, Zdzisaw E., ed. Seafood: Resources, Nutritional Composition, and Preservation. Boca Raton, Fla.; CRC Press, 1990. 248p.	
Second	Simatos, D., and J. L. Multon, eds. Properties of Water in Foods: In Relation to Quality and Stability; Proceedings . . . NATO Advanced Research Workshop on Influence of Water on Food Quality and Stability, 1983, Beaune, France. Dordrecht and Boston; M. Nijhoff; Higham, Mass; Distributors for the U.S. and Canada Kluwer Boston, 1985. 693p. (NATO ASI Series E, Applied Sciences no. 90)	
First	Simic, Michael G., and Marcus Karel, eds. Autoxidation in Food and Biological Systems; Proceedings of a Workshop on Autoxidation Processes, U.S. Army Natick Research and Development Command, Natick, Mass., Oct. 1979. New York; Plenum Press, 1980. 659p.	
Second	Simoons, Frederick J. Eat Not This Flesh; Food Avoidances in the Old World. Madison Wis.; University of Wisconsin Press, 1961. 241p.	
Third	Simopoulos, Artemis P., and Barton Childs, eds. Genetic Variation and Nutrition; Proceedings of the 1st International Conference . . . Washington, D.C., June 1989. Basel, Switzerland and New York; Karger, 1990. 300p.	Third
Third	Sinclair, H. M., and G. R. Howat, eds. World Nutrition and Nutrition Education. Oxford and New York; Oxford University Press, 1980. 226p.	Third

Developed countries ranking		Third World ranking
Second	Singh, R. Paul, and Dennis R. Heldman. Introduction to Food Engineering. Orlando, Fla.; Academic Press, 1984. 306p.	Third
Third	Singleton, Vernon L., and Paul Esau. Phenolic Substances in Grapes and Wine, and Their Significance. New York; Academic Press, 1969. 282p.	
Second	Sivetz, Michael, and Norman W. Desrosier. Coffee Technology. Westport, Conn.; Avi, 1979. 716p. (1963 ed. published as Coffee Processing Technology.)	
Third	Skinner, F. A., and J. G. Carr, eds. Microbiology in Agriculture, Fisheries, and Food. London and New York; Academic Press, 1976. 274p. (Society for Applied Bacteriology, Symposium Series no. 4)	
Second	Small, Donald M. et al. The Physical Chemistry of Lipids: From Alkanes to Phospholipids. New York; Plenum Press, 1986. 672p. (Handbook of Lipid Research no. 4)	
	Smith, Allan K. and Sidney J. Circle, ed. Soybeans: Chemistry and Technology. Rev. 2d printing. Westport, Conn.; Avi, 1978. 1 vol. (1st ed., 1972.)	Second
Second	Smith, Kenneth T., ed. Trace Minerals in Foods. New York; M. Dekker, 1988. 470p.	
Third	Smith, Philip M. The Chemotaxonomy of Plants. London; E. Arnold, 1976. 313p.	
First	Snedecor, George W., and William G. Cochran. Statistical Methods. 8th ed. Ames; Iowa State University Press, 1989. 503p. (Early eds. published as Statistical Methods Applied to Experiments in Agriculture and Biology.)	Second
First	Solms, J., D. A. Booth, R. M. Pangborn, and O. Raunhardt, eds. Food Acceptance and Nutrition. London, etc.; Academic Press, 1987. 490p.	
Third	Solms, J., and R. L. Hall, eds. Criteria of Food Acceptance: How Man Chooses What He Eats; Papers from a Symposium, Einsiedeln, Switzerland, October 1979, sponsored by the International Union of Food Science and Technology et al. Zurich; Forster, 1981. 461p.	
Third	Solomons, Noel W., and Irwin H. Rosenberg. Absorption and Malabsorption of Mineral Nutrients. New York; Liss, 1984. 314p.	
First	Sommer, Alfred. Field Guide to the Detection and Control of Xerophthalmia. 2d ed. Geneva; World Health Organization, 1982. 58p. (1st ed., 1978. 47p.)	First
First	Sommer, Alfred. Nutritional Blindness: Xerophthalmia and Keratomalacia. New York; Oxford University Press, 1982. 282p.	First
Third	Somogyi, J. C., ed. Nutritional Deficiencies in Industrialized Countries; Proceedings of the 17th Symposium of the Group of European Nutritionists, Santiago de Compostela, Oct. 1979.	

Developed countries ranking		Third World ranking
	Basel, Switzerland, etc.; S. Karger, 1981. 172p. (Bibliotheca Nutritio et Dieta no. 30)	
Third	Somogyi, J. C., and D. Hotzel, eds. Nutrition and Neurobiology; Proceedings of the 23d Symposium of the Group of European Nutritionists . . . Bonn, May 1985. Basel and New York; Karger, 1986. 224p. (Bibliotheca Nutritio et Dieta no. 38)	
Third	Somogyi, J. C., and H. R. Muller, eds. Nutritional Impact of Food Processing; Proceedings . . . 25th Symposium of the Group of European Nutritionists, Reykjavik, September 1987. Basel, Switzerland and New York; Karger, 1989. 346p.	Third
Second	Southgate, D. A. T. Determination of Food Carbohydrates. London; Applied Science Publishers, 1976. 178p.	
First	Southgate, D. A. T., J. C. Somogyi, and E. M. Widdowson. Guide Lines for the Preparation of Tables of Food Composition. Basel, Switzerland and New York; S. Karger, 1974. 57p.	Second
First	Spiller, Gene A., and Ronald J. Amen, eds. Fiber in Human Nutrition. New York; Plenum Press, 1976. 278p.	First
Second	Spiller, Gene A., and Ruth M. Kay. Medical Aspects of Dietary Fiber. New York; Plenum Medical Book Co., 1980. 299p.	
First	Sporn, Michael B., Anita B. Roberts, and DeWitt S. Goodman, eds. The Retinoids. Orlando, Fla.; Academic Press, 1984. 2 vols.	
First	Stadelman, William J., and Owen J. Cotterill, eds. Egg Science and Technology. 3d ed. Westport, Conn.; Avi, 1986. 449p. (1st ed., 1973. 314p.)	
First	Stanbury, John B., and Basil S. Hetzel. Endemic Goiter and Endemic Cretinism: Iodine Nutrition in Health and Disease. New York; Wiley, 1980. 606p. (Updates the 1960 ed., by F. W. Clements et al., published as Endemic Goitre.)	First
Third	Stanbury, Peter F., and Allan Whitaker. Principles of Fermentation Technology. 1st ed. Oxford and New York; Pergamon Press, 1984. 255p.	Second
Second	Stanley, David W., E. Donald Murray, and David H. Lees, ed. Utilization of Protein Resources. Westport, Conn.; Food & Nutrition Press, 1981. 403p.	Third
Second	Stansby, Maurice E., ed. Fish Oils; Their Chemistry, Technology, Stability, Nutritional Properties, and Uses. Westport, Conn.; Avi, 1967. 440p.	Third
Second	Stare, Fredrick J., and Margaret McWilliams. Living Nutrition. 4th ed. New York; Wiley, 1984. 640p. (1st ed., 1973. 467p.)	
Second	Stedman, Thomas L. Medical Dictionary. 25th ed. Baltimore; Williams & Wilkins, 1990. 1784p. (First published, 1911, as A Practical Medical Dictionary.)	Second
Third	Steinkraus, Keith H., ed. Industrialization of Indigenous Fermented Foods. New York; M. Dekker, 1989. 439p.	Third
Second	Steinkraus, Keith H. et al., eds. Handbook of Indigenous Fer-	Second

Developed countries ranking		Third World ranking
	mented Foods; Based on papers submitted to a Symposium Workshop . . . Bangkok, November, 1977. New York; M. Dekker, 1983. 671p.	
Second	Stephenson, Lani S. Impact of Helminth Infections on Human Nutrition: Schistosomes and Soil-Transmitted Helminths. London and New York; Taylor & Francis, 1987. 233p.	Second
Second	Stephenson, Lani S., ed. Schistosomiasis and Malnutrition. Ithaca, N.Y.; Cornell University, Program in International Nutrition, 1986. 192p. (Cornell International Nutrition Monograph Series no. 16)	Second
Third	Stephenson, Lani S., Michael C. Latham, and Ad Jansen. A Comparison of Growth Standards: Similarities Between NCHS, Harvard, Denver, and Privileged African Children and Differences with Kenyan Rural Children . . . edited by Michael C. Latham. Ithaca, N.Y.; Cornell University, Program in International Nutrition, 1983. 109p. (Cornell International Nutrition Monograph Series no. 12)	Second
First	Stewart, George F., and Maynard A. Amerine. Introduction to Food Science and Technology. 2d ed. New York; Academic Press, 1982. 289p. (1st ed., 1973. 294p.)	Second
Second	Stewart, Kent K., and John R. Whitaker, eds. Modern Methods of Food Analysis; Proceedings of a Symposium sponsored jointly by the Institute of Food Technologists and International Union of Food Science and Technology, New Orleans, June 1983. Westport, Conn.; Avi, 1984. 421p.	
	Stinnet, J. Dwight. Nutrition and the Immune Response. Boca Raton, Fla.; CRC Press, 1983. 150p.	Third
Second	Stone, Herbert, and Joel L. Sidel. Sensory Evaluation Practices. Orlando, Fla.; Academic Press, 1985. 311p.	
	Strickland, G. Thomas, ed. Hunter's Tropical Medicine. 7th ed. Philadelphia; W. B. Saunders, 1991. 1056p. (1st ed., 1945, by Thomas T. Mackie; 3d-5th eds. by George W. Hunter.)	Third
Second	Strohecker, Rolf, and Heinz M. Henning. Vitamin Assay; Tested Methods . . . trans. by D. D. Libman. Weinheim Bergstr.; Verlag Chemie, 1965. 360p. (Translation of: Vitamin-Bestimmungen.)	
Third	Stumbo, C. R. et al. CRC Handbook of Lethality Guides for Low-Acid Canned Foods. Boca Raton, Fla.; CRC Press, 1983. 2 vols.	
Second	Stunkard, Albert J., ed. Obesity. Philadelphia; Saunders, 1980. 470p.	
Third	Stunkard, Albert J., and Eliot Stellar, eds. Eating and Its Disorders. New York; Raven Press, 1984. 280p. (Research Publications, Association for Research in Nervous and Mental Disease no. 62)	
Second	Suskind, Robert M., ed. Malnutrition and the Immune Re-	Third

Developed countries ranking		Third World ranking
	sponse; Proceedings of a Conference sponsored by the Subcommittee on Nutrition and Infection of the National Academy of Sciences, the Malnutrition Panel of the U.S.-Japan Cooperative Medical Science Program, and the Kroc Foundation. New York; Raven Press, 1977. 468p. (Kroc Foundation Series no. 7)	
	Suskind, Robert M. Textbook of Pediatric Nutrition. New York; Raven Press, 1981. 662p.	Third
Third	Suskind, Robert M., and Leslie Lewinter-Suskind, eds. The Malnourished Child. New York; Raven Press, 1990. 416p. (Nestle Nutrition Workshop Series no. 19)	Third
Second	Suttie, John W., ed. Current Advances in Vitamin K Research; Proceedings of the 17th Steenbock Symposium, University of Wisconsin-Madison, June 1987. New York; Elsevier, 1988. 530p.	
Second	Suzuki, Taneko. Fish and Krill Protein: Processing Technology. London; Applied Science, 1981. 260p. (Available in Spanish: Technología de las Proteínas de Pescado y Krill. Zaragoza; Acribia, 1987. 24–*0p.)	Third
First	Szuhaj, Bernard F., and Gary R. List. Lecithins. Champaign, Ill.; American Oil Chemists' Society, 1985. 393p.	

T

Developed countries ranking		Third World ranking
Second	Talburt, William F., and Ora Smith, eds. Potato Processing. 4th ed. New York; Van Nostrand Reinhold, 1987. 796p. (1st ed., Westport, Conn.; Avi, 1959. 475p.)	
Second	Tannahill, Reay. Food in History. 2d ed. Penguin Books, 1991. 448p. (1s ed., New York; Stein & Day, 1973.)	Third
First	Tannenbaum, Steven R., ed. Nutritional and Safety Aspects of Food Processing. New York; M. Dekker, 1979. 448p.	
Second	Tanner, J. M., ed. Control of Growth. New York; Published for the British Council by Churchill Livingstone, 1981. 304p.	
Second	Tanner, W., and F. A. Loewus, eds. Plant Carbohydrates: Intracellular Carbohydrates. Berlin and New York; Springer-Verlag, 1981–1982. 2 vols. (Encyclopedia of Plant Physiology, New Ser. no. 13A-B)	Third
	Tartakow, I. Jackson, and John H. Vorperian. Foodborne and Waterborne Diseases: Their Epidemiologic Characteristics. Westport, Conn.; Avi, 1981. 300p.	Third
Second	Taylor, R. J. Food Additives. Chichester, England and New York; J. Wiley, 1980. 126p.	
Third	Teranishi, Roy, ed. Agricultural and Food Chemistry: Past, Present, Future; Papers presented at the Agricultural and Food Division sessions of the American Chemical Society's Centennial Meeting, New York, April 1976. Westport, Conn.; Avi, 1978. 458p.	

Developed countries ranking		Third World ranking
First	Teranishi, Roy, Robert A. Flath, and Hiroshi Sugisawa, eds. Flavor Research, Recent Advances. New York; M. Dekker, 1981. 381p. (Expanded and updated version of Flavor Research: Principles and Techniques.)	
First	Thorne, Stuart, ed. Developments in Food Preservation. London and Englewood, N.J.; Applied Science Publishers, 1981–1983. 4 vols.	Third
Second	Timmer, C. Peter, Walter P. Falcon, and Scott R. Pearson. Food Policy Analysis. Baltimore; Published for the World Bank by the Johns Hopkins University Press, 1983. 301p.	Second
Second	Ting, S. V., and Russell L. Rouseff. Citrus Fruits and Their Products: Analysis Technology. New York; M. Dekker, 1986. 293p.	
Second	Toledo, Romeo T. Fundamentals of Food Process Engineering. 2d ed. New York; Van Nostrand Reinhold, 1991. 602p. (1st ed., Westport, Conn.; Avi Pub. Co., 1980. 409p.)	Second
Second	Tomkins, Andrew, and Fiona Watson. Malnutrition and Infection: A Review . . . with discussions by N. S. Scrimshaw. London; Clinical Nutrition Unit, Centre for Human Nutrition, London School of Hygiene and Tropical Medicine, 1989. 136p. (Nutrition Policy Discussion Paper no. 5) (At head of title: United Nations, Administrative Committee on Coordination/Subcommittee on Nutrition)	Third
	Torrey, Barbara B., Kevin Kinsella, and Cynthia M. Taeuber. An Aging World. Washington, D.C.; U.S. Dept. of Commerce, Bureau of the Census, 1987. 85p. (International Population Reports. Series P-95 no. 78)	Third
Second	Torun, Benjamin, Vernon R. Young, and William M. Rand, eds. Protein-Energy Requirements of Developing Countries: Evaluation of New Data; Report of a Working Group, Sponsored by the International Union of Nutritional Sciences and the United Nations University World Hunger Programme. Tokyo; United Nations University, 1981. 268p. (Food and Nutrition Bulletin. Supplement no. 5)	First
Second	Tressler, Donald K. et al. The Freezing Preservation of Foods. 4th ed. Westport, Conn.; Avi, 1968. 4 vols. (First ed., 1936, as The Freezing Preservation of Fruits, Fruit Juices, and Vegetables.)	
Third	Trickett, Jill. The Prevention of Food Poisoning. 2d ed. Cheltenham; Thornes, 1986. 136p. (1st ed., 1978. 114p.)	Second
Third	Troller, John A. Sanitation in Food Processing. New York; Academic Press, 1983. 456p.	
Second	Troller, John A., and J. H. B. Christian. Water Activity and Food. New York; Academic Press, 1978. 235p.	
Second	Trowell, Hubert C. Non-Infective Disease in Africa; The Pecu-	Third

Developed countries ranking		Third World ranking
	liarities of Medical Non-Infective Diseases in the Indigenous Inhabitants of Africa South of the Sahara. London; E. Arnold, 1960. 481p.	
Second	Trowell, Hubert C., and D. P. Burkitt, eds. Western Diseases, Their Emergence and Prevention. Cambridge, Mass.; Harvard University Press, 1981. 456p.	Third
First	Trowell, Hubert C., Denis Burkitt, and Kenneth Heaton, eds. Dietary Fibre, Fibre-Depleted Foods and Disease. London and Orlando, Fla.; Academic Press, 1985. 433p.	First
Second	Trowell, Hubert C., J. N. P. Davies, and R. F. A. Dean. Kwashiorkor. London; E. Arnold, 1954. 308p.	Third
Third	Truswell, A. Stewart. ABC of Nutrition. 2d ed. London; British Medical Association, 1992. 104p. (1st ed., 1986. 93p.)	Third
	Tsang, Reginald C., and Buford L. Nichols. Nutrition During Infancy. Philadelphia and St. Louis; Hanley & Belfus Mosby, 1988. 440p.	Second
Second	Turner, Michael R., ed. Nutrition and Health: A Perspective: The Current Status of Research on Diet-Related Diseases; Proceedings of the British Nutrition Foundation 3d Annual Conference, Royal College of Physicians, London, June 1981. New York; A. R. Liss, 1982. 261p.	
Third	Turner, Michael R., ed. Preventive Nutrition and Society; Proceedings . . . 2d Annual Conference held at the Royal Society, July, 1980. London and New York; Academic Press, 1981. 228p.	
	U	
	Ukoli, F. M. A. Introduction to Parasitology in Tropical Africa. Chichester and New York; Wiley, 1984. 464p.	Third
Second	Underwood, Barbara A., ed. Nutrition Intervention Strategies in National Development. New York; Academic Press, 1983. 419p.	Second
First	Underwood, Eric J. Trace Elements in Human and Animal Nutrition. 4th ed. New York; Academic Press, 1977. 430p. (1st ed., 1956.) (Available in Spanish: Minerales en la Nutrición del Ganado. Zaragoza; Acribia, 1983. 222p.)	First
Second	United Nations. Administrative Committee on Coordination, Subcommittee on Nutrition. Update on the Nutrition Situation: Recent Trends in Nutrition in 33 Countries. Geneva, Switzerland; UN ACC/SCN, 1989. 193p. (Updates and extends information published in the ACC/SCN's First Report on the World Nutrition Situation, November 1987.)	Third
	United Nations Childrens Fund. Current Views on Nutrition Strategies: Report of an Informal Consultation in UNICEF Headquarters, New York, Sept. 1982. New York; UNICEF, 1983. 40p.	Third

Developed countries ranking		Third World ranking
Third	Urbain, Walter M. Food Irradiation. Orlando, Fla.; Academic Press, 1986. 351p.	
	U.S. Dept. of Agriculture. Composition of Foods: Raw, Processed, Prepared. Rev. ed. Washington D.C.; Agricultural Research Service, USDA, 1976. 12pts. (USDA Agricultural Handbook no. 8–1 to 8–12) (Pts. 3–7 published by Science and Education Administration, U.S. Dept. of Agriculture. Pt. 8– published by U.S. Dept. of Agriculture, Human Nutrition Information Service. A revision of the 1963 ed. by Bernice K. Watt. 189p.)	First
First	U.S. Dept. of Agriculture. Composition of Foods: Beef Products; Raw, Processed, Prepared . . . by Barbara A. Anderson and I. Margaret Hoke. Rev. ed. Washington, D.C.; USDA, Human Nutrition Information Service, 1990. 412p. (USDA Agricultural Handbook no. 8–13) (Continuation of earlier series ed., 1976, pts. 8–1 to 8–12.)	First
	U.S. Dept. of Agriculture. Composition of Foods: Beverages; Raw, Processed, Prepared . . . by Rena Cutrufelli and Ruth H. Matthews. Rev. ed. Washington, D.C.; USDA, Human Nutrition Information Service, 1986. 173p. (USDA Agriculture Handbook no. 8–14) (Continuation of earlier series ed., 1976, pts. 8–1 to 8–12.)	Second
	U.S. Dept. of Agriculture. Composition of Foods: Cereal Grains and Pasta; Raw, Processed, Prepared . . . by Dennis L. Drake, Susan E. Gebhardt, and Ruth H. Matthews. Washington, D.C.; USDA, Human Nutrition Information Service, 1989. 1 vol. (USDA Agriculture Handbook no. 8–20) (Continuation of earlier series ed., 1976, pts. 8–1 to 8–12.)	Second
First	U.S. Dept. of Agriculture. Composition of Foods: Fast Foods; Raw, Processed, Prepared . . . by Lynn E. Dickey and John L. Weihrauch. Rev. ed. Washington, D.C.; USDA, Human Nutrition Information Service, 1988. 12 pts. (USDA Agriculture Handbook no. 8–21) (Continuation of earlier series ed., 1976, pts. 8–1 to 8–12.)	
	U.S. Dept. of Agriculture. Composition of Foods: Finfish and Shellfish Products; Raw, Processed, Prepared . . . by Jacob Exler. Rev. ed. Washington, D.C.; USDA, Human Nutrition Information Service, 1987. 1 vol. (USDA Agriculture Handbook no. 8–15) (Continuation of earlier series ed., 1976, pts. 8–1 to 8–12.)	Second
	U.S. Dept. of Agriculture. Composition of Foods: Lamb, Veal, and Game Products; Raw, Processed, Prepared . . . by Barbara A. Anderson et al. Washington, D.C.; USDA, Human Nutrition Information Service, 1989. 251p. (USDA Agriculture Handbook no. 8–17) (Continuation of earlier series ed., 1976, pts. 8–1 to 8–12.)	Second

Developed countries ranking		Third World ranking
Third	U.S. Dept. of Agriculture. Composition of Foods: Legumes and Legume Products; Raw, Processed, Prepared . . . by David B. Haytowitz and Ruth H. Matthews. Washington, D.C.; ULDA, Human Nutrition Information Service, 1986. 156p. (USDA Agriculture Handbook no. 8–16) (Continuation of earlier series ed., 1976, pts. 8–1 to 8–12.)	Second
Second	U.S. Dept. of Health and Human Services. Diet and Iron Status, A Study of Relationships, United States, 1971–1974. Corr. ed. Hyattsville, Md.; U.S. Dept. of Health and Human Services, Public Health Service, National Center for Health Statistics, 1983. 83p. (Vital and Health Statistics. Series 11, Data from the National Health Survey No. 229; DHHS Publication no. 82–1679)	
Second	U.S. House of Representatives. Select Committee on Hunger and the National Commission to Prevent Infant Mortality. Infant Mortality within Minority and Rural Communities: A Global Perspective on Causes and Solutions: A Symposium. Washington, D.C.; U.S. Govt. Printing Office, 1991. 70p. (At head of title: 101st Congress, 2d Session, Committee Print.)	
Second	U.S. Senate. Select Committee on Nutrition and Human Needs. Dietary Goals for the United States. 2d ed. Washington, D.C.; U.S. Govt. Print. Off., 1977. 83p. (Reprinted: Cambridge, Mass.; M.I.T. Press, as Eating in America.)	Third
Second	U.S. Surgeon General. The Surgeon General's Report on Nutrition and Health, 1988. Washington, D.C.; U.S. Dept. of Health and Human Services, Public Health Service; Supt. of Docs., U.S. G.P.O., 1988. 727p. (DHHS, PHS Publication no. 88–50210)	Third
	V	
First	Vahouny, George V., and David Kritchevsky, eds. Dietary Fiber in Health and Disease. New York; Plenum Press, 1982. 330p.	
First	Vahouny, George V., and David Kritchevsky, eds. Dietary Fiber: Basic and Clinical Aspects; Proceedings of the 2d Washington Symposium on Dietary Fiber, April 1984, Washington, D.C. New York; Plenum Press, 1986. 566p.	First
Second	Van Arsdel, Wallace B., Michael J. Copley, and Arthur I. Morgan, eds. Food Dehydration. 2d ed. Westport, Conn.; Avi, 1973. 2 vols. (1st ed., 1963.)	Second
Second	Van Beynum, G. M. A., and J. A. Roels, eds. Starch Conversion Technology. New York; M. Dekker, 1985. 362p.	
Second	Van Straten, S., ed. Volatile Compounds in Food. 4th ed. Zeist, Netherlands; Central Institute for Nutrition and Food Research, 1977. 200p. (1st ed., 1963.)	

Developed countries ranking		Third World ranking
Third	Van Toller, S. Aging and the Sense of Smell. Springfield, Ill.; Thomas, 1985. 170p.	
Second	Vaughan, John G., ed. Food Microscopy. London and New York; Academic Press, 1979. 651p.	Second
Third	Velazquez, Antonio, and Hector Bourges, eds. Genetic Factors in Nutrition; Proceedings of an International Workshop . . . Teotihuacan, Mexico, August 1982. Orlando, Fla.; Academic Press, 1984. 441p.	Third
First	Vergroesen, A. J., and M. A. Crawford. The Role of Fats in Human Nutrition. 2d ed. London and San Diego; Academic Press, 1989. 580p. (1st ed., 1975. 494p.)	Second
	Ville de Goyet, C. de, J. Seaman, and U. Geijer. The Management of Nutritional Emergencies in Large Populations. Geneva; World Health Organization, 1978. 98p.	Third
Third	Vine, Richard P. Commercial Winemaking, Processing and Controls. Westport, Conn.; Avi, 1981. 493p.	
Second	Von Loesecke, Harry W. Bananas: Chemistry, Physiology, Technology. 2d rev. ed. New York; Interscience Publishers, 1950. 189p. (1st ed., 1949. 189p.)	Second
	W	
Second	Walford, John, ed. Developments in Food Colours. London; Applied Science, 1980. 1 vol.	
	Walker-Smith, J. A., and A. S. McNeish, eds. Diarrhoea and Malnutrition in Childhood; Proceedings of a Conference held at the Royal Commonwealth Society and St. Bartholomew's Hospital, London, November 1984. London and Boston; Butterworths, 1986. 249p. (Available in Spanish: Enfermedades del Intestino Delgado en la Infancia. Barcelona; Salvat. 272p.)	Third
Third	Wall, Joseph S., and William M. Ross, eds. Sorghum Production and Utilization: Major Feed and Food Crops in Agriculture and Food Series. Westport, Conn.; Avi, 1970. 702p.	
First	Waller, George R., and Milton S. Feather, eds. The Maillard Reaction in Foods and Nutrition; Based on a Symposium jointly sponsored by the Divisions of Agricultural and Food Chemistry, and Carbohydrate Chemistry at the 183d Meeting of the American Chemical Society, Las Vegas, Nevada, March-April 1982. Washington, D.C.; American Chemical Society, 1983. 585p. (ACS Symposium Series, x 0097–6157 no. 215)	
First	Walstra, Pieter, and Robert Jenness. Dairy Chemistry and Physics. New York; Wiley, 1984. 467p. (Available in Spanish: Química y Física Lactológica. Zaragoza; Acribia, 1986. 417p.)	
Second	Waterlow, John C., ed. Linear Growth Retardation in Less Developed Countries . . . Based on papers presented at the 14th Nestle Nutrition Workshop, Cha-am, Thailand, March 1986.	Second

Developed countries ranking		Third World ranking
	Vevey, Switzerland; Nestle Nutrition; New York; Raven Press, 1988. 295p.	
Third	Waterlow, John C., ed. Nutrition of Man. London; Published for the British Council by Churchill Livingstone, 1981. 104p.	
Second	Waterlow, John C., P. J. Garlick, and D. J. Millward. Protein Turnover in Mammalian Tissues and in the Whole Body. Amsterdam and New York; North-Holland Pub. Co., 1978. 804p.	Third
Second	Waterlow, John C., and J. M. L. Stephen, eds. Nitrogen Metabolism in Man; Proceedings of an International Symposium organized by the Rank Prize Funds, Kingston, Jamaica, November 1980. London and Englewood, N.J.; Applied Science Publishers, 1981. 558p.	
Third	Watson, Ronald R., ed. CRC Handbook of Nutrition in the Aged. Boca Raton, Fla.; CRC Press, 1985. 355p.	Third
Third	Watson, Ronald R., ed. Nutrition, Disease Resistance, and Immune Function. New York; M. Dekker, 1984. 404p. (Clinical and Experimental Nutrition no. 1)	Third
Second	Watson, Stanley A., and Paul E. Ramstad, eds. Corn: Chemistry and Technology. St. Paul, Minn.; American Association of Cereal Chemists, 1987. 605p.	
Third	Webb, Tony, and Tim Lang. Food Irradiation: The Facts. Wellingborough, Northamptonshire, U.K. and Rochester, Vt.; Thorsons, 1987. 144p.	
First	Wedzicha, B. L. Chemistry of Sulphur Dioxide in Foods. London and New York; Elsevier Applied Science, 1984. 381p.	
Second	Weichmann, J., ed. Postharvest Physiology of Vegetables. New York; M. Dekker, 1987. 597p.	Second
Second	Weinsier, Roland L., Douglas C. Heimburger, and Charles E. Butterworth. Handbook of Clinical Nutrition: Clinician's Manual for the Prevention, Diagnosis, and Management of Nutritional Problems. 2d ed. St. Louis; Mosby, 1989. 427p. (1st ed., by R. L. Weinsier and C. E. Butterworth, 1981. 231p.)	Third
First	Weiss, Theodore J. Food Oils and Their Uses. 2d ed. Westport, Conn.; Avi, 1983. 310p. (1st ed., 1970. 224p.)	First
Third	West, Bessie B., and LeVelle Wood. Foodservice in Institutions. 6th ed., rev. by Virginia F. Harger, Grace S. Shugart and June Payne-Palacio. New York; Macmillan; London; Collier Macmillan, 1988. 662p. (2d ed., New York; Wiley, 1945. 599p.)	
First	Whistler, Roy L., and James N. BeMiller, eds. Industrial Gums, Polysaccharides and Their Derivatives. 2d ed. New York; Academic Press, 1973. 807p. (1st ed., 1959. 766p.)	
First	Whistler, Roy L., James N. BeMiller, and Eugene F. Paschall, eds. Starch: Chemistry and Technology. 2d ed. Orlando, Fla.;	

Developed countries ranking		Third World ranking
	Academic Press, 1984. 718p. (1st ed., New York; Academic Press, 1965. 2 vols.)	
First	Whistler, Roy L. et al., eds. Methods in Carbohydrate Chemistry. New York; Academic Press, 1962–1983. 8 vols.	Second
Second	Whitaker, Andrew M. Tissue and Cell Culture. Baltimore; Williams & Wilkins, 1972. 119p.	
First	Whitaker, John R. Principles of Enzymology for the Food Sciences. New York; M. Dekker, 1972. 636p.	First
Third	Whitaker, John R., and Masao Fujimaki, eds. Chemical Deterioration of Proteins; Proceedings of a Symposium sponsored by the Division of Agricultural and Food Chemistry, ACS/CSJ Chemical Congress, Honolulu, April 1979. Washington, D.C.; American Chemical Society, 1980. 268p. (ACS Symposium Series no. 123)	
First	Whitaker, John R., and Steven R. Tannenbaum, eds. Food Proteins; Papers from a Symposium sponsored by the Institute of Food Technologists and the International Union of Food Science and Technology. Westport, Conn.; Avi, 1977. 603p.	
Third	White, Abraham et al. Principles of Biochemistry. 6th ed. New York; McGraw-Hill, 1978. 1492p. (1st ed., by Albert P. Mathews. Baltimore; W. Wood, 1936. 512p.)	Third
Third	White, Philip L., and Stephanie C. Crocco, eds. Sodium and Potassium in Foods and Drugs; Proceedings of a Conference . . . 1st ed. Chicago; American Medical Association, 1982. 78p.	
Third	White, Philip L., and Dean C. Fletcher, eds. Nutrients in Processed Foods. Acton, Mass.; Publishing Sciences Group, 1974. 3 vols. (Compilation of papers, discussions and recommendations from a series of Symposia, March 1971–October 1973.)	
	Whitehead, Roger G., ed. Maternal Diet, Breast-Feeding Capacity and Lactational Infertility: Report of a Joint UNU/WHO Workshop held in Cambridge, March 1981. Tokyo; United Nations University, 1983. 107p. (Food and Nutrition Bulletin. Supplement no. 6)	Third
Second	Whitney, Eleanor N., Eva May N. Hamilton, and Sharon R. Rolfes. Understanding Nutrition. 5th ed. St. Paul, Minn.; West Pub., 1990. 603p. (1st ed., 1977. 607p.)	
Third	Wilcke, Harold L., Daniel T. Hopkins, and Doyle H. Waggle, eds. Soy Protein and Human Nutrition: Proceedings of the Keystone Conference . . . Keystone, Colo., May 1978. New York; Academic Press, 1979. 406p.	Third
Second	Williams, A. A., and R. K. Atkin, eds. Sensory Quality in Foods and Beverages: Definition, Measurement and Control; Proceedings of an International Symposium . . . University of	

Developed countries ranking		Third World ranking
	Bristol, April 1982. Chichester, West Sussex, U.K.; E. Horwood; Deerfield Beach, Fla.; Verlag Chemie International, distributor, 1983. 488p. (Published for the Society of Chemical Industry, London.)	
Third	Williams, Melvin H. Nutritional Aspects of Human Physical and Athletic Performance. 2d ed. Springfield, Ill.; Thomas, 1985. 565p. (1st ed., 1976. 444p.)	
Third	Williams, Phil, and Karl Norris, eds. Near-Infrared Technology in the Agricultural and Food Industries. St. Paul, Minn.; American Association of Cereal Chemists, 1987. 330p.	
Second	Wilson, N. R. P. et al., eds. Meat and Meat Products: Factors Affecting Quality Control. London and Englewood, N.J.; Applied Science, 1981. 207p. (Available in Spanish: Carne y Productos Càrnicos. Zaragoza; Acribia, 1987. 250p.)	
Second	Winick, Myron, ed. Hunger Disease: Studies by the Jewish Physicians in the Warsaw Ghetto . . . trans. from the Polish by Martha Osnos. New York; Wiley, 1979. 261p. (Translation of Choroba Godowa.)	
Third	Winick, Myron. Malnutrition and Brain Development. New York; Oxford University Press, 1976. 169p.	Second
Third	Winikoff, Beverly, ed. Nutrition and National Policy. Cambridge, Mass.; MIT Press, 1978. 580p.	
Second	Winikoff, Beverly, Mary Ann Castle, and Virginia H. Laukaran, eds. Feeding Infants in Four Societies: Causes and Consequences of Mothers' Choices. New York; Greenwood Press, 1988. 255p.	Third
	Winkelmann, Fritz. Imitation Milk and Imitation Milk Products (Milk-Like Products) . . . Rome; Food and Agriculture Organization, 1974. 117p.	Third
Second	Wintrobe's Clinical Hematology, by G. Richard Lee 9th ed. Philadelphia; Lea & Febiger, 1991. (1st ed., by Maxwell M. Wintrobe, 1942. 703p.)	Second
Second	Wiseman, Alan, ed. Handbook of Enzyme Biotechnology. 2d ed. Chichester; E. Horwood; Chichester, England and New York; Halsted Press, 1985. 457p. (1st ed., 1975. 275p.) (Available in Spanish: Principios de Biotecnología. Zaragoza; Acribia, 1985. 256p.)	
Second	Wolf, Walter J., and J. C. Cowan. Soybeans as a Food Source. Rev. ed. Cleveland, Ohio; CRC Press, 1977. 101p.	Second
Second	Wolff, Ivan A., ed. CRC Handbook of Processing and Utilization in Agriculture. Boca Raton, Fla.; CRC Press, 1982–1983. 2 vols.	Second
Second	Wong, D. W. S. Mechanism and Theory in Food Chemistry. New York; Van Nostrand Reinhold, 1989. 428p.	Third

Developed countries ranking		Third World ranking
First	Wong, Noble P. et al., eds. Fundamentals of Dairy Chemistry. 3d ed. New York; Van Nostrand Reinhold Co., 1988. 779p. (1st ed., edited by Byron H. Webb and Arnold H. Johnson, Westport, Conn.; Avi Pub. Co., 1965. 827p.)	Second
Third	Wood, Brian J. B., ed. Microbiology of Fermented Foods. London and New York; Elsevier Applied Science, 1985. 2 vols.	
Third	Wood, George A. R., and R. A. Lass. Cocoa. 4th ed. London and New York; Longman, 1985. 620p. (1st ed., by D. H. Urquhart, 1955. 230p.) (Available in Spanish: Cacao. México; Cecsa, 1983. 368p.)	
Third	Woodroof, Jasper G., ed. Peanuts: Production, Processing, Products. 3d ed. Westport, Conn.; Avi, 1983. 414p. (1st ed., 1966. 291p.)	
Third	Woodroof, Jasper G., and Bor Shium Luh, eds. Commercial Fruit Processing. 2d ed. Westport, Conn.; Avi, 1986. 678p. (1st ed., 1975. 710p.)	
Third	Woodroof, Jasper G., and G. Frank Phillips. Beverages—Carbonated and Noncarbonated. Rev. ed. Westport, Conn.; Avi, 1981. 526p. (Earlier ed., 1974.)	
Second	World Bank. Child and Maternal Health Services in Rural India: The Narangwal Experiment. Baltimore; Published for the World Bank by Johns Hopkins University Press, 1983. 2 vols.	Third
Second	World Bank. Poverty and Hunger: Issues and Options for Food Security in Developing Countries. Washington, D.C.; World Bank, 1986. 69p.	First
Second	World Health Organization. Diet, Nutrition, and the Prevention of Chronic Diseases; Report of a WHO Study Group. Geneva; WHO, 1990. 203p. (WHO Technical Report Series no. 797)	Third
Second	World Health Organization. Fluorides and Human Health. Geneva; WHO, 1970. 364p. (WHO Monograph Series no. 59)	
Third	World Health Organization. Food Irradiation: A Technique for Preserving and Improving the Safety of Food. Geneva; WHO, 1988. 84p.	
	World Health Organization. A Growth Chart for International Use in Maternal and Child Health Care: Guidelines for Primary Health Care Personnel. Geneva; World Health Organization, 1978. 36p.	Second
	World Health Organization. International Standards for Drinking-Water. 3d ed. Geneva; WHO, 1971. 70p. (2d ed., 1963. 206p.)	Second
Second	World Health Organization. Measuring Change in Nutritional Status: Guidelines for Assessing the Nutritional Impact of Supplementary Feeding Programmes for Vulnerable Groups. Geneva; World Health Organization, 1983. 101p.	First

Developed countries ranking		Third World ranking
	World Health Organization. Milk Hygiene; Hygiene in Milk Production, Processing, and Distribution. Geneva; Published under the auspices of the Food and Agriculture Organization and WHO, 1962. 782p. (WHO Monograph Series no. 48)	Third
	World Health Organization. The Quantity and Quality of Breast Milk: Report on the WHO Collaborative Study on Breast-Feeding. Geneva; World Health Organization; Albany, N.Y.; Available from WHO Publications Centre USA, 1985. 148p.	Second
	World Health Organization. The Treatment and Prevention of Acute Diarrhoea: Practical Guidelines. 2d ed. Geneva; WHO, 1989. 49p. (1st ed. entitled: Treatment and Prevention of Acute Diarrhoea: Guidelines for the Trainers of Health Workers. 1985. 35p.)	Second
Second	World Health Organization. Expert Committee on Medical Assessment of Nutritional Status. Report. Geneva; WHO, 1963. 67p. (WHO Technical Report Series no. 258)	Third
Third	World Health Organization. Expert Committee on Trace Elements in Human Nutrition. Trace Elements in Human Nutrition; Report of a WHO Expert Committee. Geneva; WHO, 1973. 65p. (WHO Technical Report Series no. 532)	Second
	Wurtman, Richard J., and Judith J. Wurtman, eds. Control of Feeding Behavior and Biology of the Brain in Protein-Calorie Malnutrition. New York; Raven Press, 1977. 313p.	Third
Third	Wurtman, Richard J., and Judith J. Wurtman, eds. Food Constituents Affecting Normal and Abnormal Behaviors. New York; Raven Press, 1986. 253p. (Nutrition and the Brain no. 7)	Third
First	Wurtman, Richard J., and Judith J. Wurtman, eds. Nutrition and the Brain. New York; Raven Press, 1977–1986. 8 vols.	
Second	Wurzburg, O. B. Modified Starches: Properties and Uses. Boca Raton, Fla.; CRC Press, 1986. 277p.	
	X	
	Xanthou, Marietta, ed. New Aspects of Nutrition in Pregnancy, Infancy, and Prematurity; Proceedings of the International Workshop on the Composition and Physiological Properties of Human Milk, Athens, October 1986. Amsterdam and New York; Elsevier Science Publishers, 1987. 207p.	Third
	Y	
Third	Yamazaki, W. T., and C. T. Greenwood, eds. Soft Wheat: Production, Breeding, Milling, and Uses. St. Paul, Minn.; American Association of Cereal Chemists, 1981. 307p. (AACC Monographs Series no. 6)	
Second	Young, Raymond A., and Roger M. Rowell, eds. Cellulose: Structure, Modification, and Hydrolysis. New York; Wiley, 1986. 379p.	

Developed countries ranking		Third World ranking
Second	Yudkin, John, ed. Diet of Man, Needs and Wants; International Symposium organized by the Rank Prize Funds, Bath, Avon, England, April 1977. London; Applied Science Publishers, 1978. 358p.	
	Z	
Second	Zapsalis, Charles, and R. Anderle Beck. Food Chemistry and Nutritional Biochemistry. New York; Wiley, 1985. 1219p.	Second
Third	Zeitlin, Marian F., Hossein Ghassemi, and Mohamed Mansour. Positive Deviance in Child Nutrition: With Emphasis on Psychosocial and Behavioural Aspects and Implications for Development. Tokyo; United Nationas University, 1990. 153p. (Food and Nutrition Bulletin, Supplement no. 14)	Third
First	Zeuthen, P., ed. Thermal Processing and Quality of Foods. London and New York; Elsevier Applied Science, 1984. 933p.	
Third	Zuckerman, Solly. Food Quality and Safety: A Century of Progress; Proceedings of the Symposium Celebrating the Centenary of the Sale of Food and Drugs Act 1875, London, October 1975. London; H.M.S.O., 1976. 243p.	

E. The Nature of the Core Monographs

Commercial presses made a strong showing in the list of core monographs. All but two of the top ten are the same publishers identified in the literature analysis (Table 4.5). This demonstrates a remarkable concentration of primary publishing in this discipline.

Table 4.5. Commercial publishers comparison

Title in core lists	Rank	Monograph publishers cited in analysis
Academic	1	Academic
AVI	2	AVI
Elsevier	3	Wiley
M. Dekker	4	Plenum
Plenum	5	M. Dekker
CRC	6	Applied Science Publ.
Wiley	7	Elsevier
Applied Science Publ.	8	CRC
Raven	9	Raven
Van Nostrand Reinhold	10	Pergamon

The names of first, second, and third authors or editors of the core monographs were compiled. The most cited author or editor was Gordon G. Birch, listed thirteen times, all but once as an editor. He is followed by Nevin S. Scrimshaw, cited twelve times, five of them as first author. Governmental institutions most cited as author or compiler, but not as publisher, were the National Research Council of the United States National Academy of Sciences, with sixteen monographs; the World Health Organization, with eleven documents; the Food and Agricultural Organization, with eight (WHO and the FAO also have nine documents that they have authored jointly); and the United States Department of Agriculture, with seven.

Table 4.6 provides some detailed characteristics on the monographs in

Table 4.6. Characteristics of core monographs

	Core monograph list N=1,011	Comparison with citation analysis data (see Table 4.2) N=11,739
Types of publishers		
Commercial presses	73.1%	60.7%
Governments (incl. FAO & UN)	12.0	19.9
Independent organizations & societies	7.5	12.5
Universities (presses, depts., institutes)	7.4	7.8
Place of publication		
United States	63.3%	68.4%
United Kingdom	22.9	14.6
Switzerland	4.4	3.5
Netherlands	2.8	3.4
Italy	2.2	1.2
Germany	1.7	3.0
Non-English publications	.1%	.3
Non-English publications with translations into English	1.3%	
Median year of publication	1983.0	1977.4
Primary Publishers		
Academic	11.8%	11.4%
AVI	7.0	5.0
Elsevier	4.7	3.3
M. Dekker	4.6	2.5
Plenum	3.4	3.1
U. S. Government	3.2	8.8

the core list. The place of publication (the first city or country listed in the imprint of the publication) is of limited significance with the commercial press titles because of the internationalization of so many publishing houses.

F. The Top-Ranked Monographs

The following two lists of top-ranked core monographs include the top twenty-one titles in the developed countries and the top nineteen in the Third World. They are provided here for insights into the closeness and diversity of the two communities in food science and human nutrition.

Developed Countries Top Food Science and Human Nutrition Monographs

1 National Research Council (U.S.). *Recommended Dietary Allowances.* 10th ed. Washington, D.C.; National Academy Press, 1989. 284p. (1st rev. ed., 1958. 36p.)

2 Association of Official Analytical Chemists. *Official Methods of Analysis . . .* 15th ed. Washington, D.C.; Association of Official Analytical Chemists, 1990. n.p. (1st ed., 1919. 1st-10th ed. published under Association of Official Agricultural Chemists, the earlier name of the association.)

3 Shils, Maurice E., James A. Olson, and Moshe Shike, eds. *Modern Nutrition in Health and Disease.* 8th ed. Philadelphia; Lea & Febiger, 1994. 2 vols. (Early eds., edited by Michael G. Wohl and Robert S. Goodhart, as *Modern Nutrition in Health and Disease; Dietotherapy.*)

4 Joint FAO/WHO/UNU Expert Consultation. *Energy and Protein Requirements II: Report . . . Geneva*; World Health Organization, 1985. 206p. (*WHO Technical Report Series* no. 724) (Earlier ed., 1973. 118p.)

5 Furia, Thomas E., ed. *CRC Handbook of Food Additives.* 2d ed. Cleveland; CRC Press, 1972–1981. 2 vols. (Vol. 2 published in Boca Raton, Fla.; 1st ed., 1968. 771p.)

6–7 Brown, Myrtle L., ed. *Present Knowledge in Nutrition.* 6th ed. Washington, D.C.; International Life Sciences Institute-Nutrition Foundation, 1990. 532p. (Rev. ed. of *Nutrition Reviews' Present Knowledge in Nutrition.* 1st ed., 1953. 1984 ed., edited by M. A. Eastwood.)

Fennema, Owen R., ed. *Food Chemistry.* 2d ed., rev. and expanded. New York; M. Dekker, 1985. 991p. (1st ed., 1976. 792p.)

8 Augustin, Jorg, Barbara P. Klein, Deborah Becker, and Paul B. Venugopal, eds. *Methods of Vitamin Assay, for the Association of Vitamin Chemists.* 4th ed. New York; Wiley, 1985. 590p. (1st ed., New York and London; Interscience Publishers, 1947. 189p.)

9 Pomeranz, Yeshajahu, ed. *Wheat: Chemistry and Technology.* 3d ed. St. Paul,

Minn.; American Association of Cereal Chemists, 1988. 2 vols. (2d ed., 1971. 821p.)

10–11 Karmas, Endel, and Robert S. Harris, eds. *Nutritional Evaluation of Food Processing*. 3d ed. New York; Van Nostrand Reinhold, 1988. 786p. (1st ed., edited by R. S. Harris and Harry von Loesecke; New York; Wiley, 1960. 612p.)

Munro, Hamish N., and J. B. Allison. *Mammalian Protein Metabolism*. New York; Academic Press, 1964–1970. 4 vols.

12 Scriver, Charles R., John B. Stanbury, James B. Wyngaarden, and Donald S. Fredrickson, eds. *The Metabolic Basis of Inherited Disease*. 6th ed. New York; McGraw-Hill, 1989. 2 vols. (1st ed., 1960, edited by John B. Stanbury, James B. Wyngaarden, and Donald S. Fredrickson. 1477p.)

13 Wong, Noble P., et al., eds. *Fundamentals of Dairy Chemistry*. 3d ed. New York; Van Nostrand Reinhold Co., 1988. 779p. (1st ed., edited by Byron H. Webb and Arnold H. Johnson, Westport, Conn.; Avi Pub. Co., 1965. 827p.)

14 Sommer, Alfred. *Nutritional Blindness: Xerophthalmia and Keratomalacia*. New York; Oxford University Press, 1982. 282p.

15–18 Becher, Paul, ed. *Encyclopedia of Emulsion Technology*. New York; M. Dekker, 1983. 3 vols.

Maarse, Henk, ed. *Volative Compounds in Foods and Beverages*. 1st ed. New York; M. Dekker, 1991. 764p.

Stanbury, John B., and Basil S. Hetzel. *Endemic Goiter and Endemic Cretinism: Iodine Nutrition in Health and Disease*. New York; Wiley, 1980. 606p. (Updates the 1960 ed., by F. W. Clements et al., published as *Endemic Goiter*.)

Zeuthen, P., ed. *Thermal Processing and Quality of Foods*. London and New York; Elsevier Applied Science, 1984. 933p.

19 McCance, R. A. and E. M. Widdowson. *McCance and Widdowson's The Composition of Foods*. 5th ed., rev. and extended, by B. Holland et al. London; Royal Society of Chemistry and Ministry of Agriculture, Fisheries and Food, 1991. 462p. (1st suppl., by A. A. Paul; 2d suppl., by S. P. Tan; listed separately.)

Third World Top Food Science and Human Nutrition Monographs

1 National Research Council (U.S.). *Recommended Dietary Allowances*. 10th ed. Washington, D.C.; National Academy Press, 1989. 284p. (1st rev. ed., 1958. 36p.)

2 Shils, Maurice E., James A. Olson, and Moshe Shike, eds. *Modern Nutrition in Health and Disease*. 8th ed. Philadelphia; Lea & Febiger, 1994. 2 vols. (Early eds., edited by Michael G. Wohl and Robert S. Goodhart, as *Modern Nutrition in Health and Disease; Dietotherapy*.)

3 Brown, Myrtle L., ed. *Present Knowledge in Nutrition*. 6th ed. Washington, D.C.; International Life Sciences Institute-Nutrition Foundation, 1990. 532p. (Rev. ed. of *Nutrition Reviews' Present Knowledge in Nutrition*. 1st ed., 1953. 1984 ed., edited by M. A. Eastwood.)

4 Fennema, Owen R., ed. *Food Chemistry*. 2d ed., rev. and expanded. New York; M. Dekker, 1985. 991p. (1st ed., 1976. 792p.)

5–6 Bailey, Alton E., and Daniel Swern, eds. *Bailey's Industrial Oil and Fat Products . . .* by Marvin W. Formo et al. 4th ed. New York; Wiley, 1979. 3 vols. (1st ed., by A. E. Bailey, New York; Interscience Publishers, 1945. 735p.)

Hetzel, Basil S., John T. Dunn, and John B. Stanbury, eds. *The Prevention and Control of Iodine Deficiency Disorders*; Based on the Inaugural Meeting of the ICCIDD, Kathmandu, Nepal, Narch 1986. Amsterdam and New York; Elsevier, 1987. 354p. (*Major Health Issues* no. 2)

7 U.S. Dept. of Agriculture. *Composition of Foods: Raw, Processed, Prepared.* Rev. ed. Washington, D.C.; Agricultural Research Service, USDA, 1976. 12 pts. (*USDA Agriculture Handbook* no. 8–1 to 8–12) (Pts. 3–7 published by Science and Education Administration, U.S. Dept. of Agriculture. Pt. 8– published by U.S. Dept. of Agriculture, Human Nutrition Information Service. A revision of the 1963 ed. by Bernice K. Watt. 189p.)

8–10 Liener, Irvin E., ed. *Toxic Constituents of Animal Foodstuffs*. New York; Academic Press, 1974. 222p.

McLaren, Donald S., ed. *Nutrition in the Community: A Critical Look at Nutrition Policy, Planning, and Programmes*. 2d ed. Chichester and New York; Wiley, 1983. 472p. (1st ed., Wiley, 1976. 393p.)

Rechcigl, Miloslav, ed. *Handbook of Nutritive Value of Processed Food*. Boca Raton, Fla.; CRC Press, 1982. 2 vols.

11 Stanbury, John B., and Basil S. Hetzel. *Endemic Goiter and Endemic Cretinism: Iodine Nutrition in Health and Disease*. New York; Wiley, 1980. 606p. (Updates the 1960 ed. published as *Endemic Goiter*.)

12–13 Association of Official Analytical Chemists. *Official Methods of Analysis . . . 15th ed.* Washington, D.C.; Association of Official Analytical Chemists, 1990. n.p. (1st ed., 1919. 1st-10th ed. published under Association of Official Agricultural Chemists, the earlier name of the association.)

Vahouny, George V., and David Kritchevsky, eds. *Dietary Fiber in Health and Disease*. New York; Plenum Press, 1982. 330p.

14 Berg, Alan, N. S. Scrimshaw, and D. L. Call, eds. *Nutrition, National Development, and Planning*; Proceedings of a National Confernece. Cambridge, Mass.; MIT Press, 1973. 401p.

15–18 Augustin, Jorg, Barbara P. Klein, Deborah Becker, and Paul B. Venugopal, eds. *Methods of Vitamin Assay, for the Association of Vitamin Chemists*. 4th ed. New York; Wiley, 1985. 590p. (1st ed., New York and London; Interscience Publishers, 1947. 189p.)

Austin, James E., and Marian F. Zetlin. *Nutrition Intervention in Developing Countries: An Overview*; Prepared by the Harvard Institute for International Development. Cambridge, Mass.; Oelgeschlager, Gunn & Hain, 1981. 227p.

Pomeranz, Yeshajahu, ed. *Wheat: Chemistry and Technology*. 3d ed. St. Paul, Minn.; American Association of Cereal Chemists, 1988. 2 vols. (2d ed., 1971. 821p.)

Sebrell, W. H., and Robert S. Harris, eds. *The Vitamins: Chemistry, Physiology, Pathology, Methods*. 2d ed. New York; Academic Press, 1967. 7 vols. (Vols. 1–5 edited by W. H. Sebrell and R. S. Harris; v. 6–7 edited by P. Gyorgy and W. N. Pearson. Vols. 6–7 are rev. ed. of *Vitamin Methods*, by P. Gyorgy, 1950–51.)

19 Alleyne, G. A. O. et al. *Protein-Energy Malnutrition*. London; E. Arnold, 1977. 244p.

20–21 Aykroyd, Wallace R., Joyce Doughty, and Ann Walker. *Legumes in Human Nutrition*. Rev. ed. Rome; Food and Agriculture Organization, 1982. 152p. (*FAO Food and Nutrition Paper* no. 20) (1964 ed., by W. R. Aykroyd and Joyce Doughty. 138p.)

Scrimshaw, Nevin S., Carl E. Taylor, and John E. Gordon. *Interactions of Nutrition and Infection*. Geneva; World Health Organization, 1968. 329p. (*WHO Monograph Series* no. 57)

Eight titles appear in both lists, with two of these eight in the top three. This is evidence of a remarkable unanimity of opinion, considering that these rankings come from two distinct groups which neither saw each other's list nor had any interchange or discussion.

The top title for both lists was the U.S. National Research Council's *Recommended Dietary Allowances*, now in its tenth edition. The titles that appear uniquely in the Third World list relate to nutrition. Food scientists and human nutritionists seem to believe strongly in new editions, since fourteen of the top nineteen titles in the developed countries list are multiple or revised editions, as are thirteen of the twenty-one in the Third World list. This is highly understandable, since revised editions incorporate new knowledge from expanding research on food composition and nutrients. Multiple authorship or editorship seems standard, since only eight titles bear a single author or editor. As might be expected, most of the titles revolve around food composition and nutritive values.

Commercial firms published over half of these top-ranked titles: eleven in the developed countries list and twelve in the Third World list. Associations and societies are well represented with five and three titles respectively.

5. Primary Journals and Serials

JENNIE BROGDON
Rockville, Maryland

WALLACE C. OLSEN
Mann Library, Cornell University

Evaluative studies conducted during the past twenty years concerned with the journal literature of food science and human nutrition are not common. Information on the relationship of journals and monographs is provided in Chapters 3 and 4. Most studies are either mainly listings of monograph and journal titles or are examinations of very specific subjects within the field. There are three recent listings of value, however.[1]

A few qualitative studies that rank titles for their importance to food science or human nutrition have been published in the past twenty years. One study ranked the top sixty-two food science and technology journals obtained by a citation analysis of three journals published in 1980; it included information on half-life, Bradford scattering, and other data.[2] Another article identified the nineteen most significant journals for nutrition research from an analysis of data in the 1986 *Science Citation Index* (SCI).[3] This article also included information on language, country of publication, impact factor, and journal half-life for each of the nineteen journals. An earlier study ranked thirty-eight human nutrition titles obtained by a citation analysis of two United States titles published in 1970.[4] Other data such as

1. (a) Syd Green, *Keyguide to Information Sources in Food Science and Technology* (London: Mansell, 1985). (b) Kathy L. Fair and Carolyn Havens, "Nutrition Journals," *The Serials Librarian* 20 (212) (1989): 89–105. (c) Renee Bush, "An Annotated Bibliography of Journals in Nutrition," *Serials Review* 4 (1988): 35–55.

2. B. S. Maheswarappa and K. Surya Rao, "Journal Literature of Food Science and Technology: A Bibliometric Study," *Annals of Library Science and Documentation* 29 (3) (1982): 126–134.

3. Eugene Garfield, "Journal Citation Studies, 49: The Diverse Yet Essential Nutrients in the Information Diet of Nutrition Researchers," in *Science Literacy, Policy, Evaluation, and Other Essays* (Philadelphia: ISI Press, 1990), p. 451. Originally published as "Current Comments," *Current Contents* 28 (July 11, 1988).

4. Helen Grybowski, "Human Nutrition," in T. D. Wilson and Esther Herman, eds., *Fundamentals of Documentation: Students' Papers* (College Park, Md.: School of Library and Information Services, University of Maryland, 1973), pp. 138–156.

language, form of publication, type of publisher, and Bradford multiplier were also included.

A. Source Documents and Methodology

The fifty monographs used as source documents for the citation analysis for monographs (compare Chapter 4) also provided data on journals, periodicals, serials, and report series. The same methods, definitions, and caveats apply to the journal and serial data as outlined for monographs in Chapter 4. All journals, annuals, and selected serials cited in the source documents were recorded and tabulated by title and date of publication. Each time an article within a journal or serial was cited, a count was made for the journal or serial title. A total of 61,875 citations were analyzed in this way of which 47,000 were to journals.

Proceedings volumes listed as journals or serials require clarification. Of the numerous proceedings identified, approximately 85% were tallied and evaluated as monographs because they had distinctive titles, short term or non-continuous editors, or concentrated on a specialized aspect or area of food science or human nutrition. Proceedings volumes were counted as journals or serials when they represented the continuing deliberations of an organization or a society, with no varying subject focus or title other than *Proceedings* or *Transactions*. An example is the *Proceedings of the Nutrition Society*, which runs consistently under the same title each year and includes technical papers on a variety of subjects, as well as happenings at annual meetings and societal operations.

The nearly 47,000 citations to journals obtained in the citation analysis provided statistically valid data on the most valuable titles for the academic community working in food science and human nutrition. When choosing the documents to be analyzed, careful consideration was given to the teaching and research needs of this community. This study thus varies from many citation studies by accommodating college instructional needs.

Data from the citation analysis has been correlated with other data where valid and insightful, and a final list of recommended titles is provided.

B. Journal Results

Table 4.1 (Chapter 4) indicates that 75.6% of the references in the analyzed documents were to journal articles. This is similar to that reported for all of agriculture, and for four other disciplines analyzed in the Core

Agricultural Literature Project (pages 51,55). Indeed, a similar percentage is found in most fields of contemporary science, where a representation of journal literature under 75% would be unusual.

Analysis included calculations of the citing half-life of the journal articles. As noted in Chapter 4, the half-life is the median age of fifty percent of all citations, calculated from the year that the source document was published. This is a measure of how long publications remain relevant and provides a relative guide to the currency of the literature. The half-life for all the journal articles analyzed in the source documents was 9.7 years, whereas those articles concentrating on food science had a half-life of 11.01 years. This is substantially longer than the half-life of 7 years reported by B. S. Maheswarappa and K. Surya Rao in their study of food science and technology journals.[5] It also indicates that the food science literature has a slower turnover than the human nutrition literature which had a half-life of 7.0 years. Eugene Garfield reported in 1988 a citing half-life of 7.6 years from nutrition citations in journals.[6] These variations derive from the differing nature of the literature used in the core citation analysis. In this study, unlike others, the literature was not restricted to journal source documents only.

There were 1,337 different journal or serial titles identified in the 46,760 article citations. The number of titles is substantially greater than in most of the agricultural subjects analyzed to date, and is the result of the diversity of the two subject areas and the low overlap rate between them. The large number of journals may also have been affected, less significantly, by the large quantity of citations analyzed. Of the 1,337 titles 775 or 57.7% were cited four times or fewer. Only 3.7% of all titles accounted for 45.4% of the citations (Table 5.1). The remaining 25,519 citations were scattered in

Table 5.1. Citations to top ranked journal titles

Journal titles (N=1,337)			Citations (N=46,760)	
Number of titles	% of all Titles		% of all journal citations	Number
Top 10	0.8	=	26.3	12,282
Top 20	1.5	=	34.5	16,116
Top 30	2.2	=	38.1	17,826
Top 40	3.0	=	42.1	19,694
Top 50	3.7	=	45.4	21,241

5. Maheswarappa, "Journal Literature."
6. Garfield, "Journal Citation Studies, 49."

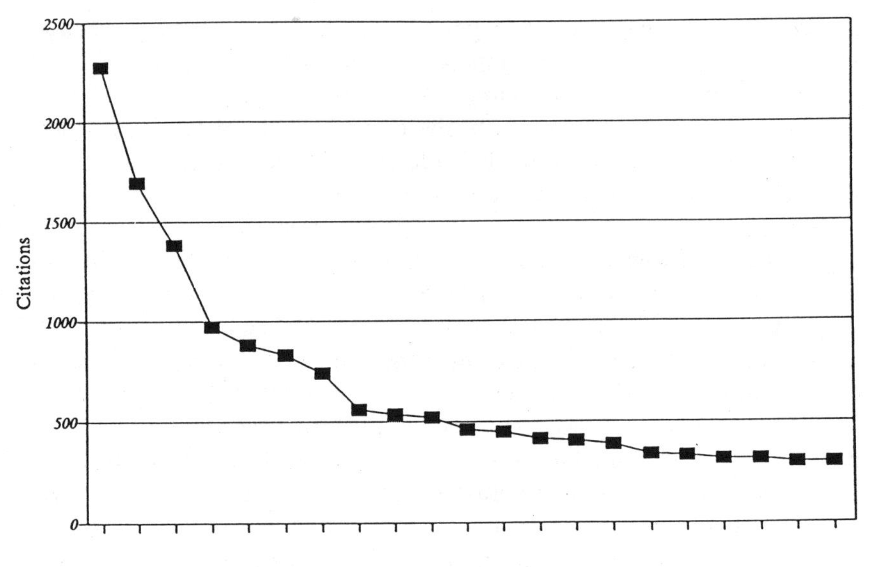

Figure 5.1. Influence of top 21 titles.

the remaining 1,287 titles. Figure 5.1 demonstrates the influence of the top twenty-one titles as well as the standard pattern in a Bradford scattering.[7] The top sixty-one journals in the Core Project citation analysis are listed and ranked in Table 5.2. The same journals are also ranked using citation data from the *Science Citation Index's, Journal Citation Reports.*[8] These sixty-one journals account for 50% of all journal citations in the analysis. They include titles relevant both to developed countries and to the Third World. A Third World concern is particularly evident in the human nutrition area, where titles related to tropical nutrition appear.

The journals fall into three broad subject categories based on where the majority of a title's articles fit best:

Strongly nutrition	25 titles
Food science and technology	22
Equally divided	14

7. (a) S. C. Bradford, "Sources of Information on Specific Subjects," *Engineering* 137 (1934): 85–86. (b) S. C. Bradford, "Sources of Information on Specific Subject Charts," *Journal of Information Science* 10 (4) (1985): 176–180.

8. Data were taken from *Journal Citation Reports*, issued annually from data gathered for the *Science Citation Index.*

Table 5.2. Major Core Project analysis journal rankings, and *Science Citation Index* rankings

		Science Citation Index[a]	
	Core citation analysis	Rank based on average number of citations	Impact factor
American Journal of Clinical Nutrition	1	28	25
Journal of Food Science	2	38	49
JAOCS; Journal of the American Oil Chemists' Society	3	44	52
Food Technology (Chicago)	4	49	48
Archives of Disease in Childhood	5	37	34
Lancet	6	7	2
Journal of Agricultural and Food Chemistry	7	35	35
Journal of Nutrition	8	32	31
Journal of Biological Chemistry	9	1	8
New England Journal of Medicine	10	8	1
Science	11	5	4
Journal of the Science of Food and Agriculture	12	45	51
Applied and Environmental Microbiology	13	33	28
Nature	14	2	3
British Medical Journal	15	13	18
Journal of Chromatography	16	21	33
Journal of Clinical Investigation	17	9	7
Federation Proceedings	18	22	61
Journal of the American Dietetic Association	19	51	53
Journal of the American Chemical Society	20	4	11
Journal of Food Protection	21	51	47
Biochemical Journal	22	10	14
Biochimica et Biophysica Acta	23	6	23
American Journal of Physiology	24	11	16
British Journal of Nutrition	25	41	32
Journal of Pediatrics	26	24	21
JAMA; Journal of the American Medical Association	27	15	13
Journal of the Association of Official Analytical Chemists	28	42	41
Proceedings of the National Academy of Sciences (U.S.A.)	29	3	5
Cereal Chemistry	30	47	45
Agricultural and Biological Chemistry	31	39	46
Gastroenterology	32	19	9
Analytical Chemistry	33	17	15
Journal of Dairy Science	34	34	42
Phytochemistry	35	31	36
Annals of the New York Academy of Sciences	36	20	43
Proceedings of the Society of Experimental Biology and Medicine	37	26	38

Table 5.2. (Continued)

	Core citation analysis	*Science Citation Index*[a] Rank based on average number of citations	Impact factor
Annals of Internal Medicine	38	18	6
Metabolism	39	36	26
Pediatrics	40	27	20
International Journal of Food Science and Technology (Incl. *Journal of Food Technology*)	41	55	55
Journal of Bacteriology	42	16	19
Journal of Applied Bacteriology	43	48	40
Lipids	44	40	29
CRC Critical Reviews in Food Science and Nutrition	45	59	39
Zeitschrift fur Lebensmittel-Untersuchung und -Forschung	46	53	50
Transactions Royal Society of Tropical Medicine and Hygiene	47	46	37
Cancer Research (& Supplement)	48	12	12
Cereal Foods World	49	62	59
Lebensmittel-Wissenschaft + Technologie	50	56	60
Food Chemistry	51	60	56
Journal of Tropical Pediatrics	52	58	62
Infection and Immunity	53	23	17
Journal of Texture Studies	54	57	57
Proceedings Nutrition Society	55	52	24
Acta Paediatrica Scandinavica (& Supplement)	56–57	43	44
Archives of Biochemistry and Biophysics	56–57	61	58
The Journal of Laboratory and Clinical Medicine	58	29	27
Nutrition Reviews (& Supplement)	59	54	54
Journal of the National Cancer Institute	60	25	22
Journal of Applied Physiology	61	14	30

[a]Data gathered for the Core journals from *SCI Reports* for the years 1979, 1982, 1985, and 1988, were averaged for both the number of citations and the impact factor.

These sixty-one titles identified in the Core Agricultural Literature Project were examined using the yearly summary citation data provided by *Science Citation Index*. *SCI* data were gathered for the number of times each title was cited in the *SCI* database for four selected years and then averaged. These titles were then ranked. Impact factors, as computed by *SCI* for the same four years, were also obtained for the same journals and these were averaged and ranked. There is a rather dramatic difference in rankings between the *SCI* data and that of the Core Project citation work. The discrepancy arises because most of the articles published in journals like *Science, JAMA*, and the *Journal of Biological Chemistry* are not related to human nutrition or food science. *Science*, for example, is cited in numerous scientific journals each year in fields unrelated to food science and human nutrition, which pushes its rank very high. For the same reason, many of the medically oriented journals rank high in the *SCI* data since they are so encompassing of the medical subjects they include.

C. Separate Rankings for Food Science and Human Nutrition

Because food science and human nutrition are two distinct (although overlapping) subjects, each was considered separately and concentrations and correlations within each were sought. This was done by dividing the source documents into three groups: documents clearly within the food science field, documents clearly within human nutrition, and documents bridging the two. Of the fifty source documents,

28	were assigned to food science only,
16	were assigned to human nutrition only, and
6	were assigned to both categories.

Therefore thirty-four source documents were tabulated and assigned to food science amd twenty-two provided data for human nutrition.

To find the primary rankings in journals for the developed countries only, the thirty-four and twenty-two source documents were divided into areas of geographic influence. In the case of food science, only four of the thirty-four titles were concerned directly with the Third World. The reverse was true in human nutrition, where sixteen applied to the Third World and nine to the developed countries. Most of the source documents were large and provided adequate data for valid statistical rankings.

Table 5.3 provides the ranking from the Core Project citation analysis for the food science literature of primary value to the developed countries and to the Third World. The Third World titles were ranked separately from the others, which introduced some titles not in the major citation list (Table 5.2). An additional column provides data from a 1980 bibliometric study of journal literature in food science and technology. This study provides an additional ranking for titles high in the list.[9] The Third World titles from the

9. Maheswarappa, "Journal Literature."

Table 5.3. Food science journal rankings

	Core Project Citation Analysis		
	Developed countries	Third World	1980 Study[a]
Journal of Food Science	1	1	1
JAOCS; Journal of the American Oil Chemists' Society	2	14	10
Food Technology (Chicago)	3	4	2
Journal of Agriculture and Food Chemistry	4	20	4
Applied and Environmental Microbiology	5	2	16–24
Journals of the Science of Food and Agriculture	6	9	5
Journal of Food Protection	7	3	15
Journal of Chromatography	8	—	11
Nature	9	23–24	26
Journal of the American Chemical Association	10	—	30–31
Science	11	15–16	30–31
Journal of Association of Official Analytical Chemists	12	11–12	8
Journal of Biological Chemistry	13	15–16	12
Biochemical Journal	14	—	27
Cereal Chemistry	15	—	7
Journal of Dairy Science	16	—	18
Analytical Chemistry	17	—	38
Agricultural and Biological Chemistry	18	—	24
Phytochemistry	19	—	20–21
International Journal of Food Science and Technology	20	17–19	6
Biochimica et Biophysica Acta	21	—	22
Journal of Applied Bacteriology	22	5	20–21
Journal of Bacteriology	23	6	25
Zeitschrift fur Lebensmittel–Untersuchung und –Forschung	24	—	—
Journal of Texture Studies	25	—	40
CRC Critical Reviews in Food Science and Nutrition	26–27	—	—
Lebensmittel–Wissenschaft + Technologie	26–27	—	41
Food Chemistry	28	—	—
Journal of Nutrition	29	26	19
American Journal of Clinical Nutrition	30	10	28
Acta Horticulturae	31	—	—
Proceedings National Academy of Sciences (U.S.A.)	32–33	—	—
Lipids	32–33	—	—
Cereal Foods World	34	—	—
Journal of Dairy Research	35	—	—
Fleischwirschaft	36	—	—
Archives of Biochemistry and Biophysics	37	—	—
Meat Science	38	—	—
Analytical Biochemistry	39	—	—
Nippon Suissan Gakkaishiz	—	7	—
Infection and Immunity	—	8	—
Advanced Food Research	—	11–12	—

Canadian Journal of Microbiology	—	13	—
Bacteriological Review	—	17–19	—
Annual Review of Microbiology	—	17–19	—
Journal of Clinical Microbiology	—	21–22	—
Canadian Institute of Food Science and Technology Journal	—	21–22	—
Journal of General Microbiology	—	23–24	—

[a]B.S. Maheswarappa and K. Surya Rao, "Journal Literature of Food Science and Technology: A Bibliographic Study," *Annals of Library Science and Documentation* 29 (3) (1982): 126–134.

Core Project citation analysis had valid data through the top twenty-four titles, which provided nine additional titles not represented in the valid list for developed countries.

The human nutrition journal data came from twenty-two source documents. These included thirteen assigned to the Third World literature only, six to the developed countries, and three additional to both. The nutrition source documents tended to be rather voluminous, particularly those for the developed countries. As a result approximately 65% of all citations in the total analysis came exclusively from the human nutrition source documents. Table 5.4 lists these primary journals from the Core Project citation analysis along with data from two other studies. Two of the titles, *Journal of Agricultural and Food Chemistry* and *Journal of the Science of Food and Agri-*

Table 5.4. Human nutrition journal rankings

	Core Project Citation Analysis			
	Developed countries	Third World	Grybowski (1970)[a]	Classics[b]
American Journal of Clinical Nutrition	1	1	1	12–15
Lancet	2	3	6	5–8
Journal of Nutrition	3	4	3	3
New England Journal of Medicine	4	5	18	12–15
Journal Clinical Investigation	5	6	5	12–15
Journal of Biological Chemistry	6	7	4	1
American Journal of Physiology	7	13	9	16–22
British Medical Journal	8	8	35	—
Science	9	10	22	5–8
Gastroenterology	10	16	—	—
JAMA; Journal of the American Medical Association	11	15	21	9–11
Journal of the American Dietetic Association	12	11	17	—

Table 5.4. (Continued)

	Core Project Citation Analysis			
	Developed countries	Third World	Grybowski (1970)[a]	Classics[b]
Federation Procedings (Superseded by *FASEB Journal*)	13	12	11	—
Pediatrics	14–15	14	—	—
British Journal of Nutrition	14–15	17	10	—
Journal of Pediatrics	16	9	28	—
Annals of Internal Medicine	17	18–19	—	—
Journal of Food Science	18	—	—	—
Biochimica et Biophysica Acta	19	26	19	—
Nature	20–21	23	14	12–15
Annals of the New York Academy of Sciences	20–21	28	23	—
Metabolism	22	18–19	7	—
Proceedings of the Society of Experimental Biology and Medicine	23	25	2	9–11
Food Technology (Chicago)	24	—	—	—
Proceedings National Academy of Sciences (U.S.A.)	25–26	24	—	5–8
Biochemical Journal	25–26	30	24	2
Nutrition Reviews (& Supplement)	27	36	—	—
Human Biology	28	31	26	—
The Journal of Laboratory and Clinical Medicine	29	21	12	16–22
Annual Review of Nutrition	30	37	—	—
American Journal of Medicine	31	32	16	—
Acta Paediatrica Scandinavica (& Supplement)	32	29	—	—
Clinical Science	33	38	—	—
Cancer Research (& Supplement)	34	27	—	—
Journal of the National Cancer Institute	35	34	—	—
Journal of Agricultural and Food Chemistry	36	—	—	—
Proceedings of the Nutrition Society	37	33	—	—
Archives of Disease in Childhood	—	2	—	—
Journal of Tropical Pediatrics	—	20	—	—
Transactions of the Royal Society of Tropical Medicine and Hygiene	—	22	—	—
Ecology of Food and Nutrition	—	35	—	—
Journal of the American Chemical Society	—	—	—	4
Archives of Internal Medicine	—	—	8	—

[a]Helen Grybowski, "Human Nutrition," in T. D. Wilson and Esther Herman, eds., *Fundamentals of Documentation: Students' Papers* (College Park, Md.: School of Library and Information Service, University of Maryland, 1973), pp. 138–156.

[b]Classics n = 189; for an explanation of classics, see Chapter 3, page 50.

culture, appear on a list of sixty-six core journals for all of agriculture as determined by *SCI* data in 1989.[10]

Titles were included from the Core Project citation analysis when the data was statistically adequate and valid, which meant that only thirty-seven titles were listed. Ties to the biological, physiological, and medical worlds are clear for both the developed and Third World countries. Again, the tropical influence is clear with the Third World literature. The other two studies are remarkably similar, showing only two unusual variations: *Journal of the American Chemical Society* and *Archives of Internal Medicine*. These are the result of a slightly different subject focus and changes over twenty years.

The commonality of titles between developed and Third World titles is demonstrated in Figure 5.2.

Several observations are evident from these data when they are compared with data from the entire citation analysis and the full titles lists. First, Third World literature is in its infancy in food science. There is a clear dependency on international journals for the scientific literature applicable to the Third World. This observation should not be read as denigrating local, site-specific food science literature, from the Third World, but these titles often have only limited application for other Third World countries. The reverse appears to be true for the literature of the developed countries,

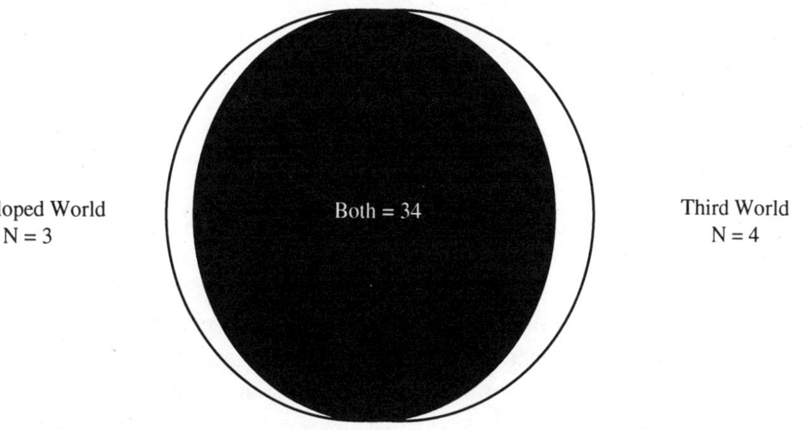

Figure 5.2. Commonality and difference of human nutrition journals.

10. Eugene Garfield, "Journal Citation Studies, 53: Agricultural Sciences, Most Fruitful Journals and High Yield Research Fields," in *Journalology, KeyWords Plus™, and Other Essays* (Philadelphia: ISI Press, 1991), pp. 455–467. Originally published as "Current Comments 51," *Current Contents* (December 17, 1990).

which has direct application in the Third World. Second, only a small number of nutrition journals appear in the food science ranking. Almost all pertain to the Third World only. Third, the twenty highest ranking titles for developed countries in the Core Project analysis rank highly in other estimates as well. There is fair unanimity of agreement.

The Core Project titles show a heavy reliance on United States journals and also those from Great Britain. These two countries have been and probably still are the world's leaders in scientific human nutrition research and journal publishing. Only a half-dozen general science and agricultural journals are included as primary titles. The difference from the food science literature is clear.

In looking separately at the primary journals in these two subject areas, only eleven journals appear in both lists. This demonstrates little coincidence in the journal literature and the valuable core journals in the two areas. The titles in both the food science and human nutrition primary analysis lists are

American Journal of Clinical Nutrition
Biochemical Journal
Biochimica et Biophysica Acta
Food Technology (Chicago)
Journal of Agricultural and Food Chemistry
Journal of Biological Chemistry
Journal of Food Science
Journal of Nutrition
Nature
Proceedings of the National Academy of Sciences (U.S.)
Science

D. Recommended Current Core Journals for Food Science and Human Nutrition

Data from the Core Project citation analysis served as base information and the primary influence in determining core journal titles. High rankings in other sources of information were correlated and their influences weighed. This recommended core list does not match exactly the titles in the earlier tables. The most common reason for dropping a title is that it is no longer published. The earlier rankings covered a period from 1950 through 1991, a forty-two year span. Data for a title which showed a downward trend in publishing importance in the last ten years were taken into account, as were influences from other studies. It is necessary to provide a balance between the two major subject areas, considering that only eleven titles are highly ranked in each. The developed world list and the Third World journals are scaled separately in order to provide information specific to each. The overlap between the lists is great, however. Top-ranked titles are listed with a 1, second-ranked with a 2.

Core Journals in Food Science and Human Nutrition

	Developed Countries	Third World
Acta Paediatrica Scandinavica. Vol. 54. (1965)+. Stockholm; Almquist & Wiksell. Bimonthly. (Continues *Acta Paediatrica*.)	2	2
Advances in Food and Nutrition Research. Vol. 33. (1989)+. New York; Academic Press. Annual. (Formerly *Advances in Food Research*.)	–	1
Agricultural and Biological Chemistry. Nippon Nogei-Kagakkai. Vol. 25. (Jan. 1961)+. Tokyo; Nippon Nogei-Kagakkai. Monthly. (Continues *Nippon Nogei-Kagakkai Bulletin*).	2	–
American Journal of Clinical Nutrition. Vol. 2. (July/Aug. 1954)+. Bethesda Md.; American Society for Clinical Nutrition. Monthly. (Formerly *Journal of Clinical Nutrition*.)	1	1
American Journal of Physiology. Vol. 1 (1898)+. Bethesda, Md.; American Physiology Society. Monthly.	1	2
Analytical Chemistry. Vol. 19. (Jan. 1947)+. Washington, D.C.; American Chemical Society. Semimonthly. (Continues *Industrial and Engineering Chemistry*.)	2	–
Annals of Internal Medicine. Vol. 1. (July 1927)+. Philadelphia, Pa.; American College of Physicians. Monthly.	2	2
Annals of the New York Academy of Sciences. Vol. 1. (July 1877)+. New York; New York Academy of Sciences. Approx. 20 vols. per year.	2	–
Annual Review of Microbiology. Vol. 1 (1947)+. Palo Alto, Calif.; Annual Reviews Inc. Annual.	–	2
Applied and Environmental Microbiology. Vol. 31 (1976)+. Washington D.C.; American Society for Microbiology. Monthly. (Formerly *Applied Microbiology*.)	1	2
Archives of Disease in Childhood. Vol. 1 (1926)+. London; British Medical Association. Bimonthly.	–	1
Archives of Biochemistry and Biophysics. Vol. 1. (1942)+. New York; Academic Press. Fourteen a year.	2	–
Bacteriology Review. Vol. 1. (Dec. 1937)+. Baltimore; American Society for Microbiology. Annual.	–	2

	Developed Countries	Third World
Biochimica et Biophysica Acta. Vol. 1 (1947)+. Amsterdam; Elsevier. Monthly.	1	2
Biochemical Journal. Vol. 1 (1906)+. London; Biochemical Journal. Semimonthly.	1	2
British Journal of Nutrition. Vol. 1 (1947)+. Cambridge; Sponsored by The Nutrition Society, Cambridge University Press. Bimonthly.	2	2
British Medical Journal. Vol. 1 (1957)+. London; British Medical Association. Weekly.	1	2
Canadian Journal of Microbiology. Vol. 1. (Aug. 1954)+. Ottawa, Ont.; National Research Council Canada. Monthly.	–	2
Cancer Research. Vol. 1. (Jan. 1941)+. Baltimore, Md.; Waverly Press. Semimonthly.	2	2
Cereal Chemistry. Vo. 1. (Jan. 1924)+. St. Paul, Minn.; American Association of Cereal Chemists. Bimonthly.	2	–
Cereal Foods World. Vol. 20. (Jan. 1975)+. St. Paul, Minn.; American Association of Cereal Chemists. Monthly. (Continues *Cereal Science Today*.)	2	–
CRC Critical Reviews in Food Science and Nutrition. Vol. 12. (June 1980)+. Boca Raton, Fla.; CRC Press. Bimonthly. (Continues *Critical Reviews in Food Science and Nutrition*.)	2	–
FASEB Journal. Vol. 1. (July 1987)+. Bethesda, Md.; Federation of American Societies for Experimental Biology. Monthly. (Supersedes *Federation Proceedings*.)	1	1
Food Chemistry. Vol. 1. (July 1976)+. Barking, Essex.; Applied Science Publishers. Quarterly.	2	–
Food Technology. Vol. 1. (1947)+. Chicago, Ill.; Institute of Food Technologists. Monthly.	1	1
Gastroenterology. Vol. 1. (1943)+. Baltimore, Md.; American Gastroentology Association. Monthly.	2	–
Infection and Immunity. Vol. 1. (Jan. 1970)+. Washington, D.C.; American Society for Microbiology. Monthly.	–	2
International Journal of Food Science and Technology. Vol. 22. (1987)+. Oxford; Blackwell Scientific. Bimonthly. (Supersedes *Journal of Food Technology*.)	2	2
Journal of Agricultural and Food Chemistry. Vol. 1. (1953)+. Washington, D.C.; American Chemical Society. Bimonthly, 1960+.	1	2
Journal of Applied Bacteriology. Vol. 17. (April 1954)+. London; Academic Press. Quarterly. (Continues *Society for Applied Bacteriology Proceedings*.)	2	2
Journal of Bacteriology. Vol. 1. (Jan. 1985)+. Baltimore, Md.; American Society for Microbiology. Monthly.	2	2
Journal of Biological Chemistry. Vol. 1. (1905)+. Bal-	1	2

	Developed Countries	Third World
timore, Md.; American Society of Biological Chemists. Three times a month.		
Journal of Chromatography. Vol. 1. (1958)+. Amsterdam; Elsevier. Biweekly.	2	–
Journal of Clinical Investigation. Vol. 1. (1924)+. New York; Publ. by Rockefeller University Press for American Society for Microbiology. Monthly.	1	2
Journal of Dairy Science. Vol. 1. (May 1917)+. Champaign, Ill.; American Dairy Science Association. Monthly.	2	–
Journal of Food Protection. Vol. 40. (1977)+. Ames, Iowa; International Association of Milk, Food, and Environmental Sanitarians. Monthly. (Formerly *Journal of Milk and Food Technology*.)	2	2
Journal of Food Science. Vol. 26. (1961)+. Chicago, Ill.; Institute of Food Technologists. Bimonthly. (Formerly *Food Research*.)	1	1
Journal of Nutrition. Vol. 1. (1928)+. Bethesda, Md.; American Institute of Nutrition. Monthly.	1	1
Journal of Pediatrics. Vol. 1. (1932)+. St. Louis, Mo.; C.V. Mosby. Monthly	2	1
Journal of Texture Studies. Vol. 1. (Nov. 1969)+. Westport, Conn.; Food & Nutrition Press. Quarterly.	2	–
Journal of the American Chemical Society. Vol. 1. (1879)+. Washington D.C.; American Chemical Society. Biweekly.	2	–
Journal of the American Dietetic Association. Vol. 1. (1925)+. Chicago, Ill.; American Dietetic Association. Monthly.	1	2
Journal of the American Medical Association (JAMA). Vol. 1 (1883)+. Chicago, Ill.; American Medical Association. Four issues per month.	2	2
Journal of the American Oil Chemists' Society (JAOCS). Vol. 24. (1947)+. Champaign, Ill.; American Oil Chemists' Society. Monthly. (Formerly *Oil and Soap*.)	1	–
Journal of the Association of Official Analytical Chemists. Vol. 49. (1966)+. Washington, D.C.; Association of Official Analytical Chemists. Bimonthly. (Formerly *Journal of the Association of Official Agricultural Chemists*.)	2	2
Journal of the National Cancer Institute (JNCI). Vol. 1. (Aug. 1940)+. Bethesda, Md.; U.S. Government Printing Office. Annual.	2	2
Journal of the Science of Food and Agriculture. Vol. 1. (1950) +. London; Society of Chemical Industry. Monthly.	1	2
Journal of Tropical Pediatrics. Vol. 26. (Feb. 1980)+. London; Oxford University Press. Bimonthly. (Continues	–	2

	Developed Countries	Third World
Journal of Tropical Pediatrics and Environmental Child Health.)		
Lancet. Vol. 1. (1823)+. London; Lancet Limited. The North American ed. began with no. 7453. (July 1966)+. Boston; Little, Brown. Weekly.	1	1
Lebensmittel-Wissenschaft+Technologie. Vol. 1. (1968)+. Zurich; Forster Verlag. Bimonthly.	2	–
Lipids. Vol. 1. (Jan. 1966)+. Chicago, Ill.; American Oil Chemists' Society. Monthly.	2	–
Metabolism; Clinical and Experimental. Vol. 1. (1952)+. New York; Grune & Stratton. Monthly.	2	2
Nature. Vol. 1. (1869)+. London; Macmillan Journals. Weekly.	1	2
New England Journal of Medicine. Vol. 198. (1928)+. Boston; Massachusetts Medical Society. Weekly. (Formerly *Boston Medical and Surgical Journal*.)	1	2
Nippon Eiyo Shokuryo Gakkaishi = Journal of Japanese Society of Nutrition and Food Science . Vol. 36. (1983)+. Tokyo; Da Gakkai. (Continues *Eiy o to Shokury o*). Bimonthly.	–	1
Nutrition Reviews (&Suppl). Vol. 1. (1942)+. New York; Sponsored by International Life Science Institute, Nutrition Foundation. Monthly.	2	–
Pediatrics. Vol. 1. (1948)+. Evanston, Ill.; American Academy of Pediatrics. Monthly.	1	2
Phytochemistry. Vol. 1. (Oct. 1961)+. Oxford; Pergamon Press. Monthly.	2	–
Proceedings of the National Academy of Sciences. Vol. 1. (1915)+. Washington, D.C.; National Academy of Sciences. Monthly.	2	2
Proceedings of the Nutrition Society. Vol. 1. (1944)+. Cambridge, England; Nutrition Society. Three issues a year.	2	2
Proceedings of the Society for Experimental Biology and Medicine. Vol. 1. (1903)+. New York; The Society. Monthly.	2	2
Science. Vol. 1. (1895)+. Washington, D.C.; American Association for the Advancement of Science. Weekly.	1	2
Transactions of the Royal Society of Tropical Medicine and Hygiene. Vol. 1. (1907)+. London; The Society. Bimonthly.	–	2
Zeitschrift für Lebensmittel-Untersuchung und -Forschung. Vol. 1. (1943)+. Berlin; Springer Verlag. Monthly.	2	–

The crossover in subject matter between the literatures of food science and human nutrition is extensive, but only thirteen of the sixty-four journals in the core list can be counted as having equal content in both areas. Twenty-seven center on human nutrition and twenty-three on food science. A wide array of countries are represented as places of publication:

United States	42 titles
United Kingdom	14
Netherlands	2
Japan	2
Canada, Germany, Sweden, and Switzerland	1 each

This represents a remarkable diversity of places of publication, even though two-thirds are published in the United States.

Of the sixty-four titles, thirty-nine (62%) are published directly by societies or non-profit associations. Two additional titles are published by university presses for societies. Food science and human nutrition have a higher percentage of core titles published by societies than other disciplines in the Core Project. In fact, thirty-one different societies are represented as sponsors or publishers. The American Society for Microbiology publishes four of the titles, and the American Chemical Society three. Four additional societies in the United States publish two titles each.

An analysis of 480 human nutrition citations published in two journals in 1968 found that societies, associations, and independent organizations were the chief producers of periodicals, publishing 68% of the total. Commercial publishers were second at 15%.[11] The commercial publishing influence is relatively slight, with only nineteen titles. Elsevier is the only commercial publisher with two titles in the list. The Canadian government has one title and the United States government has two.

Of the sixty-four titles, fifty-five are core titles in the developed countries, and forty-five are core in the Third World. Thirty-six are core in both, which means that 56.3% of this core journal literature is valuable to both communities. Only nine of the forty-four Third World titles rank as of top importance. This lack of diversity in Third World titles probably reflects an uneven developmental stage which is not extensive outside the developed world or the international agencies.

E. New Journal Titles

Growth of specialized journals in food science and human nutrition is demonstrated by the number of titles which have begun publication since

11. Grybowski, "Human Nutrition."

1980. With one exception, they are not represented among the top-ranked titles, since they titles relatively new and have not yet been cited frequently.

These titles are provided as a reference list which, although not exhaustive, covers most new scholarly journals or serials. Popular literature, such as most newsletters, are excluded; titles which began before 1980 but changed names are not included.

New Food Science and Human Nutrition Journals, 1980–

Acta Biotechnologica. Vol. 1 (1981)+ Berlin; Akademie-Verlag. Four issues yearly.

Advances in Food Science. Vol. 1 (1992)+ Greenwich, Conn.; JAI Press. Annual.

Annals of Nutrition and Metabolism: European Journal of Nutrition, Metabolic Diseases and Dietetics. (1981)+ Basel and New York; Karger. Bimonthly.

Annual Review of Nutrition. Vol. 1 (1981)+ Palo Alto, Calif.; Annual Reviews Inc.

Appetite: The Journal for Research on Intake, and Dietary Practices, Their Control and Consequences. Vol. 1 (1980)+ London and New York; Academic Press. Quarterly.

Arteriosclerosis. Vol. 1 (1981)+ Dallas, Texas; The American Heart Association, Inc. Bimonthly.

ASEAN Food Journal. Vol. 1 (1985)+ Kuala Lumpur, Malaysia; ASEAN Food Handling Bureau. Four no. yearly.

BioFactors. Vol. 1 (1988)+ Oxford and Washington, D.C.; IRL Press. Quarterly.

Bioscience Reports. Vol. 1 (1981)+ London; The Biochemical Society. Monthly.

Biotechnology Progress. Vol. 1 (1985)+ New York; American Institute of Chemical Engineers. Quarterly.

Brauwelt International. Vol. 1 (1985)+ Nurnberg; H. Carl. Semiannual.

Clinical Consultations in Nutritional Support. Vol. 1 (1981)+

Clinics in Laboratory Medicine Vol. 1 (1981)+ Philadelphia, Pa.; W. B. Saunders Co. Quarterly.

Clinical Nutrition. Vol. 1 (1984)+ Philadelphia, Pa.; W. B. Saunders Co. Irregular.

Clinical Nutrition: Official Journal of the European Society of Parenteral and Enteral Nutrition. Vol. 1 (1982)+ Edinburgh and New York; Churchill Livingston. Four issues yearly.

Clinical Reviews in Allergy. Vol. 1 (1983)+ New York; Elsevier Biomedical. Four issues yearly.

Clinics in Applied Nutrition. Vol. 1 (1991)+ Reading, Mass.; Andover Medical Publishers. Quarterly.

Comments on Inorganic Chemistry Vol. 1 (1981)+ London and New York; Gordon and Breach Sicence. Bimonthly.

Cryoletters. Vol. 1 (1979)+ Cambridge; Science and Technology Letters. Monthly.

Drug-Nutrient Interactions: A Journal of Research in Nutritional Pharmacology and Toxicology. Vol. 1 (1981)+ New York; A. R. Liss. Quarterly.

Ecology of Disease (Oxford). Vol. 1 (1982)+ Oxford and New York; Pergamon Press. Quarterly.

Eating Disorders Review. Vol. 1 (1993) + Chichester, England; John Wiley. Three no. yearly. (continues *British Review of Bulimia & Anorexia Nervosa*.)
The EMBO Journal. Vol. 1 (1982) + Oxford; IRL Press. Monthly
The FASEB Journal (Federation of American Societies for Experimental Biology). Vol. 1 (1987) + Bethesda, Md.; The Federation. Monthly. Supercedes its *Federation Proceedings*.
Ferment. Vol. 1 (1988) + London; Institute of Brewing. Bimonthly.
Flavour and Fragrance Journal. Vol. 1 (1986) + Chichester, U.K. and New York; J. Wiley & Sons. Quarterly.
Food Additives: Contaminants, Analysis, Surveillance, Evaluation. Vol. 1 (1984) + Philadelphia, Pa.; Taylor & Francis. Monthly.
Food and Bioproducts Processing. Vol. 1 (1991) + Rugby, England; The Institution of Chemical Engineers. Four issues yearly.
Food and Drug Law Reports. No. 1 (1989) + Washington, D.C.; Food and Drug Law Institute. Monthly.
Food and Foodways. Vol. 1 (1985) + New York; Harwood. Quarterly.
Food Biotechnology. Vol. 1 (1987) + New York; M. Dekker. Twice a year.
Food Business Annual. Vol.1 (1991) + New Berlin, WI.; FRI Enterprises. Annual.
Food Control. Vol. 1 (1990) + Guildford, U.K.; Butterworths. Quarterly.
Food Hydrocolloids. Vol. 1 (1986) + Washington, D.C.; IRL Press. Six no. yearly.
Food Microbiology. Vol. 1 (1984) + London; Academic Press. Quarterly.
Food Nutrition and Agriculture Vol 1 (1991) + (also in French and Spanish). Rome; Food and Agriculture Organization of the United Nations. Three issues yearly.
Food Quality and Preference. Vol. 1 (1988) + Harlow, U.K.; Longman Scientific & Technical. Quarterly.
Food Reviews International. Vol. 1 (1985) + New York; Marcel Dekker. Three issues yearly.
Food Structure Vol. 1 (1982) + Chicago; Scanning Microscopy International. Quarterly. (formerly Food Microstructure).
FSIS Food Safety Review. Vol. 1 (1991) + Washington, D.C.; USDA, Food Safety Inspection Service. Quarterly.
International Journal of Eating Disorders. Vol. 1 (1981) + New York; Van Nostrand Reinhold. Quarterly.
International Journal of Food Microbiology. Vol. 1 (1984) + Amsterdam; Elsevier Science Publishers. Six no. yearly.
Issues in Food Science
Italian Journal of Food Science. Vol. 1 (1989) + IJFS; Rivista Italiana di Scienza Degli Alimenti. Pinerolo, Italy: Chiriotti Editori. Quarterly.
Journal of Adolescent Health. Vol. 1 (1980) + New York; Elsevier North Holland. Bimonthly.
Journal of the American College of Nutrition. Vol. 1 (1982) + New York; A. R. Liss. Quarterly.
Journal of Aquatic Food Product Technology. Vol. 1 (1992) + Binghamton, New York; Haworth Press. Quarterly.
Journal of Cereal Science. Vol. 1 (1983) + London and New York; Academic Press. Quarterly.
Journal of Clinical Oncology; Official Journal of the American Society of Clinical Oncology. Vol. 1 (1983) + Monthly.

Journal of Food Composition and Analysis. Vol. 1 (1987)+ San Diego; Academic Press. Four issues yearly.

Journal of Food Lipids. Vol. 1 (1993)+ Trumbull, Conn; Food and Nutrition Press. Quarterly.

Journal of Food Physics. Vol. 1 (1988)+ Budapest; University of Horticulture and Food Industry. Annual.

Journal of Food Products Marketing. Vol. 1 (1992)+ Binghamton, NY; Food Products Press. Quarterly.

Journal of Food Service Systems. Vol. 1 (1981)+ Westport, Conn; Food and Nutrition Press. Quarterly.

Journal of Human Nutrition and Dietetics. Vol. 1 (1988)+ Oxford; Blackwell Scientific Publications. Bimonthly.

Journal of Hypertension. Vol. 1 (1983)+ London and New York; Grower Medical. Bimonthly.

Journal of Industrial Irradiation Technology. Vol. 1 (1983)+ New York; Marcel Dekker, Inc. Four issues yearly.

Journal of Industrial Microbiology. Vol. 1 (1986)+ The Netherlands; Elsevier Science. Bimonthly.

Journal of Human Lactation. Vol. 1 (1985)+ Charlottesville, Va.; International Lactation Consultant Association. Quarterly.

Journal of Microbiology Methods. Vol. 1 (1983)+ The Netherlands; Elsevier. Bimonthly.

Journal of Micronutrient Analysis. Vol. 1 (1985)+ Essex; Elsevier Applied Science. Quarterly.

Journal of Nutrition for the Elderly. Vol. 1 (1980)+ New York; Haworth Press. Quarterly.

Journal of Nutrition, Growth and Cancer. Vol. 1 (1983)+ Westport, Conn.; Food & Nutrition Press. Quarterly.

Journal of Nutritional Biochemistry. Vol. 1 (1990)+ Stoneham, Mass.; Butterworth Publishers. Monthly

Journal of Nutritional Immunology. Vol. 1 (1991)+ Binghamton, New York; Haworth Medical Press. Quarterly.

Journal of Nutritional Medicine. Vol. 1 (1990)+ Abington, England; Carfax Pub. Co. Quarterly.

Journal of Packaging Technology. Vol. 1 (1987)+ Mahwah, New Jersey; Technical Publications. Bimonthly.

Journal of Pediatric Gastroenterology and Nutrition. Vol. 1 (1982)+ New York; Raven Press. Quarterly.

Journal of Pediatric and Perinatal Nutrition. Vol. 1 (1987)+ Binghamton, New York; Haworth Press. Semiannual.

Journal of Rapid Methods and Automation in Microbiology. Vol. 1 (1992)+ Trumbull, Conn.; Food & Nutrition Press, Inc. Quarterly.

Journal of Sensory Studies. Vol. 1 (1986)+ Westport, Conn.; Food & Nutriton Press. Quarterly.

Lebensmittel und Biotechnologie. Vol. 1 (1984)+ Austria; Fachverlan Wein. Four no. yearly.

Letters in Applied Microbiology. Vol. 1 (1985)+ London; Blackwell Scientific Publ. Monthly.

Life Chemistry Reports. Vol. 1 (1982)+ Chur, New York; Harwood Academic. Irregular.

Lymphokine Research Vol. 1 (1982)+ New York; Mary Ann Liebert, Inc. Quarterly.

Magnesium. Vol. 1 (1982)+ Basel and New York; Karger. Bimonthly.

Magnesium Bulletin. Vol. 1 (1981)+ Heidelberg; Fischer. Irregular.

Molochnoe imiasnoe skotovodstvo. Vol. 1 (1983)+ Moskva; Kolos. Monthly.

Nutrition. Vol. 1 (1987/88)+ Guilford, Conn.; Dushkin Publ., Group. Annual.

Nutrition. Vol. 1 (1987)+ Toronto, Ontario; Druid Publ. Corp. Annual. (Suppl. to *Paediatric Medicine*)

Nutrition (Burbank, California). Vol. 1 (1985)+ Burbank, Calif.; Nutrition. Bimonthly. (Continues *Nutrition International*)

Nutrition and Behavior. Vol. 1 (1982)+ New York; Alan R. Liss. Quarterly.

Nutrition and Health. Vol. 1 (1982)+ Berkhamsted, England; AB Academic Publishers. Quarterly.

Nutrition Clinical Dietetica Hospitalaria. Vol. 1 (1981)+ Madrid; Grutesa. Quarterly.

Nutrition Clinics. Vol. 1 (1986)+ Philadelphia; George F. Stickley Co. Bimonthly.

Nutrition Clinique et Metabolisme Vol. 1 (1987)+ Paris; Arnette. Four no. yearly.

Nutrition Forum. Vol. 1 (1984)+ Philadelphia; George F. Stickley Co. Monthly.

Nutrition In Clinical Practice. Vol. 1 (1986)+ Baltimore; Williams & Wilkins for America Society for Parental and Enteral Nutrition. Bimonthly.

Nutrition, Metabolism and Cardiovascular Diseases: NMCD. Vol. 1 (1991)+ Heidelberg; Springer International. Four issues yearly.

Nutrition News. Vol. 1 (1985)+ Hyberbad, India; National Institute of Nutritional Council of Medical Research. Bimonthly.

Nutrition Research. Vol. 1 (1981)+ New York; Pergamon Press. Bimonthly. and *Supplement* 1985+; each issue has a distinctive title.

Nutrition Research Reviews. Vol. 1 (1988)+ Cambridge and New York; Cambridge University Press. Annual.

Nutrition Support Services. Vol. 1 (1981)+ North Hollywood, Calif.; Nutrition Support Services, Inc. Monthly.

Nutrition Update. Vol. 1 (1983)+ New York; J. Wiley & Sons. Annual.

Packaging Technology and Science. Vol. 1 (1988)+ Chichester, England; J. Wiley & Sons. Quarterly.

Parasitology Today. Vol. 1 (1985)+ Amsterdam; Elsevier Science Publ. Monthly.

Perspectives in Applied Nutrition. Vol. 1 (1993)+ Chicago, Ill.; Mosby. Quarterly.

Practical Diabetes. Vol. 1 (1984)+ Petersfield, Hants; Asgard Publ. Co. Bimonthly.

Prenatal Diagnosis. Vol. 1 (1981)+ Chichester and New York; Wiley. Bimonthly.

Refrigerated & Frozen Foods. Vol. 1 (1990)+ Northbrook, Ill.; Stagnito Publ. Co. Monthly.

Regulatory Toxicology and Pharmacology. Vol. 1 (1981)+ New York; Academic Press. Quarterly.

Sciences des Aliments. Vol. 1 (1981)+ Paris; Lavoisier Abonnements. Biennial.

Special Topics in Endocrinology and Metabolism. Vol. 1 (1980)+ New York; A. R. Liss, Inc. Annual.

Topics in Clinical Nutrition. Vol. 1 (1986)+ Gaithersburg, Md.; Aspen Publ. Inc. Quarterly.

Trends in Biotechnology. Vol. 1 (1983)+ Amsterdam; Elsevier Science Publ. Monthly.

Trends in Food Science and Technology. Vol. 1 (1990)+ Cambridge; Elsevier. Monthly.
Vignevini. Vol. 1 (1974)+ Bologna; Edagricole. Bimonthly.

Additional Selected Reference

Mundy, C. C., "Accessing the Literature of Food Science," *Trends in Food Science & Technology* 2 (11) (1991): 272–276.

6. Databases of Nutrient Composition, Dietary Intake, and Food Adulteration

JEAN A. T. PENNINGTON
U. S. Food and Drug Administration

Food composition and consumption databases have many and varied uses among nutrition professionals in government, clinical, institutional, industrial, and academic settings. Food composition databases are used by government agencies to determine the safety and nutritional quality of food supplies. They are used in clinical and institutional settings to plan and evaluate single meals and daily diets. Databases are used to develop therapeutic diets modified in one or more nutrients for patients with special nutritional requirements. In academic settings, food composition databases are used to instruct students about the nutrient and contaminant content of foods and food groups. Databases are also used to develop nutrition education materials and programs for students and consumers. Food composition databases may be used in industry settings to develop new products and to assist with nutrition labeling and dietary claims.

The information in food composition and consumption databases is merged and used to assess the dietary status of individuals (patients, students), subjects participating in research trials or studies, or other population groups. Information on dietary status may be used to determine relationships between diet and disease in clinical and epidemiologic research studies. Information on dietary status is also useful for identifying population groups in need of nutrition intervention and for the development of policies concerning nutrient fortification.

A. Nutrient Composition Databases

Nutrient composition databases, both hard copy and machine-readable versions, are available in almost every country. Many are developed and managed by government agencies. Others are developed and used by academic institutions, food service departments, and the food industry. Commercial enterprises adopt and sell database systems or services for professional or personal use. The content of databases is variable in terms of the types and number of foods and nutrients. Also variable are the organizational structure of the database, the quality of the data, and the completeness of the database (i.e., number of missing values).

Information and directories are available to assist potential users in finding and selecting appropriate databases. The National Nutrient Databank Conference[1] holds annual meetings and produces a directory of databases in the United States and Canada. The current directory lists 51 databases and provides information on the number of foods and nutrients, cost, availability, computer compatibility, and available software.[2] The *INFOODS International Directory of Food Composition Tables* provides citations for 196 national and 8 international databases.[3] The Food and Agricultural Organization (FAO) of the United Nations produced the first international directory in 1975.[4] Additional information about food composition databases is available for the United States,[5] Europe,[6] Nordic countries,[7] Eastern Europe,[8] Latin America and the Caribbean Islands,[9] and Asia.[10]

1. S. P. Murphy, ed., "Nutrient Databases for the 1990's: Excellence in Diversity," in *Proceedings of the 16th National Nutrient Databank Conference* (Ithaca, N.Y.: The CBORD Group, 1991).

2. J. L. Smith, ed., *Nutrient Databank Directory*, 8th ed. (Newark: University of Delaware, 1992).

3. D. Heintze, W. M. Rand, and J. C. Klensin, *INFOODS International Directory of Food Composition Tables*, 2d ed. (Cambridge: Massachusetts Institute of Technology, 1988).

4. Food and Agricultural Organization of the United Nations, *Food Composition Tables: Updated Annotated Bibliography* (Rome: FAO, 1975).

5. D. M. Hildebrandt, *Computer Programs and Databases in the Field of Nutrition*, 5th ed. (Seattle: Computing Information Center, University of Washington, 1988).

6. (a) "The Establishment of Eurofoods," in C. E. West, ed., *Eurofoods: Towards Compatibility of Nutrient Data Banks in Europe* [*Annals of Nutrition & Metabolism* 29 (Suppl. 1) (1985): 7–8]. (b) "Review of Food Composition Tables and Nutrient Data Banks in Europe," in West, *Eurofoods*, pp. 11–38. (c) L. Arab, M. Wittler, and G. Schettler, *European Food Composition Tables in Translation* (Berlin: Springer, 1987). (d) C. E. West, ed., *Inventory of European Food Composition Tables and Nutrient Database Systems* (Uppsala: National Food Administration, 1989).

7. A. Moller, "NORFOODS Computer Group," in A. P. Simopoulos and R. R. Butrum, eds., *International Food Data Bases and Information Exchange, Concepts, Principles and Designs* (Basel: Karger, 1992 [*World Review of Nutrition and Dietetics* 68], pp. 104–120.)

8. J. H. Dobrzycki and M. Los-Kuczera, "Food Composition Tables and Food Composition Analysis in East Europe," in Simopoulos and Butrum, *International Food Data Bases*, pp. 136–156.

9. R. Bressani and M. Flores, "Past and Present Activities in Food Composition Tables in Latin America and the Caribbean Islands," in Simopoulos and Butrum, *International Food Data Bases*, pp. 121–135.)

10. (a) A. Valyasevi, *Proceedings of the First ASIAFOODS Conference* (Bangkok: 1985). (b) P. Puwastein, "Issues and Problems in Using Food Composition Data in Asia," in *Proceedings of the 16th National Nutrient Databank Conference*, pp. 157–163.

Several professional groups meet regularly to discuss issues relating to developing, maintaining, and improving food composition databases. These groups include the National Nutrient Databank Conference in the United States,[11] EUROFOODS in Europe,[12] NORFOODS in the Nordic countries,[13] LATINFOODS in Latin America,[14] and ASIAFOODS in Asia.[15]

Types of Food Composition Databases

Food composition databases may be classified according to (1) the groups that develop and manage them (government agencies, academic institutions, hospitals, food services, food companies, restaurants, commercial enterprises), (2) their purpose (reference, study-specific, research, national monitoring of food supplies and public health, diet assessment, menu planning, patient monitoring and assessment, consumer use, multipurpose), (3) the type of data they contain (original analyses, compilations, aggregations), or (4) the physical form in which they are available to users (hard copy, computer disc or tape).[16] Databases developed for research or commercial use may be expansions or modifications of a more generic national database developed by a government agency. This is the case in the United States, where many of the academic, hospital, and commercial databases are derived from the *USDA Standard Reference Data Tape* with added data from industry.[17]

The purpose of a database is the main factor in determining its organizational structure and contents in terms of foods and nutrients. Databases used to determine dietary status of individuals or population groups should include complete nutritional profiles for all nutrients to be assessed. Reference databases are authoritative collections of data derived from laboratory analyses. They may include data aggregations but not imputations; missing values are left blank. Hospital and other food service databases (e.g.,

11. Murphy, "Nutrient Databases for the 1990's."
12. (a) "Establishment of Eurofoods." (b) "Review of Food Composition Tables." (c) Arab, Wittler, and Schettler, "European Food Composition." (d) West, *Inventory of European Food Composition.*
13. Moller, "NORFOODS Computer Group."
14. Bressani and Flores, "Past and Present Activities in Food."
15. Valyasevi, "Proceedings of the First ASIAFOODS Conference."
16. (a) W. M. Rand, C. T. Windham, B. W. Wyse, and V. R. Young, *Food Composition Data, A User's Perspective* (Tokyo: United Nations University Press, 1988). (b) W. M. Rand, J. A. T. Pennington, S. P. Murphy, and J. C. Klensin, *Compiling Data for Food Composition Data Bases* (Tokyo: United Nations University Press, 1991).
17. (a) Smith, "Nutrient Databank Directory." (b) United States Department of Agriculture, *Nutrient Data Base for Standard Reference* (Springfield, Va.: National Technical Information Service, 1990 [Release no. 9]).

school lunch, congregate meals for the elderly, prisons) designed for menu planning and patient diet assessments include the institutional foods and recipe items prepared by the kitchen staff. Food company and restaurant databases contain the proprietary products prepared and sold by the company or restaurant.

Nutrient Database Concerns

Some areas of concern regarding databases include data quality, documentation, nutrient variation, food descriptions, database organization, updating, and user knowledge.[18]

Data Quality

Issues relating to data quality are discussed by M. Feinberg et al.,[19] J. O'Brien,[20] and D. A. T. Southgate and H. Greenfield.[21] A database should ideally contain average nutrient values that are representative of foods for a given location on a year-round basis. For example, a United States database should contain nutrient values representative of foods commonly sold in grocery stores across the country on a year-round basis. The sampling scheme used to collect the foods to be analyzed is crucial in obtaining representative values. Agricultural experts and statisticians should be consulted to determine when and where to collect the foods, how many cases (lots, cans, etc.) of each food to collect, and how to composite the foods for analysis. Other data quality issues include the use of approved analytical methods, the use of good laboratory procedures, and the analyses of standard reference materials along with foods.

The names of the nutrients in a database should be consistent with what was measured analytically. Because countries may define nutrients differently and may use different analytical methods, specific information about nutrient names and methods should be provided in the documentation to the

18. (a) Rand, "Compiling Data for Food Composition Data Bases." (b) J. A. T. Pennington, "Development and Use of Food Composition Data and Databases," in E. R. Monsen, ed., *Research, Successful Approaches* (Chicago: The American Dietetic Association, 1991).

19. M. Feinberg, J. Ireland-Ripert, and J. C. Flavier, "Validated Data Banks on Food Composition: Concepts for Modeling Information," in Simopoulos and Butrum, *International Food Data Bases*, pp. 49–93.

20. J. O'Brien, "Problems in Nutritional Analysis," *Trends in Food Science & Technology* 2 (1991): 283–285.

21. D. A. T. Southgate and H. Greenfield, "Principles for the Preparation of Nutritional Data Bases and Food Composition Tables," in Simopoulos and Butrum, *International Food Data Bases*, pp. 27–48.

database. This is especially important if data from databases in different countries are to be exchanged and incorporated. For example, the United States and the United Kingdom have different definitions and methods for determining carbohydrate, dietary fiber, and energy values.

If food composition data are gathered from several sources and aggregated, the information must be reviewed carefully (by food names and descriptions, sampling scheme, number of samples, and analytical method) to determine if, indeed, the data apply to the same food and which values should be used in the database. It might be necessary to weight the values based on market share or perhaps on the number of samples from each source. Databases used for dietary assessment should ideally have no missing values because the use of incomplete databases may result in underestimation of daily intakes. Database developers may impute values that are missing on the basis of information available for similar foods or by using recipe formulations. Rand et al. provide guidelines for imputation and recipe calculations.[22] Imputed and calculated values in a database should be clearly identified and replaced by analytical values when they become available.

Documentation

Database compilers should document the sources of data and the decisions made in deriving values. Because it is difficult to provide documentation directly with a computerized database, it is usually necessary to keep a separate document with notes, imputations, recipes, etc. This documentation should be made available to database users upon request. Documentation is also useful when a database is updated, since this enables the database manager to compare current decisions with previous ones. Rand et al. discuss issues related to database documentation.[23]

Nutrient Variation

Ideally, food composition databases should allow space for information about the number of samples analyzed and the variance (e.g., a standard deviation) around the mean value. An indication of the variance gives the user some idea of the confidence to be put in the mean value. It also reminds the user that printed values are not exact. Professionals in the field of nutrition are generally aware of the many causes for nutrient variation (ge-

22. Rand et al., *Compiling Data for Food Composition Data Bases.*
23. Rand et al., *Compiling Data for Food Composition Data Bases.*

netic, environmental, processing, sampling, analytical); however, they sometimes are unaware of the magnitude of the variation. Uninitiated users are apt to assume that the values printed in a database are absolute. Unfortunately, standard deviations are less meaningful when applied to nutrient values based on calculations (e.g., energy or carbohydrate by difference), and they may be difficult to apply to values compiled or aggregated from various sources.

Food Descriptions

Appropriate and adequate food descriptions are essential to locate and enter foods in databases and to retrieve information about foods from them. Discussions of food descriptors are found in McCann et al.,[24] Pennington and Butrum,[25] and Truswell et al.[26] A database should be internally consistent with descriptive terms (brand names, processing terms, and cooking terms) and abbreviations to assist the user in developing retrieval terms and organizing retrieved information. If consistent terminology is used, the user, when viewing a computer printout or hard copy database, can more readily discern the foods available in the database and the subtle differences among similar foods. Table 6.1 provides examples of variations of descrip-

Table 6.1. Various permutations of descriptive terms for several foods

apricots, cnd, med syrup, Del Monte
Del Monte canned apricots in medium syrup
medium syrup canned apricots, Del Monte
canned apricots, Del Monte, with medium syrup
beef hot dogs, Oscar Mayer
franks, beef, Oscar Mayer
Oscar Mayer frankfurters, all beef
all beef weiners, Oscar Mayer
baked potato with cheese, Stouffers, frozen
potato, baked with cheese topping, frzn, Stouffers
Stouffers cheese potato, frozen
cheese topped potato, frozen, Stouffers

24. A. McCann, J. A. T. Pennington, E. D. Smith, J. M. Holden, D.Soergel, and R. C. Wiley, "FDA's Factored Food Vocabulary for Food Product Description," *Journal of the American Dietetic Association* 88 (1988): 336–341.

25. J. A. T. Pennington and R. R. Butrum, "Food Descriptions Using Taxonomy and the 'Langual' System," *Trends in Food Science & Technology* 2 (1991): 285–288.

26. A. S. Truswell, D. J. Bateson, K. C. Madafiglio, J. A. T. Pennington, W. M. Rand, and J. C. Klensin, "Committee Report: INFOODS Guidelines for Describing Foods: A Systematic Approach to Describing Foods to Facilitate International Exchange of Food Composition Data," *Journal of Food Composition and Analysis* 4 (1991): 18–38.

tive terms for several foods. The practices used to establish consistency within a database should be documented, and the database (especially new or updated entries) should be reviewed for consistency. For foods that have more than one name, a preferred name should be selected and cross-referenced to other names.

LANGUAL is a standard food description language originally developed for use by the United States Food and Drug Administration (FDA).[27] It describes foods from 15 factors (Figure 6.1) and allows for efficient computerized retrieval of foods based on various descriptive terms for these factors. LANGUAL is currently used in databases in several countries other than the United States. The International Interface Standard, developed under contract by the US FDA,[28] includes the LANGUAL descriptors plus some additional descriptive terms (Figure 6.1). The purpose of the interface is to improve international exchange of data by providing clear descriptions of foods. It provides a means of retrieval among food-related databases based on the descriptive characteristics of foods.

Database Organization

Food composition databases are usually organized into a hierarchy of food groups, subgroups, and further subdivisions. This organization is particularly important with hard copy databases, where it assists users in locating foods. Food groupings based on food type (e.g., fish, eggs, poultry, meat, nuts, fruits, vegetables, grain products) are usually straightforward and internationally understood. Food groupings based on food use (e.g., beverage, snack, dessert, breakfast cereal, entree, fast food) are culture-dependent. A hard copy database that is intended for international use might best be organized alphabetically or by food type, rather than by food use.

With expansions in food technology, food groupings have become complex, and the boundaries between the groups have become increasingly fuzzy. Many products seem to fall into several food groups, and it is difficult to classify mixed dishes which may contain grain products, vegetables, cheese sauce, and/or animal flesh. For example, frozen asparagus with cheese in a pastry shell might be grouped with vegetables, grain products, or entrees.

Nonetheless, food groupings are important and should be retained for national use. The way people think about foods and classify them determines, in part, when and how they eat them. An understanding of dietary

27. (a) McCann et al., "FDA's Factored Food Vocabulary." (b) Pennington and Butrum, "Food Descriptions Using Taxonomy."

28. J. A. T. Pennington and T. C. Hendricks, "Proposal for an International Interface Standard for Food Databases," *Food Additives and Contaminants* 9 (1992): 265–275.

INTERNATIONAL INTERFACE STANDARD FOR FOOD DATABASES
FACTORS
1. Product Type
2. Food Source
3. Part of Plant or Animal
4. Physical State, Shape or Form
5. Extent of Heat Treatment
6. Cooking Method
7. Treatment Applied
8. Preservation Method
9. Packing Medium
10. Container or Wrapping
11. Food Contact Surface
12. Consumer Group/Dietary Use
13. Geographic Places and Regions
a. Area of origin (grown/produced)
b. Area of processing
c. Area of consumption
14. Cuisine
15. Adjunct Characteristics of Food
INGREDIENTS
May Include Quantities and/or Recipe Procedures
FOOD DATA
Food Composition Data
• Date and location of collection
• Sampling scheme
• Number of samples
• Analytical methods
• Nutrient values (mean ± SD, median, range)
Food Consumption Data
• Population surveyed
• Number of people
• Number of days of diet records
• Methods of assessing consumption
• Demographic variables (age, sex, region, race, income, urbanization, season, disease status, smoking status, pregnancy, lactation, activity level)
• Food composition database used to assess intakes
• Daily intakes of individual foods
FOOD/FOOD PRODUCT IDENTIFICATION (NAME/NUMBER)
FOOD NAME SYNONYMS
In the Same or Other Languages
OTHER FOOD DESCRIPTORS
Language of Food Name (e.g., English, French, Spanish)
Latin Food Name (genus & species)
Variety/Cultivar
Agricultural Production Conditions
• Season
• Climate
• Year of harvest/production
• Soil type
• Fertilizer treatment
• Pesticide treatment
Maturity/Ripeness
Grade
Animal Feed Supplements
Color
Percent Refuse
Storage Conditions
• Length (time)
• Temperature
• Humidity
• Location
Location(s) of Preparation/ Manufacture/Preservation/ (e.g., home, industry, institutional kitchen, restaurant)
Manufacturer/Institution/Restaurant Name & Address
Serving Portion Size & Weight (g)
Specific Uses of the Food (e.g., holidays, religious events)
Other Coding Systems (e.g., EUROCODE 2)
DATA SOURCE(S)
Literature Citations
Databases (hardcopy/computerized)
Food Labels
Laboratory Data

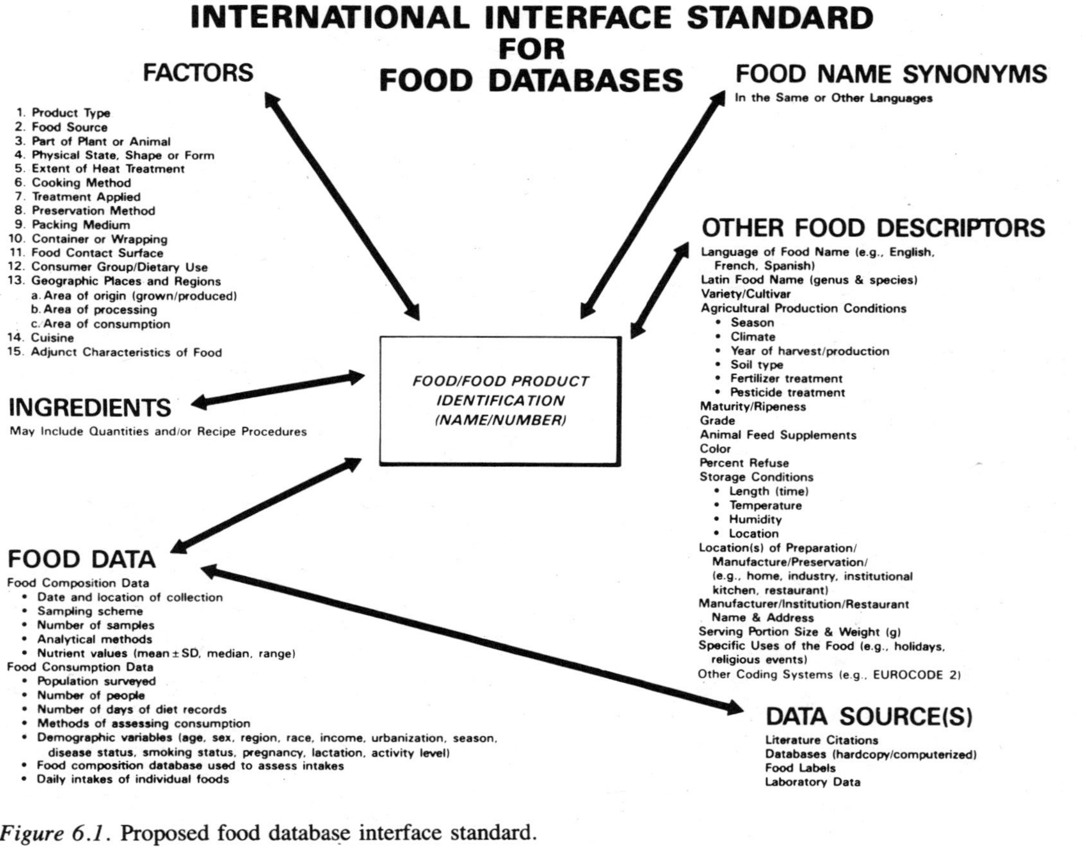

Figure 6.1. Proposed food database interface standard.

Source: Reproduced from J. A. T. Pennington and T. C. Hendricks, "Proposal for an International Interface Standard for Food Databases," *Food Additives and Contaminants* 9 (1992): 265–275, with the approval of the authors and Taylor and Francis.

patterns is important for assessing the relationships between diet and health and disease. EUROFOODS has provided a food grouping hierarchy called EUROCODE for use with western European foods.[29] The "product type" factor in LANGUAL represents a United States food grouping system. EUROCODE and other food grouping systems can be used with the International Interface Standard (Figure 6.1). This allows retrieval of information based on characteristics inherent to the food as well as retrievals based on the use of the food in cultures with different food groupings.

Updating

Periodic updates of a database are essential so that it reflects the current food supply. Updates include changing values for products and adding and deleting foods and nutrients. The changes may result from improved analytical methods or product reformulations. It is important to document the dates and reasons for changes. A copy of a database used with a specific food consumption survey should be "frozen" (no updates) to allow researchers access to it if they find an error, want to do some time trend analyses, or simply want to review at various issues. Another copy of the database could be updated, if desired, to accommodate an upcoming survey.

User Knowledge

Database users should be provided with information about the database, such as its organizational structure, foods and nutrients included, and software capabilities. This information could also mention concerns about nutrient variation, warn against assessing dietary status from a one-day record, and provide other information to guide the user. New users may not read the information at first, but they may come back to it when problems arise. The latest edition of *McCance and Widdowson's The Composition of Foods* provides information on sources of data, evaluation of data, definitions of nutrients, nutrient variation, and bioavailability; it also includes a section entitled "Potential Pitfalls When Using the Tables."[30] The Australian database[31] has explanatory sections dealing with data sources, sampling, analytical methods, and nutrient variability.

29. "EUROCODE 2 System," in *Development of a Merged Food Composition Database* (Final Report to the European Community, DG XIII, February 1986), pp. 132–155.

30. B. Holland, A. A. Welch, I. D. Unwin, D. H. Buss, A. A. Paul, and D. A. T. Southgate, ed., *McCance and Widdowson's The Composition of Foods*, 5th ed. (Cambridge, U.K.: The Royal Society of Chemistry and Ministry of Agriculture, Fisheries and Food, 1991).

31. R. English and J. Lewis, *Nutritional Values of Australian Foods* (Canberra: Australian Government Publishing Service, 1992).

B. Nonnutrient Composition Databases

Nonnutrient food components include direct food additives (butylated hydroxytoluene, butylated hydroxyanisole, nitrites, flavors, colors, aluminum compounds), naturally occurring components (plant hormones, nitrites, phytate, oxalate, mercury, solanine), pesticide residues, veterinary residues (hormones), and indirect food additives (packaging materials, lead).[32] The FAO has set Acceptable Daily Intakes (ADI) for some of these substances.[33]

Nonnutrient databases are often generated as part of food monitoring programs. Louekari and Salminen[34] summarized six food monitoring programs which included analyses for nonnutrients. The Australian National Residue Survey covers cadmium, lead, arsenic, mercury, selected pesticides, and more than a hundred other compounds. The Danish Food Monitoring System includes heavy metals, pesticides, mycotoxins, and nitrate. The Finnish Survey of Foods of Animal Origin covers cadmium, lead, mercury, selected pesticides, and residues of animal medications. The Netherlands nutrition surveillance program includes trace elements, nitrogen, organochlorine and organophosphorus compounds, and pesticides. The United Kingdom Food Surveillance program covers mercury, cadmium, and lead. The United States Total Diet Study includes toxic elements, radionuclides, industrial chemicals, and pesticides.

Nonnutrient Database Concerns

Databases for nonnutrients are less well developed than those for nutrients because they have not been so routinely analyzed, there are so many of them, and the levels in foods may be highly variable (more so than nutrients). The presence of a nonnutrient may be dependent on environmental accidents, processing variables, brand specificity (e.g., a food additive), or defined by regulations that differ among countries. The presence of a non-

32. (a) G. B. Guest and S. C. Fitzpatrick, "Estimating the Dietary Intake of Veterinary Drug Residues," in I. Macdonald, ed., *Monitoring Dietary Intakes* (New York: Springer-Verlag, 1991), pp. 204–212. (b) L. L. Katan, "Packaging Materials," in Macdonald, *Monitoring Dietary Intakes*, pp. 221–227. (c) K. Louekari and S. Salminen, "Non-Nutrient Databases," *Trends in Food Science & Technology* 2 (1991): 289–292. (d) National Research Council, Food and Nutrition Board, Committee on Food Protection, *Toxicants Occurring Naturally in Foods*, 2d ed., (Washington, D.C.: National Academy Press, 1973).

33. *Pesticide Residues in Foods 1991: Report of the Joint Meeting of the FAO Panel of Experts on Pesticide Residues in Food and the Environment and a WHO Expert Group on Pesticide Residues* (Rome: Food and Agriculture Organization of the United Nations, 1991).

34. Louekari and Salminen, "Non-Nutrient Databases."

nutrient is more likely to follow a "hit or miss" situation, which makes database development difficult. For example, if there are many misses (i.e., zeros) and only a few hits, it may be inappropriate to average the results. Ranges of nonnutrients are not useful in this situation. The question remains as to what data to put into the database. Should it be an average of all results (with all the misses) or an average of only the hits? A plot of distributions would probably be more informative.

Regulatory agencies in charge of food monitoring programs may develop sampling schemes skewed to increase the number of hits. The data resulting from these programs will not be representative of the food supply, although the monitoring agency may increase its chances of finding violations. The information in nonnutrient databases should be clearly identified as being based on sampling geared to finding representative levels or to improving public health (i.e., focused on foods with potential problems).

Foods included in monitoring programs are often selected because of their importance in the diet (i.e., foods regularly consumed in large quantities) and because high concentrations of nonnutrients have been observed in previous studies. Criteria for selecting nonnutrients to be monitored and stored in databases have been proposed by the United Nations Environment Program.[35] These include toxicity (potential risk), frequency of known intoxications, persistence, and quantities discharged into the environment. EUROFOODS has begun work on the selection and classification of substances for inclusion in nonnutrient databases.[36] The duplicate portion technique may be appropriate for evaluating the diets of groups who have an unusually high risk of exposure or who live in contaminated areas.[37]

Some of the nutrient database concerns mentioned previously also apply to nonnutrient databases. Ideally, nonnutrient databases should use the same food names and descriptors and be maintained on the same systems as nutrient databases. Dietary changes that attempt to reduce exposure to nonnutrients may have an impact on nutrient intakes. For example, changes in dietary patterns to decrease exposure to aluminum (e.g., by decreasing intake of baked products and processed cheese) might affect dietary intakes of calcium and iron. Replacing one type of food additive with another (e.g., using iodates instead of bromates as dough conditioners) could affect nutri-

35. *Assessment of Chemical Contaminants in Food* (Geneva: Global Environment Monitoring System. United Nations Environment Program; Food and Agriculture Organization, World Health Organization, 1988).

36. W. Becker and E. Danfors, eds., *Proceedings of the 4th EUROFOODS Meeting* (Uppsala: National Food Administration, 1990).

37. *Guidelines for the Study of Dietary Intakes of Chemical Contaminants; GEMS: Global Environmental Monitoring System* (Geneva: World Health Organization, 1985 [WHO Offset Publication no. 87]).

ent and nonnutrient intakes, depending on the chemical compound included in the additives. Databases with both nutrients and nonnutrients on the same computer system can be used to determine the effects of potential changes in diet, in food processing, or agricultural practices on nutrient and nonnutrient intakes for various age-sex groups in a population.

C. Food Consumption Databases

Many countries have government agencies that conduct national or regional food consumption surveys to assess the dietary status of the population or selected population groups. The collection of demographic information (age, sex, race, urbanization, income, etc.) allows for the information on dietary status to be linked to these variables. This allows subgroups at risk of nutritional problems to be identified and helps define public health programs to serve those in need.

Government agencies or academic institutions may conduct smaller studies of specific population groups to assess the intake of food, nutrients, or other food components. The purpose may be to assess public health, to research relationships between diet and disease, or to identify subjects needing dietary intervention.

Assessment of dietary intake of nutrients or nonnutrients requires the merging of a food composition database with a food consumption database. Food consumption databases provide a list of the foods consumed and quantities ingested by each individual included in a survey or study. A code number or some other identifier is used to link each food consumed to the same food in a food consumption database.

Before food consumption surveys or studies are conducted, a food composition database, linked to the survey tool, is usually in place. The food composition database may be increased or modified as necessary during or after the study so that it reflects the foods consumed by the participants and includes the nutrients important to the study.

Methods to Assess Food Intake

Methods to determine individual food intakes include diet histories, 24-hour recalls, dietary records, food frequencies, weighed intakes, and duplicate portions.[38] A system to conduct 24-hour recalls on-line at a computer

38. (a) *Guidelines for the Study of Dietary Intakes*. (b) J. H. Hankin, "Dietary Intake Methodology," in Monsen, *Research, Successful Approaches*, pp. 173–194. (c) C. Medlin and J. D. Skin-

terminal was developed by the Nutrition Coordinating Center at the University of Minnesota and used successfully in the Third Health and Nutrition Examination Survey in the United States.[39] This system probes for details about the foods consumed by asking about added fat, type of fat, added salt, etc.

Other methods for obtaining information on food consumption include food balance sheets, national food disappearance data with corrections for exports and waste, and household inventories (food disappearance in a home divided by the number of persons in the household). These methods may be used with national surveys to assess the adequacy of the food supply. The information derived from them is usually expressed per capita and cannot be linked to specific population subgroups by age, sex, or other variables.

Concerns about Food Consumption Databases

The assessment of food intake is the weakest link in the attempt to establish relationships between diet and health and disease. The goal of dietary intake studies is usually to capture a picture of "usual" food intake. Unfortunately, the methods currently used rely either on selective memory of foods previously eaten or on record-keeping, both of which tend to cause changes in food intake patterns. Twenty-four hour recalls and food frequencies rely on memory to recall the specific foods and quantities eaten on the previous day or the frequency of types of foods consumed in the previous three months or other time period, respectively. This is difficult, especially for the young, the elderly, and those who take no active role in food purchase or preparation. Parents or caregivers generally need to respond for children and for some elderly persons.

Food diaries, weighed intakes, and duplicate portions may also alter the usual eating patterns. The recording and weighing of foods has the effect of decreasing food intake and changing food selections to more healthful or appropriate foods. The honesty of the participant in reporting or recording

---

ner, "Individual Dietary Intake Methodology: 50–Year Review of Progress," *Journal of the American Dietetic Association* 88 (1988): 1250–1257. (d) J. A. T. Pennington, "Commentary on Diet and Health; Associations Between Diet and Health: The Use of Food Consumption Measurements, Nutrient Databases, and Dietary Guidelines," *Journal of the American Dietetic Association* 88 (1988): 1221–1224. (e) J. A. T. Pennington, "Methods for Obtaining Food Consumption Information," in Macdonald, *Monitoring Dietary Intakes*, pp. 3–8.

39. M. McDowell, R. R. Briefel, R. A. Warren, I. M. Buzzard, D. Feskanich, and S. N. Gardner, "The Dietary Data Collection System: An Automated Interview and Coding System for NHANES III," *Proceedings of the 14th National Nutrient Databank Conference* (New York: CBORD Group, 1990), pp. 125–131.

dietary intake is also sometimes suspect. Some participants unfortunately try to please the investigator by consuming (or claiming to consume) more healthy foods, fewer alcoholic beverages, and fewer desserts and snacks for the days of the study. Assessing the dietary intake of an individual requires more days of dietary recalls or records than assessing the dietary intake of a group of people. A one-day recall or record from a large group of people is sufficient to assess the group dietary profile. The dietary status of an individual is determined by repeated recalls or records (e.g., 7–14 days), depending upon the nutrients of concern. Some nutrients require more days of dietary intake to assess their status.[40]

Although continued improvements in food composition databases are important, the methods for assessing food intake must also improve if accurate associations are to be drawn between diet and health. Efforts are underway to improve dietary assessment methods. The first International Conference on Dietary Assessment Methods was held in St. Paul, Minnesota, in September 1992, and a second in Boston in 1994.

D. Implications

Computerization

Computerization of food composition and consumption data has become essential to minimize errors, reduce time-consuming calculations, and provide fast retrievals of information. Computerization allows for ease in updating databases (adding and deleting foods and nutrients or changing values). Also available with many databases are software components providing for recipe calculations, product reformulations, dietary assessments, comparisons of daily intakes with recommended intakes, and suggestions for patients or clients on improving diets.

Computer technology cannot, however, compensate for inaccuracies in food intake data or food composition data or for inappropriate standards of intake of physiological measures. The design of studies requires decisions about which specific tools to use, and the results derived from studies are, in part, dependent on the tools selected. To avoid erroneous conclusions, care must be taken to make appropriate decisions at each of the various steps in a study. The comparison of values or results from different studies requires additional considerations, because the studies being compared may

40. C. T. Sempos, A. C. Looker, C. L. Johnson, and C. E. Woteki, "The Importance of Within-Person Variability in Estimating Prevalence," in Macdonald, *Monitoring Dietary Intakes*, pp. 99–109.

have used different food consumption methods, food composition databases, dietary standards, and/or statistical analyses.[41]

Food Description

Common to the three types of databases described here and to other food-related databases (e.g., food production, sales, cost, and distribution) is the importance of the food name and its descriptors. Foods in databases must be adequately, appropriately, and consistently described if information is to shared and linked among databases, data are to be retrieved from databases, and conclusions are to be made about the relationship of diet to health and disease. A system for naming and describing foods using LANGUAL has been described by D. Soergel et al.[42]

Generic foods are needed in some databases. When included, they should be described as clearly as possible. They are used in food consumption databases for survey participants who have difficulty in remembering details about what or how much they ate. Thus, there is need for generic terms such as steak, apple, sandwich, beef stew, milk, etc., which are not further described. The food composition database for food consumption surveys must also include these foods. Their nutritional profiles can be based on the most similar commonly consumed items in the database (e.g., red Delicious apple or whole milk) or weighted averages of nutrient values for all types of steaks, milks, apples, sandwiches, or beef stews. The serving portion may default (if the survey participant cannot remember the amount consumed) to a standard or average serving based on previous surveys.

Basic to sharing and exchanging data about food composition and food consumption are several questions. How do we know if two or more foods in different databases are really the same? Having the same name (or synonym) and descriptive characteristics is a good start. We need to consider national regulations that pertain to fortification, nutrition labeling, use of food additives, and food standards as well as cultural issues relating to processing, preparation, and cuisine. The use of LANGUAL and the International Interface Standard may help to answer some of these questions. Another question is, Are the nutrients or contaminants really the same? Are we talking about the same chemical molecule and did we measure it in the same way? Finally, Is the sample we analyzed representative of our country and will it be representative of another country?

41. Pennington, "Commentary on Diet and Health."

42. D. Soergel, J. A. T. Pennington, A. McCann, J. M. Holden, E. C. Smith, and R. C. Wiley, "Improving Access to Food Data: A System Model for a Food Database Network," *Journal of the American Dietetic Association* 92 (1992): 78–82.

Retrieval

It is important to be able to retrieve information about nutrient and non-nutrient composition and food consumption from databases to address questions of food safety, nutritional quality, or dietary status. Retrievals may be based on nutrients, contaminants, descriptive characteristics of foods, or consumption patterns. Retrievals based on descriptive characteristics are possible with the use of LANGUAL descriptive terms and with additional descriptive terms in the International Interface Standard. Possible retrievals from food composition and consumption databases are lists of

foods containing more than 1 mg aluminum per 100 g
foods that contribute 15% or more of the recommended allowance for iron in the diets of women 20–35 years of age
canned foods containing corn
foods derived from or containing peanuts, consumed by pregnant women
records for persons who met recommended calcium allowances but did not consume milk or cheese products
consumers (by specified age-sex groups, in decreasing order) of aspartame, cholesterol, saturated fatty acids, etc.
consumers (by specified age-sex groups, in decreasing order) of soups, fried chicken, cakes, chocolate chip cookies, etc.

Diet and Health

Government and academic institutions in various countries are reaching conclusions about recommended dietary allowances for nutrients, acceptable daily intakes of contaminants, relationships between diet and disease, and dietary guidelines to improve the health of population groups. The nutrition community is interested in the conclusions reached in other countries and the bases for them. Data about food composition and results from food consumption surveys need to be shared and exchanged nationally and internationally. We have begun to share and exchange information from studies concerning relationships between diet and diseases such as heart attacks, cancer, strokes, and diabetes. We do not know if the conclusions reached in one country are valid in other countries. We need to retain important cultural distinctions regarding food processing, preparation, and consumption. We need to identify unique differences in food composition among countries and food consumption patterns among population groups to determine what effect (if any) these differences have on health status. Sharing information on the results of food composition and food consumption studies may prevent needless repetition of studies previously completed and allow researchers to address more urgent questions. Sharing information may also allow those of us in more technically developed countries to join together to solve nutrition-related crises in Third World countries.

7. Reference Update

ROBYN C. FRANK
National Agricultural Library, U.S. Department of Agriculture

Since the early 1970s, the number of food and nutrition reference works published has risen dramatically. Increased public awareness of the causal relationship between diet and health as well as increased funding for human nutrition research have resulted in new and sometimes conflicting research results and a confused and often misinformed public. Reference works are updated frequently in order to present the latest scientific findings that support dietary recommendations.

The *Guide to Sources for Agricultural and Biological Research* is the most recent major compilation of reference tools for food science and human nutrition. It was published in 1981 and edited by J. Richard Blanchard and Lois Farrell (University of California Press). This immense work serves as the basic guide to the literature of the agricultural sciences. The book's Chapter F, compiled by Phyllis Reich, is on food science and nutrition and is organized as follows: literature guides and bibliographies of bibliographies, abstracts and indexes, bibliographies, reviews, dictionaries and encyclopedias, directories, handbooks, manuals, texts, food tables, dietary requirements, legislation, regulations, standards, food inspection, patents, and statistics.

This chapter update lists major reference works in the fields of food science and human nutrition published since 1980. At first glance, this listing may appear to be incomplete, but the intent of this chapter is to supplement, not supersede, the Blanchard and Farrell work. Those titles which have been updated in this chapter bear a reference number preceded by the *F* corresponding to those in Chapter F in Blanchard and Farrell. Several monographic works listed here are also listed in Chapter 4; they are identified in this chapter by *CORE* in their citations. Most citations have annotations.

Most of the reference materials cited in this chapter are directed toward researchers, academicians, advanced students, policy makers, and health professionals. The area of food service management is not within the scope of this work, but a few general titles are included. In general, consumer-oriented and practical application materials have not been included.

Reference materials are listed under the following headings:

A. Literature Guides
B. Abstracts and Indexes
C. Bibliographies
D. Reviews
E. Dictionaries and Encyclopedias
F. Directories
G. Handbooks, Manuals, and Texts
    General
    Food Science/Technology
    Food/Nutrition Policy
    Human Nutrition
    Food Service Management
H. Food Tables
I. Dietary Requirements and Recommendations
J. Legislation, Regulations, Standards, and Inspection
K. Statistics, Surveys, and Reports

Current awareness services, which keep researchers and pratitioners abreast of new developments or publications in their specific fields, were not included under the abstracts and indexes section. Current awareness services may include recent accession lists, clipping services, selective dissemination of information (SDI), and table of contents services. Many major database producers such as *BIOSIS, Chemical Abstracts*, and the National Technical Information Service provide current awareness services in specific areas of interest. Also, many professional journals include book and article reviews. These journals were also excluded from this update.

The inclusion of titles in this list is a bit more restrictive than in Blanchard and Farrell, since some of the important titles appear in the core monographic lists in Chapter 4 of this book. In this reference listing, there is a bias toward United States food science and human nutrition publications, although many of the major new tools for the Third World are identified. Some items were not included because they did not present the latest dietary recommendations. As with any compilation of this type, some items may have been overlooked.

The author thanks to Sandy Facinoli, Shirley King Evans, and Rebecca Thompson at the National Agricultural Library for their assistance and support in preparing this chapter.

A. Literature Guides

Green, Syd. *Key Guide to Information Sources in Food Science and Technology.* London and New York: Mansell Publishing Limited, 1985. 231p.
This extensive work with a British perspective is directed toward librarians and food science and technology researchers, educators, and students. The author traces the history and scope of food science and technology presenting it primarily a narrative form. The bulk of the volume covers food science and technology literature, including reference works, journals, bibliographic databases, general works, specialized information, and non-book materials. A directory of food science and technology organizations is provided.

Haselbauer, Kathleen J. *Research Guide to the Health Sciences: Medical, Nutritional and Environmental.* New York: Greenwood Press, 1987. 655p.
Directed toward health professionals, this book lists reference works and information sources in the health sciences. The chapter on nutrition, dietetics, and food science includes bibliographies, indexes, abstracts, databases, dictionaries, encyclopedias, directories, food composition tables and dietary standards, statistical surveys, handbooks and sourcebooks, textbooks and treatises, reviews, and suggested popular works for the lay public. Remaining chapters deal with other health science subjects such as oncology, psychology, etc.

Prytherch, Raymond John and Suzanne Stanley. *Food, Cookery, and Diet: An Information Guide.* Aldershot, Hants, England; and Brookfield, VT: Gower, 1989. 109p.
Written for food service professionals, students, and amateurs, this volume examines the body of literature published about food, the production and processing of food, preparation and cookery, and the effect of food components on human metabolism.

Special Libraries Association. *Tools of the Profession.* 2nd edition. Washington, DC: Special Libraries Association, 1991. 192p.
The chapter (29 pages) on food, agriculture, and nutrition identifies the key resources used by librarians and information professionals working in the food industry, agribusiness, academia, government, and nonprofit organizations. Heavy emphasis on food industry topics.

Szilard, Paula. *Food and Nutrition Information Guide.* Littleton, CO: Libraries Unlimited, 1987. 358p.
Identifies standard reference materials as well as diet manuals, nutrition and food consumption surveys, government publications, food standards, regulation, and food service. Provides useful tips on how to locate food information in libraries and databases.

B. Abstracts and Indexes

Foods Adlibra. Minneapolis, MN: Foods Adlibra Publications, 1974–. Semimonthly.
Contains abstracts of current food industry literature covering the topics of food

technology, food packaging, new food products, world food economics, nutrition, marketing, and patents.

Leatherhead Food RA Abstracts from Current Scientific and Technical Literature. Surrey, U.K.: Leatherhead Food Research Association, 1947–. Monthly.
Contains the nearly 1,700 abstracts that are added each month to the bibliographic database (FROSTI) produced by the Leatherhead Food Research Association.

C. Bibliographies

BioSciences Information Service of Biological Abstracts. *International Bibliography of Eating Disorders, 1977–1986*. Philadelphia: BIOSIS, 1987.
Includes over 2,500 technical references covering eating disorders. The categories range from behavioral biology to metabolism and public health.

Food and Agriculture Organization of the United Nations. *Nutritional Implications of Food Aid: An Annotated Bibliography*. Rome: Food and Agriculture Organization of the United Nations, 1985. 118p. (FAO Food and Nutrition Papers no. 33)
This annotated bibliography lists research reports, evaluation studies, and reviews of operational aspects of the nutritional impact of food and programs throughout the world. In general, all of the entries stress the difficulty in measuring the nutritional impact of supplementary feeding programs.

Food and Agriculture Organization of the United Nations. Statistics Division. *Bibliography of Food Consumption Surveys*. Rome: Food and Agriculture Organization of the United Nations, 1987. 49p. (FAO Food and Nutrition Papers no. 18, rev. 2.)
Includes household budget and food consumption surveys conducted in different countries from 1970–1985. For more detailed methodological and statistical texts, cross-references are made to issues of the *Review of Food Consumption Surveys*, FAO, Rome.

Freedman, Robert L. *Human Food Uses: A Cross-Cultural Comprehensive Annotated Bibliography*. Westport, CT: Greenwood Press, 1981. 552p. (*Supplement*. 1983. 387p.)
Various aspects of food in human culture are covered for the use of scholars, scientists, and professionals in the area of health care delivery. The extensive bibliography is organized by cultural terms, and listed entries (numbering 9,097) are also listed alphabetically by author. All but a few of the 4,025 entrees in the *Supplement* are annotated. The majority of the citations are in English, although major works and some lesser-known material are represented for most of the world's more common languages.

Kader, Adel A. and Christi M. Heintz. *Gamma Irradiation of Fresh Fruits and Vegetables: An Indexed Reference List (1965–1982)*. Davis: University of California, Dept. of Pomology, 1983. 55p.
A bibliography of 648 titles covering the literature in this subject.

MacLeod, Scott. *Food Systems in Asia: A Select Bibliography on Changing Food Habits in Asia*. Vancouver: Institute of Asian Research, 1989. 73p. (New Directions in Asian Development Working Paper no. 1.)

Newman, Jacqueline M. *Melting Pot: An Annotated Bibliography and Guide to Food and Nutrition Information for Ethnic Groups in America*. New York: Garland Publishing, 1986. 194p.
Directed toward food sociologists and food and nutrition professionals, this book contains annotated references concerning the food habits, customs, behaviors, nutrition, and health-related dietary concerns of the principal U.S. ethnic groups. Includes lists of cookbooks that give advice on ingredients, food preparation techniques, and food practices of each ethnic group.

Orta, John. *Computer Applications in Nutrition and Dietetics: An Annotated Bibliography*. New York: Garland Publishing, 1988. 242p. (Garland Reference Library of Social Science Vol. 428)
Contains 201 annotated entries concerning the use of computer programs and databases in nutrition-related areas. The entries are grouped into six principal categories: normal nutrition, clinical nutrition, community nutrition, management activities (functions, labor relations, information systems including nutrient analysis databases), food service operations, and computer-assisted nutrition and dietetic education.

U. S. Department of Agriculture. National Agricultural Library. *Quick Bibliography Series/Special Reference Briefs Series*. Beltsville, MD: National Agricultural Library.
Quick Bibliographies lists citations from AGRICOLA. *Special Reference Briefs* are selected from several sources. Current food and nutrition titles include *Cultural Perspectives on Food and Nutrition* (April 1992, 81p.); *Food Service Management: Printed Material and Audiovisuals* (April 1992, 94p.); *Infant Nutrition* (January 1987–March 1991, 281 citations); *Nutrition and AIDS* (May 1991, 23p.).

United States Agency for International Development. Office of Nutrition. U.S. Department of Agriculture. Office of International Cooperation and Development. Technical Assistance Division. Nutrition Economics Group. *Food Consumption and Nutrition Effects of International Development Projects and Programs: An Annotated Bibliography*. Washington, DC: U.S. Government Printing Office, 1983. 100p.
Deals with the impact of agricultural policies on nutrition in developing countries. It is divided into three main categories: (1) causes and solutions of malnutrition problems from a technical or policy perspective; (2) effects of particular development programs and policies on nutrition; and (3) guidelines and methodologies for exploring the nutritional impact of development projects.

University of Wisconsin-Madison. Food Research Institute. *Food Safety 1990: An Annotated Bibliography of the Literature*. Boston: Butterworth-Heinemann, 1991.
Unlike most annotated bibliographies, this book has chapters containing interpretations of the literature. Each chapter is followed by a bibliography. Topics cover diet and health, safety of food components, and foodborne microbial illness.

D. Reviews

Advances in Food and Nutrition Research. Vol. 33–. San Diego: Academic Press, 1989–. (Continues *Advances in Food Research.*) Annual. CORE [F148]
The expanded title recognizes the integral relationships betweeen food science and nutrition and presents reviews of topics in both areas. The change encourages nutritionists and food scientists to become more familiar with relevant advances in interrelated areas. Important for biochemists, chemists, food scientists, nutritionists, and others interested in analysis.

Advances in Meat Research. Vol. 1–. Westport, CT: AVI Publishing, 1985–. (A VNR/AVI Book. Available from: Van Nostrand Reinhold, Florence, KY.)
Each monograph presents up-to-date information on a specific theme related to meat research, e.g.; meat and poultry microbiology, restructured meat and poultry products, and collagen.

Annual Review of Nutrition. Vol. 1–. Palo Alto, CA: Annual Reviews, 1981–.
Composed of contributed review papers. Each volume focuses on basic research, clinical science, and epidemiology/public health issues related to human nutrition.

AVI Food Products Formulary Series. 4 vols. Westport, Conn.: AVI Publishing, 1974–1982. CORE

Bristol-Myers Squibb/Mead Johnson Nutrition Symposia. Vol. 8–. San Diego: Academic Press, 1990–. (Continues *Bristol-Myers Nutrition Symposia.*)
Volumes focus on specific topics such as malnutrition. Exemplary titles are *Chronic Diet-Associated Infantile Diarrhea, New Techniques in Nutrition Research,* and *Nutrition and the Origins of Disease.*

Contemporary Issues in Clinical Nutrition. Edited by Richard Rivlin. New York: John Wiley and Sons, 1981.
Each annual volume focuses on a specific topic such as *Nutrition and Diabetes, Nutrition and the Skin,* and *Vitamins and Cancer Prevention.*

Current Topics in Nutrition and Disease. Edited by Antony A. Albanese. Vol. 1–. New York: Liss, 1977–.
Titles cover specific topics such as *New Protective Roles for Selected Nutrients, Mineral Homeostatics in the Elderly, Fat Distribution During Growth and Later Health Outcomes,* and *Essential and Toxic Trace Elements in Human Health and Disease.*

Ellis Horwood Series in Food Science and Technology. New York: Van Nostrand Reinhold.
A monographic series that focuses on a specific food science issue in each volume. Topics covered include food production and food policy trends. One volume is entitled *Directory of Food and Nutrition,* by Jean Adrian, Gilberte Legrand, and Regine Frangne.

Ethnic and Regional Food Practices: A Series. Chicago, IL: American Dietetic Association, 1989–.
Includes the 1986 Exchange Lists that have been expanded to encompass regional and ethnic specialties along with cultural and dietary customs. Topics cover Mexican-American, Chinese- American, and Jewish food practices.

Food and Nutrition in History and Anthropology. Edited by J. Robson. New York: Gordon and Breach, Science Publishers, 1980–.

Titles include Vol. 1, *Food, Ecology, and Culture*, J. Robson (1980, 144p.); Vol. 2, *Famine*, J. Robson (1981, 170p.); Vol. 3, *Infant Care and Feeding in the South Pacific*, L. Marshall (1985, 356p.); Vol. 4, *Food Energy in Tropical Ecosystems*, D. J. Cattle (1985, 290p.); Vol. 5, *The Infant Feeding Triad*, B. Popkin et al. (1986, 248p.); Vol. 6, *The Effects of Undernutrition on Children's Behavior*, D. Barrett and D. Frank (1987, 348p.); Vol. 7, *Africa Food Systems in Crisis, Part One: Microperspectives*, R. Huss-Ashmore and S. H. Katz (1989, 340p.).

Frankle, Reva T. and Mei-Uih Yang. *Obesity and Weight Control: The Health Professional's Guide to Understanding and Treatment*. Rockville, MD: Aspen Publishers, 1988. 465p.

Covers contemporary weight control topics including scientific rationale, state-of-the-art treatment, weight control in the life cycle, and nutrition-related disease.

Hathcock, John N., ed. *Nutrition: Basic and Applied Science*. New York: Academic Press, 1986.

A reference source of current knowledge on specific topics. Titles include *Nutrition Toxicology* and *Vitamin A Deficiency and Its Control*.

Montville, Thomas J. *Food Microbiology*. 2 vols. Boca Raton, FL: CRC Press, 1987.

A two-volume reference set for food microbiologists that deals with the physiology of foodborne microbes at the molecular level, addressing the regulation of important intracellular processes, ranging from osmoregulation of bacterial cells to germination of spores. The intricacies and potential of new methods in microbiological assays and their scientific bases are also examined.

Morley, John E. et al., eds. *Geriatric Nutrition: A Comprehensive Review*. New York: Raven Press, 1990. 503p.

Discusses the realities and fallacies related to the role of nutrition in the aging process, nutritional deficiencies of the elderly, and the effects of age-associated diseases on nutrients. Special topics such as as nutrition and behavior and malnutrition in nursing homes are also covered.

Nestlé Nutrition S.A. *Nestlé Nutrition Workshop Series*. New York: Raven Press.

Each volume focuses on a specific perinatal or infant nutrition topic such as food allergies, weaning, and intrauterine growth retardation.

Priest, F. G. and I. Campbell. *Brewing Microbiology*. London: Elsevier Applied Science, 1987. 275p.

Progress in Clinical and Biological Research. Vol. 1–. New York: Liss, 1975–.

Covers several nutrition topics in titles such as *The Maillard Reaction in Aging, Diabetes, and Nutrition; Dietary Fat and Cancer; Nutrition and Aging;* and *Mutagens and Carcinogens in the Diet*.

E. Dictionaries and Encyclopedias

Adrian, J., G. Legrand, and R. Frangne. *Dictionary of Food and Nutrition*. Transl. by B. Weitz. Chichester, England and Weinheim, Germany; VCH Verlagsgesellschaft mbH, 1988. 233p. (Published as *Dictionnaire de Biochimie et de Nutrition*. Paris; Technique et Documentation, 1981).

Allison, Sonia. *The Cassell Food Dictionary*. Cassell, U.K.: Sterling Publishing Company, 1991. 512p.

Anderson, Kenneth N. and Lois E. Anderson. *The International Dictionary of Food & Nutrition*. New York: John Wiley, 1993. 330p.
Includes over 7,500 definitions of food ingredients, garnishes, sauces, entrees, and appetizers that are useful and may appear on menus and shopping lists. Terms appear in over forty languages. Cross-references are shown to help guide the reader to further information.

Anderson, Kenneth N. and Lois Harmon. *The Prentice-Hall Dictionary of Nutrition and Health*. Englewood Cliffs, NJ: Prentice-Hall, 1985. 257p.
A comprehensive dictionary covering the chemical composition of natural and synthetic foods, food additives and food safety laws, current concepts of clinical nutrition research, the physical effects of dietary deficiency and inborn errors of metabolism, and related basic data about human body form and function. Contains mini-articles to describe the roles of vitamins, minerals, fats, proteins, and carbohydrates in human health.

Bakker, Marilyn. *The Encyclopedia of Packaging Technology*. Herndon, VA: Institute of Packaging Professionals, 1986. 746p.
A comprehensive reference source covering information and statistics related to packaging, including food packaging.

Bender, Arnold E. *Dictionary of Nutrition and Food Technology*. 6th ed. London and Boston: Butterworths, 1990. 336p. CORE [F159]
Includes United Kingdom and United States recommended intakes of nutrients.

C.A.B. International. *CAB Thesaurus*. 2 vols. Wallingford, Oxon, U.K.: C.A.B. International, 1990. 1207p.
Contains over 50,000 terms covering agriculture and related topics. This edition includes both British and American spellings and represents input from the U.S. National Agricultural Library (NAL), which has adopted the *CAB Thesaurus* as its authority for indexing journal records into the AGRICOLA database.

Claudio, Virginia S. and Rosalinda T. Lagua. *Nutrition and Diet Therapy Dictionary*. 3d ed. New York: Van Nostrand Reinhold, 1991. 355p. [F185]
Approximately 4,000 terms used in nutrition and diet therapy are featured. Emphasis is placed on the relationship between basic nutrition and disease.

Considine, Douglas M. and Glenn D. Considine. *Foods and Food Production Encyclopedia*. New York: Van Nostrand Reinhold, 1982. 2305p.
An extensive amount of data on food, food science, food production, and food technology is presented. The subject areas are broad and highly interdisciplinary and include explanations of the natural food-growth cycle, nurturing of plants and animals, and processing of raw food materials into refined and complex products. Food production equipment, chemicals for promoting plant growth and

controlling pests, food additives, and worldwide food production statistics also are included along with numerous pictures, graphs, and charts.

Ensminger, Audrey. *A Nutrition Encyclopedia*. Clovis, CA: Pegus Press, 1986. 1178p.

A comprehensive encyclopedia covering over 2,700 topics for health and nutrition students, consumers, health professionals, and food producers.

Lück, Erich et al. *Four Language Dictionary of Food Technology: English, German, Spanish, French (Viersprachiges Wörterbuch der Lebensmittel)*. Hamburg: B. Behr's Verlag, 1992. 656p.

Title and contents in four languages. Includes the most important terms of food technology, food science, and nutrition with an eye to European unification. Four alphabetical indexes (one for each language) contain all the language synonyms.

Gould, Wilbur A. *Glossary for the Food Industries*. Baltimore, MD: CTI Publications, 1990. 118p.

This handy reference tool contains abbreviations/acronyms, terms and terminology, useful conversion tables, measurements, and other useful data for the food industry.

Hamilton, Eva May Nunnelley and Sareen Annora Stepnick Gropper. *The Biochemistry of Human Nutrition: A Desk Reference*. St. Paul, MN: West Publishing, 1987. 324p.

Biochemical concepts essential to an understanding of nutrition are explained in easily understood terms in this reference text for professionals and students. Discussions generally are limited to widely accepted information on a given subject; references are included on recent research and more controversial issues related to each topic.

Hui Y. H., ed. *Encyclopedia of Food Science and Technology*. 4 vols. New York: John Wiley and Sons, 1991. 3016p.

This work is directed toward students and professionals in food science and technology and related fields. It presents a comprehensive examination and explanation of the fundamentals of food science and technology, including major food crops and their processing, food additives, food engineering, food constituents, key organizations in food science, specific food products, and cultural information on food consumption. Contains 380 signed articles by over 100 contributors. A useful index and numerous "see" references located among the entries assist the reader in locating information quickly.

Igoe, Robert S. *Dictionary of Food Ingredients*. 2d ed. New York: Van Nostrand Reinhold, 1989. 225p. [F233]

Details the functions, chemical properties, and applications of over 1,000 approved food ingredients.

International Food Information Service Thesaurus: The Companion Thesaurus to Food Science & Technology Abstracts. 3d ed. Reading, U.K.: International Food Information Service, 1992. [F025, I044]

A searching aid for *FSTA* in all its formats. It is based on a list of terms used in *FSTA* from 1969 to the present day. This new thesaurus contains 7375 terms, of which 1142 are non-descriptors. Descriptors are placed within numbered hierarchies of broader and narrower terms. References to related terms are given together with appropriate "use for" and "use" instructions. Includes scope notes to aid with meanings and history notes where changes have been made.

International Foodservice Manufacturers Association. *The IFMA Encyclopedia of the Foodservice Industry*. 7th ed. Deerfield, IL: International Foodservice Manufacturers Association, 1992. [F273]

Contains market data, statistics, and an extensive resource list of organizations and materials related to the food service industry.

Johnson, Frank E. *The Professional Wine Reference*. New York: Beverage Media, 1983. 401p.

Directed towards the wine trade and consumers, this handbook of wine facts is organized in an alphabetical listing. Separate sections on varietal wines and wine character listings are included.

Ketz, Hans Albrecht and Friedbert Baum. *Nutrition Lexicon* (Ernährungslexikon. 1. ed.). Leipzig: Fachbuchverlag, 1986. 610p.

Komp, Joel T. *Thesaurus of Food Terms*. Maple Grove, MN: Komputer Foods, 1988. 200p.

This thesaurus is used to index the *Foods Adlibra* database.

Lang, Jenifer Harvey. *Larousse Gastronomique, The New American Edition of the World's Greatest Culinary Encyclopedia*. New York: Crown Publishers, 1988.

A classic culinary encyclopedia written in English and French. (Uniform title: *Nouveau Larousse Gastronomique*)

Leatherdale, Donald. *Agrovoc: A Multilingual Thesaurus of Agricultural Terminology: English Version*. Rome: Apimondia, by arrangement with the CEC, 1982. 530p.

A multilingual thesaurus of agricultural terminology that is used to index records for the AGRIS databank. Available in English, French, German, Italian, and Spanish. Contains approximately 23,000 terms (13,000 allowable descriptors and 10,000 note descriptors).

Leung, Albert Y. *Encyclopedia of Common Natural Ingredients Used in Food, Drugs, Cosmetics*. New York: Wiley, 1980. 409p.

This reference book is a compendium of over 500 materials of natural origin used in foods, drugs, and cosmetics. Each entry provides a general description, chemical composition, pharmacology or biological activities, uses, commercial preparations, and references. Natural ingredients are defined as those not produced by chemical synthesis; they can be active (nutrients or drugs) or inactive (preservatives or flavorings).

Lück, Erich. *Wörterbuch der Lebensmittel, Ernährung und Kochkunst* (Dictionary of Food, Nutrition and Cookery). Hamburg: B. Behr's Verlag, 1983. 392p.

An English/German dictionary of food, nutrition, and cookery terminology.

Macrae, Robert, Richard K. Robinson, and Michele J. Sadler. *Encyclopaedia of Food Science, Food Technology, and Nutrition*. 8 vols. San Diego: Academic Press, 1993.

A comprehensive reference tool featuring more than 500 subject entries, contributed by over 1,500 experts from 50 countries, covering all aspects of food science, food technology, and nutrition. Includes entries for all the major commodities, with articles covering the technical aspects of production and processing, chemical composition and analysis, and nutritional significance. Also covers the physiological and sociological aspects of nutrition, the nutritional influences of health and disease, and the areas of clinical nutrition and dietetics. Contains a subject index with more than 50,000 entries and a directory of contributors.

Ockerman, Herbert W. *Food Science Sourcebook*. 2d ed. 2 vols. New York: Van Nostrand Reinhold, 1991. (Original title: *Source Book for Food Scientists*. AVI, 1978.) CORE [F355]

This two volume second edition is divided into two parts: (1) terms and descriptions; (2) food composition, properties, and general data. This set includes research from the twelve years between the editions. The text provides current data and relevant facts in the field of food science and technology.

Tver, David F. and Percy Russell. *The Nutrition and Health Encyclopedia*. 2d ed. New York: Van Nostrand Reinhold, 1989. 639p.

Alphabetically arranged entries cover the topics of body chemistry and composition; major foods, food additives and food toxins; nutrition-related diseases; and metabolic functions.

Winick, Myron. *The Columbia Encyclopedia of Nutrition*. New York: Perigee Books, 1989. 349p.

Based on scientific and clinical research, this text presents information on important topics in human nutrition. The focus is on areas where diet is a risk factor for certain diseases.

F. Directories

Barile, Mary Margaret. *Just Cookbooks*. Arkville, NY: Heritage Publications, 1990. 135p.

A directory for cookbook collectors containing information on antique cookbooks, newsletters, bookstores, consultants, publishers, recipe software, and mail order sources.

Federation of American Societies for Experimental Biology. Life Sciences Research Office. *Nutrition Monitoring in the United States: The Directory of Federal Nutrition Monitoring Activities*. Hyattsville, MD: U.S. Department of Health and Human Services, U.S. Department of Agriculture, September 1989. (DHHS Publication Series no. (PHS) 89–1255–1.)

Covers the recognized components of nutrition monitoring, namely nutrition and health status measurements, food and nutrient consumption measurements, food composition measurements, dietary knowledge and attitude assessment, and food supply determinations. Surveys identifying socio-demographic measurements and economic indicators are included.

Fenton, Thomas P. and Mary J. Heffron. *Food, Hunger, Agribusiness: A Directory of Resources*. Maryknoll, NY: Orbis Books, 1987. 131p.

Aimed at a broad audience, this directory contains a selected list of organizations, books, periodicals, pamphlets, articles, audiovisuals, and curricula on the topics of food, hunger, and agribusiness. This publication is a part of a series on Third World regions and issues.

Food and Agriculture Organization of the United Nations. *Directory of Food and*

Nutrition Institutions in the Near East. Rome: Food and Agriculture Organization of the United Nations, 1987. 87p. (*FAO Food and Nutrition Papers* no. 40.)

Frank, Robyn C. and Holly B. Irving. *Directory of Food and Nutrition Information for Professionals and Consumers*. 2d ed. Phoenix: Oryx Press, 1992. 322p. (Former title: *Directory of Food and Nutrition Information Services and Resources*.)
This comprehensive directory identifies key sources of food and nutrition information for nutritionists, dietitians, health professionals, educators, librarians, and consumers. It contains chapters on organizations, academic programs, microcomputer software, databases, key reference materials, professional and consumer journals, museums and special collections, cookbooks, hotlines, area agencies, and producers of books and audiovisuals.

Heintza, Denise, John C. Klensin, and William M. Rand. *INFOODS: International Directory of Food Composition Tables*. Cambridge: Massachusetts Institute of Technology, 1988. 20p.
This directory is intended to continue the FAO publication, *Food Composition Tables: Updated Annotated Bibliography*. This edition lists only titles, compilers, and publishers, but is very useful.

Miller, Duncan and Morag Soranna, comp., *Directory of Food Policy Institutes = Répertoire des Organismes Traitant des Questions Alimentaires*. Guildford Surrey, U.K.: Butterworth Scientific, 1981. 100p.
Published for the Development Centre of the Organisation for Economic Cooperation and Development, Paris, this directory provides information on the priorities and activities of food policy institutes in all areas of the world. Descriptions are in English and French. Lists one or two institutes in developing countries with ten African countries listed. Greatest coverage for Germany, Japan, the United Kingdom, and the United States.

Smith, Jack L. *Nutrient Data Bank Directory*. 8th ed. Newark: University of Delaware, 1992. 132p. (Available from: University of Delaware, Department of Nutrition and Dietetics, Alison Hall, Newark, DE 19715–3360.)
Provides basic descriptive information, scope, program language, and type of computer for 112 U.S. nutrient databases. A separate table lists the food constituents of nutrient databases, characteristics of the databases, and features of computer software.

G. Handbooks, Manuals, Texts

General

Adams, Leon David and Bridgett Novak. *The Wines of America*. 4th ed. New York: McGraw-Hill, 1990. 528p.
An historical overview of wine growing and the wine industry in America. Includes a brief chronology of wine in North America.

American Home Economics Association. *Handbook of Food Preparation*. 8th ed. Washington, DC: American Home Economics Association, 1980. 160p. [F275]
The classic reference for those who work with or teach food preparation. In-

cludes description and properties of foods, buying guides, essentials of recipe construction, cooking times, food preservation, and a glossary.

Aurand, Leonard W., Edwin A. Woods, and Marion R. Wells. *Food Composition and Analysis*. New York: Van Nostrand Reinhold, 1987. 690p.
Chapters cover food laws/standards, sampling and proximate analysis, methods of analysis, specific nutrients, flavoring and coloring agents, food groups, and food deterioration, preservation, and contamination.

Birch, G. G. and M. G. Lindley. *Alcoholic Beverages*. London and New York: Elsevier, 1985. 232p.
Describes the science and technology of alcoholic beverages. Both hard liquor and wines are covered. The physiological effects of alcohol abuse and alcohol dependence syndrome are discussed.

Booth, R. Gordon. *Snack Food*. New York: Van Nostrand Reinhold, 1990. 416p.
This reference text discusses all types of snack food and the many facets of the snack food industry.

Farrell, Kenneth T. *Spices, Condiments, and Seasonings*. New York: Van Nostrand Reinhold, 1990. 414p.
Provides an extensive account of the major spices, extractives, and seasoning technologies.

Judge, Edward E. and Sons, Inc., *Almanac of the Canning, Freezing, and Preserving Industries*.
75th ed. Westminster, MD: Edward E. Judge and Sons, 1991. [F208]

Marmion, Daniel M. *Handbook of U.S. Colorants: Foods, Drugs, Cosmetics, and Medical Devices*. 3d ed. New York: Wiley, 1991. 573p.
A collection of information on the use of color additives in the food, cosmetic, and medical industries. New developments as well as background information are included.

Martin, Roy E. and George J. Flick. *The Seafood Industry*. New York: Van Nostrand Reinhold, 1990. 445p.
Covers seafood classification, biology, products, by-products, processing, packaging, retail merchandising, labeling, plant cleaning and sanitation, transportation, distribution, and warehousing.

National Association of Meat Purveyors. *The Meat Buyers Guide*. McLean, VA: The Association, 1988. 188p.
Directed toward foodservice buyers, educators, and students, this reference guide provides information on meat standards and meat purchase specifications. Further processed by- products are included. Glossary.

Pennington, Neil L. and Charles W. Baker, eds. *Sugar: A User's Guide to Sucrose*. New York: Van Nostrand Reinhold, 1990. 352p.
A comprehensive reference on sucrose sources, production, and utilization.

Rechcigl, Miloslav, Jr., ed. *CRC Handbook of Foodborne Diseases of Biological Origin*. Boca Raton, FL: CRC Press, 1983. 518p.
Directed toward food scientists, dietitians, nutritionists, and epidemiologists, this is a book of review articles by experts.

Rosengarten, Frederic. *The Book of Edible Nuts*. New York: Walker, 1984. 384p.

Simoons, Frederick J. *Food in China: A Cultural and Historical Inquiry*. Boca Raton, FL: CRC Press, 1991. 559p.

This text covers the history and cultural aspects of food and cuisine in the regions of China. Notes on food, nutrition, and health in traditional China are included.

Food Science/Technology

Aitken, A. et al. *Fish Handling & Processing*. 2d ed. Aberdeen: Ministry of Agriculture, Fisheries & Food, Torry Research Station; Edinburgh: H.M.S.O., 1982. 191p.

American Oil Chemists' Society. *Official Methods and Recommended Practices of the American Oil Chemists' Society*. 4th ed. Champaign, IL: American Oil Chemists' Society, 1990. 1050p. CORE [F356]

Ashurst, P. R. *Food Flavourings*. Glasgow: Blackie, 1991. 310p.
This book is intended to be a practical companion to the flavorist, the applications technologist, and the technical sales person. The book covers three major areas: marketing flavorings, raw materials of the industry (essential oils, natural extracts, fruit juices and synthetic ingredients), and main user industries (beverages, confectionery, bakery, dairy).

Bailey, Alton Edward et al. *Bailey's Industrial Oil and Fat Products*. Ed. Daniel Swern. 4th ed. 3 vols. New York: Wiley, 1979–1985. CORE [F281]

Baur, Fred J., ed. *Insect Management for Food Storage and Processing*. St. Paul, MN: American Association of Cereal Chemists, 1984. 384p.
Examines sanitation and prevention measures to minimize the occurrence of insects in the food industry.

Birch, G. G. and M. G. Lindley, eds. *Low-Calorie Products*. London and New York: Elsevier Applied Science, 1988. 287p. (Sole distributor in the United States and Canada, Elsevier Science Pub. Co.)
This text is intended for food scientists, nutritionists, food manufacturers, psychologists, sociologists, sensory evaluation experts, chemists, and all those concerned with the composition of foods. Provides information on the use of intense and bulk sweetners, fibre, hydrocolloids, and low-calorie fats in the formulation of low-calorie products.

Canadian International Grains Institute. *Grains and Oilseeds: Handling, Marketing, Processing*. 3d ed. Winnipeg: The Institute, 1982. 1006p.

Chan, Harvey T., Jr. *Handbook of Tropical Foods*. New York: M. Dekker, 1983. 639p. (*Food Science* no 9.)
A resource book providing the most recent and available knowledge on selected tropical foods such as cassava, yams, fermented fish products, and rice. Explores crops such as amaranth which have promising value.

Chen, James C. P. *Meade-Chen Cane Sugar Handbook: A Manual for Cane Sugar Manufacturers and Their Chemists*. 11th ed. New York: Wiley, 1985. 1134p. [F345]

Dickinson, Eric, ed. *Food Polymers, Gels and Colloids*. Cambridge: Royal Society of Chemistry, 1991. 450p. (Special Publication no. 82.)
Provides a comprehensive and up-to-date account of current activity in the field and covers such topics as interactions and aggregation behavior of proteins and polysaccharides in solution, formation and stability of emulsions and foams, in-

terfacial behavior of food surfactants and macromolecules, and structure and rheology of solutions, gels, and glasses.

Fennema, Owen R. *Food Chemistry*. New York: M. Dekker, 1985. 991p. (*Food Science and Technology Series* no 15.) CORE

This textbook for upper-division undergraduate students provides comprehensive coverage of the subject of food chemistry. Topics include the major and minor food constituents, food dispersions, edible animal tissues and fluids, edible plant tissues, and interactions among food components. A new edition is due in late 1994.

Frazier, William Carroll and Dennis C. Westhoff. *Food Microbiology*. 4th ed. New York: McGraw-Hill, 1988. 539p.

Intended for students and field workers with emphasis on food organisms, preparation, preservation, spoilage, and relationships to diseases. Minimum concern with technology. A chapter on food irradiation has been included.

Furia, Thomas E. *CRC Handbook of Food Additives*. 2d ed. 2 vols. Boca Raton, FL: CRC Press, 1980. CORE [F312]

Covers enzymes, vitamins, amino acids, antimicrobial food additives, antioxidants as food stabiliers, acidulants in food processing, gums, starch in the food industry, natural and synthetic flavoring, nonnutritive sweeteners, color additives, and phosphates in food processing.

Furia, Thomas E. and Nicolo Bellanca. *Fenaroli's Handbook of Flavor Ingredients*. 2d ed. Boca Raton, FL: CRC Press, 1990. CORE

Over 250 natural flavors are discussed including their physical, chemical, and organoleptic characteristics.

Garifullovich, S. G. *Physical Principles of Infrared Irradiation of Foodstuffs*. New York: Hemisphere Publishing Corporation, 1991. 398p.

This updated and revised edition explains the physical principles of infrared irradiation and how they should be applied in the thermal processing of foodstuffs.

Gould, Wilbur A. and Ronald W. Gould. *Total Quality Assurance for the Food Industries*. Baltimore, MD: CTI Publications, 1988. 394p. CORE

This text describes the basic priniciples of total quality assurance for management and staff. Various attributes and characteristics of food product quality and quality evaluation methods are reviewed.

Heath, Henry B. *Sourcebook of Flavors*. Westport, CT: AVI Publishing, 1981. 863p. (A VNR/AVI Book. Available from: Van Nostrand Reinhold, Florence, KY.)

Examines plant, natural, and synthetic flavouring materials; food colorants; manufacturing methods; toxicology; and regulations.

Herschdoerfer, S. M. *Quality Control in the Food Industry*. 2d ed. 4 vols. London and Orlando, FL: Academic Press, 1984–1987. CORE

Volume 1 discusses general aspects of quality control such as health problems in food, statistical methods in quality control, and national and international standards. The remaining three volumes consider quality control in specific food industries such as dairy products and fruits and vegetables.

Third International Conference on Food Science and Technology Information; *Proceedings* . . . in Budapest, Oct. 1989. Budapest, AGROINFORM, 1990. 290p. (*FSTA Reference Series* no. 10)

Jackisch, Philip. *Modern Winemaking*. Ithaca, NY: Cornell University Press, 1985. 289p.

Directed toward amateur and small commercial winemakers, this text contains general information on winemaking, winemaking practices, specific types of wines, and using and evaluating finished wines.

Jackson, E. B. *Sugar Confectionery Manufacture*. New York: Van Nostrand Reinhold, 1990. 424p.

A state-of-the-art reference covering the sugar confectionery industry. Covers raw materials, manufacturing techniques, and other general technical information.

Jay, James M. *Modern Food Microbiology*. 3d ed. New York: Van Nostrand Reinhold, 1986. 642p.

This text is designed for a second or subsequent course in microbiology in liberal arts, food science, nutrition, or related course programs. Coverage includes (1) history of food microbiology, (2) sources and types of microorganisms in food and parameters that affect the growth and activity of the food flora, (3) methods of determining microorganisms and/or their products in foods, (4) microbial food spoilage and preservation methods, (5) indicator and foodborne pathogens, and (6) psychotrophs, thermophiles and radiation-resistant microorganisms. The appendix includes a schematical depiction of the relationship between the common genera of foodborne bacteria.

Kapsalis, John G. *Objective Methods in Food Quality Assessment*. Boca Raton, FL: CRC Press, 1987. 275p. CORE

An authoritative, comprehensive reference text for food analysts and researchers, this book addresses the broad area of measurements of foods in order to assess their quality and acceptability. The text is organized under three central themes: general concepts of sensory evaluation, food wholesomeness, and quantitative standardization of food quality assessments.

Lewis, Richard J. *Food Additives Handbook*. New York: Van Nostrand Reinhold, 1989. 592p.

Covers chemicals intentionally added to foods; chemical contaminants of foods, and flavors and coloring agents.

Lopez, Anthony. *A Complete Course in Canning and Related Processes*. 12th ed. 3 vols. Baltimore, MD: The Canning Trade, 1987. CORE [F292]

A technical reference book and textbook for students of food technology, food plant managers, product research and development specialists, food brokers, food equipment manufactures and salesmen, and food industry suppliers.

McGinnis, Richard A., ed. *Beet-Sugar Technology*. Fort Collins: CO: Beet Sugar Development Foundation, 1982. 855p.

Aimed toward factory technologists, workers, and students of the sugar industry, this text covers all phases of beet-sugar manufacturing with the exception of organization, financing, and marketing.

Morrison, Rosanna Mentzer and Tanya Roberts. *Food Irradiation: New Perspectives on a Controversial Technology: A Review of Technical, Public Health, and Economic Considerations*. Washington, DC: Congress of the United States, Office of Technology Assessment, 1985. Unpaged.

A comprehensive report for food technologists on a variety of issues concerning the commercial use of food irradiation, including its technical effects on food, the extent of demand for its benefits, the cost of food irradiation technology, its competitiveness with alternative preservatives and fumigants for ensuring food safety, its approval by regulatory agencies; and the acceptability of food irradiation to food consumers. An outlook summary for food irradiation in the United States and its related public policy issues is appended.

National Research Council. Food and Nutrition Board. Committee on Codex Specifications. *Food Chemicals Codex*. 3d ed. Washington, DC: National Academy Press, 1981. 766p. CORE [F353]
An important resource on the quality and purity of food-grade substances. The standards for chemical purity and methods for testing the purity levels of almost 800 substances are covered.

National Research Council. Food and Nutrition Board. Committee on Food Chemicals Codex. *Food Chemicals Codex: Supplements to the Third Edition*. Washington, DC: National Academy Press, 1983. (First Supplement 1983, 34p.; Second Supplement 1986, 58p.; Third Supplement 1992, 90p.) CORE [F353]
A compendium of standards and specifications for food-grade chemicals used as food additives.

Okos, Martin R., ed. *Physical and Chemical Properties of Food*. St. Joseph, MI: American Society of Agricultural Engineers, 1986. 407p. CORE
Eleven review papers that present data and mathematical relationships concerning such topics as changes in the quality of stored frozen foods and the colligative properties of foods.

Ott, Dana B. *Applied Food Science Laboratory Manual*. New York: Pergamon Press, 1987. 213p.
This manual covers basic food concepts in an applied manner utilizing the scientific method. It is intended for the upper-level food science, dietetic, and/or food and nutrition undergraduate who has a background in general and organic chemistry.

Paine, F. A. and H. Y. Paine, eds. *A Handbook of Food Packaging*. 2d ed. New York: Van Nostrand Reinhold, 1992. 504p.
This handbook approaches the development of the right package for a particular food in a particular market from the viewpoint of the food technologist, the packaging engineer, and the marketing professional.

Pyler, Ernst John. *Baking Science & Technology*. 3d ed. 2 vols. Merriam, KS: Sosland Publishing, 1988. 1346p.
Presents the present status of knowledge in baking science, ingredient development, and new technologies utilized in food production and processing.

Rees, J. A. G. and J. Bettison, eds. *Processing and Packaging of Heat Preserved Foods*. New York: AVI Publishing, 1991. 250p.
Covers the principles of heat preservation, heat processing equipment; aseptic processing and packaging; packaging in metal, glass, and plastic containers; leaker spoilage of foods in containers; effect of heat preservation on product quality; and recommendations for good manufacturing practices of heat-preserved foods.

Reuter, Helmut. *Aseptic Packaging of Food*. Herndon, VA: Institute of Packaging Professionals, 1989. 269p.

Covers the principles and modern international practices of aseptic packaging of food and beverages.

Rizvi, Syed S. H. and Gauri S. Mittal. *Experimental Methods in Food Engineering*. New York: Van Nostrand Reinhold, 1992. 289p.

The basic purpose of this book is to enhance the "teachability" of food engineering laboratory courses offered at the university and college level.

Russell, N. J. and G. W. Gould, eds. *Food Preservatives*. New York: AVI Publishing, 1991. 290p.

This book, intended for technologists in quality control and product development and for academic institutions, provides basic information and guidance on the effective use of food preservatives in industry, with chapters on the applications and basic modes of action of major antimicrobial food additives.

Schwimmer, Sigmund. *Source Book of Food Enzymology*. Westport, CT: AVI Publishing, 1981. 967p. CORE

A fundamental reference with information on enzymes and their function in relation to food characteristics.

Scott, R. *Cheesemaking Practice*. 2d ed. London and New York: Elsevier Applied Science Publishers, 1986. 529p. CORE

The author stresses the art of cheesemaking and points out advances made in the science of cheesemaking. The appendix includes selected cheese recipes.

Stauffer, John E. *Quality Assurance of Food: Ingredients, Processing, and Distribution*. Westport, CT: Food and Nutrition Press, 1988. 304p.

This book describes the scope, applications, and benefits of quality assurance in food processing operations. Topics include good manufacturing practice, hazard analysis and critical control points, kosher certification, packaging, labeling, and product recall.

U.S. Department of Agriculture. Food Safety and Inspection Service. *Chemistry Laboratory Guidebook: Revised Basic*. 1 vol. Washington, DC: U. S. Government Printing Office, 1986–. (loose-leaf).

This reference book contains methods suitable for the analysis of the natural constituents, additives, and biological and environmental residues that may occur in meat and poultry products.

Watson, Ernest L. and John C. Harper. *Elements of Food Engineering*. 2d ed. New York: Van Nostrand Reinhold, 1988. 308p.

Covers the fundamental concepts of food engineering, including thermodynamics, mass balance, and fluid flow.

Webster, Francis H., ed. *Oats: Chemistry and Technology*. St. Paul, MN: American Association of Cereal Chemists, 1986. 433p.

Directed toward cereal chemists, students, and industrial processors, this monograph provides an in-depth reference on oat chemistry and technology. Color flourescent micrographs and separate sections on dietary fiber, flavor, and phenol chemistry are also included.

Wheaton, Frederick W. and Thomas B. Lawson. *Processing Aquatic Food Products*. New York: Wiley, 1985. 518p.

Covers traditional and newer processing methods of seafood products.

Wierbicki, Eugen. *Ionizing Energy in Food Processing and Pest Control*. Ames, IA: Council for Agricultural Science and Technology, 1986–89.

Vol. I, *Wholesomeness of Food Treated with Ionizing Energy* (Council for Agricultural Science and Technology Report no. 109, 50p.) reviews research conducted on the toxicological safety, nutritional quality, and microbiological safety of foods treated with ionizing energy.
Vol. II, *Applications* (Council for Agricultural Science and Technology Task Force Report no. 115, June 1989, 98p.) discusses the radiation chemistry of food components, the effect of irradiation on various foods, and the packaging and consumer acceptance of irradiated foods.

Woodroof, Jasper Guy and Bor Shiun Luh, eds. *Commercial Fruit Processing*. Westport, CT: AVI Publishing, 1986. 678p. CORE
A reference text for the industry and technologists that details and illustrates the broad range of technological processes and processing factors involved in the commercial production of fruits.

Zapsalis, Charles and R. Anderle Beck. *Food Chemistry and Nutritional Chemistry*. New York: Macmillan, 1986. 1219p. CORE
A comprehensive textbook that integrates food chemistry, biochemistry, and nutrition. The basic chemistry of food constituents, the integrated metabolism of all food constituents, and information on molecular genetics are covered.

Food/Nutrition Policy

Berg, Alan. *Malnutrition: What Can Be Done?; Lessons From World Bank Experience*. Baltimore: Johns Hopkins University Press, 1987. 139p.
A reference text for professionals involved in supplemental feeding programs and food and nutrition policy in developing countries, this book reports the results of four major nutrition projects (in Indonesia, Brazil, Colombia, and India) carried out in collaboration with the World Bank. It also discusses over fifty nutrition components that have been incorporated into the design of agricultural, urban development, and health projects. Nutrition research and analyses supported and conducted by the World Bank also are discussed.

Cohen, Marc J. and Richard A. Hoehn. *Hunger 1992: Second Annual Report on the State of World Hunger*. Washington, DC: Bread for the World, Institute on Hunger and Development, 1991. 217p.

Croll, E. *Food Supply in China and the Nutritional Status of Children*. Geneva: UNRISD, 1986. 111p.
This preliminary assessment of the food supply and nutrition in the People's Republic of China focuses on steps taken to increase food production, nutrition education efforts, and adjustments to family food allocations to assure the improved nutritional status of children.

Falkner, Frank. *Infant and Child Nutrition Worldwide: Issues and Perspectives*. Boca Raton, FL: CRC Press, 1991. 297p.
This volume provides a contemporary and historical overview of infant nutrition in Europe, North America, and the Third World.

Foster, Phillips. *The World Food Problem: Tackling the Causes of Undernutrition in the Third World*. Boulder, CO: Lynne Rienner Publishers, 1992. 367p.

Covers the definition and facts related to malnutrition as well as its causes. Various policy approaches to undernutrition are addressed.

Kennedy, E. T., P. Pinstrup-Andersen, and R. Adams. *Nutrition-Related Policies and Programs: Past Performance and Research Needs*. Washington, DC: International Food Policy Research Institute, 1983. 104p.

This monograph for nutrition policy makers presents the results of a review of existing knowledge of nutrition-related government interventions. It identifies areas where nutrition-related policy research is urgently needed and likely to be useful in the formulation of future government interventions.

Sahn, David E., Richard Lockwood, and Nevin S. Scrimshaw. *Methods for the Evaluation of the Impact of Food and Nutrition Programmes*. Tokyo: United Nations University Press, 1991. 291p.

Sasson, A. *Feeding Tomorrow's World*. Paris: UNESCO, 1990. 805p.

This publication presents scientific and technical information on the world food and nutrition situation within the context of a broad human ecology standpoint. Subjects covered include human nutrition, food production and trade, and international cooperation.

U.S. Congress. House Select Committee on Hunger. *A Review of Selected Studies on World Hunger: Staff Report*. Washington, DC: U.S. Government Printing Office, 1985. 102p.

A reference document for food and nutrition program managers and policy makers. The report addresses (1) the extent of U.S. hunger and the effectiveness of U.S. food and nutrition programs; and (2) the extent of world hunger and major international programs and policies designed to reduce world hunger. The report is based on a comprehensive review of major studies on domestic and international hunger conducted over the past ten years. An annotated bibliography of 383 studies is included.

U.S. Congress. Senate Committee on Agriculture, Nutrition, and Forestry. *The Food Stamp Program: History, Description, Issues, and Options*. Washington, DC: U.S. Government Printing Office, 1985. 409p.

The food stamp program is the second-largest federally funded welfare program in existence in the United States and the largest in USDA. Covers legislative history, day-to-day operations, issues for Congress, and policy alternatives.

Human Nutrition

Akre, J., ed. *Infant Feeding: The Physiological Basis*. Geneva: WHO, 1990. 108p.

Written in English and French, this review covers the scientific basis for preparing guidelines on infant feeding, utilizing local foods. Local customs are incorporated into the recommendations.

American Dietetic Association. *Manual of Clinical Dietetics*. 3d ed. Chicago, IL: The Chicago Dietetic Association and The South Suburban Dietetic Association, 1991. 639p.

Covers all aspects of nutrition management throughout the life cycle. New sections on nutrition support of AIDS patients, high-fiber diets, eating disorders, and sports nutrition are included.

Breneman, James C. *Handbook of Food Allergies*. New York: Marcel Dekker, 1987. 297p.

The immunology of food allergy and food antigens are presented along with such effects as migraines and arthritis in food-intolerant persons. Approved and unapproved methods of diagnosis and treatment are described. Over 800 bibliographic citations and over 200 recipes for patients are included.

Briggs, George M. and Doris Howes Calloway. *Nutrition and Physical Fitness*. 11th ed. New York: Holt, Rinehart, and Winston, 1984. 699p.

An introductory college text designed to provide basic knowledge and a foundation for independent and advanced study.

Burton, Benjamin T. and Willis R. Foster. *Human Nutrition*. New York: McGraw-Hill, 1988. 624p. (Formerly titled *The Heinz Handbook of Nutrition: A Textbook of Nutrition in Health and Disease*.)

An authoritative and concise textbook that presents mainstream scientific and clinical thought on all areas of nutrition, from basic physiology and the biochemistry of food intake to therapeutic diets and the psychology of appetite.

Clydesdale, F. M. and F. J. Francis. *Food, Nutrition and Health*. Westport, CT: AVI Publishing, 1985. 293p.

Focuses on the relationship between the nature of food and its effects on human nutrition and overall health.

Cornatzer, W. E. *Role of Nutrition in Health and Disease*. Springfield, IL: Thomas, 1989. 423p.

This book presents a concise review of the role of each nutrient in health and disease.

Ehrlich, Ann B. *Nutrition and Dental Health*. Albany, NY: Delmar, 1987. 295p.

Directed toward dental health professionals, this text provides basic information on nutrition and its impact on dental health. Other topics covered include specialized nutritional needs, major nutritional disorders, the role of nutrition in preventive dentistry, and special diets for dental patients.

Food and Agriculture Organization of the United Nations. Nutrition Programmes Service. *Selecting Interventions for Nutritional Improvement: A Manual*. Rome: Food and Agriculture Organization of the United Nations, 1983. 79p. (Nutrition in Agriculture no. 3.)

This manual for dietitians and clinical nutritionists from the FAO Food Policy and Nutrition Division advances a systematic method of selecting effective nutritional interventions for malnourished people in rural areas.

Garrison, Robert H., Jr. and Elizabeth Somer. *The Nutrition Desk Reference*. New Canaan, CT: Keats, 1990. 306p.

Aimed toward health professionals and other interested readers, this text provides basic nutrition information as well as the latest findings in nutrition research. A chapter on nutrition and drugs covers drug-nutrient interactions and the relationship between nutrition, alcoholism, and drug abuse.

Grand, Richard J., James L. Sutphen, and William H. Dietz. *Pediatric Nutrition: Theory and Practice*. Boston: Butterworths, 1987. 852p.

This comprehensive reference text provides both theoretical and practical guidelines by which practitioners can provide children with appropriate nutritional care. Topics covered include nutritional biochemistry, digestion and enteral physiology, perinatal nutrition, the role of nutrition in behavior and growth, clinical nutrition and nutritional interventions, nutritional applications in inborn metabolic errors, enteral and total parenteral feedings, and the role of nutrition and special diets in the community.

Hunt, Sara M. and James L. Groff. *Advanced Nutrition and Human Metabolism*. St. Paul, MN: West Publishing, 1990. 517p.

An advanced text for students and a current reference to the science of nutrition, nutrition physiology, and metabolism.

Johnston, Francis E., ed. *Nutritional Anthropology*. New York: A. R. Liss, 1987. 304p.

Written by an anthropologist, this book focuses on the role food and nutrition plays in man's biology, behavior, and culture. Nutrition is presented as both a science and a process from the perspective of anthropology.

Kittler, Pamela Goyan and Kathryn P. Sucher. *Food and Culture in America: A Nutrition Handbook*. New York: Van Nostrand Reinhold, 1989. 384p.

The traditional and contemporary food habits of various ethnic, religious, and geographical groups are examined.

Pemberton, Cecilia M. *Mayo Clinic Diet Manual: A Handbook of Dietary Practices*. 6th ed. Toronto and Philadelphia: B. C. Decker, 1988. 597p.

This manual provides details on the use of nutrition and diet in the management and therapy of diseases. The manual is intended to be a comprehensive and expanded resource for healthful nutrition from infancy through adulthood and for the evaluation and management of problems in clinical nutrition.

Roe, Daphne A. *Diet and Drug Interactions*. New York: Van Nostrand Reinhold, 1989. 222p.

This text provides information on the mechanisms responsible for food and formula interference with drug absorption and metabolism, on compatibility reactions, on effects of drugs on nutritional states, and of nutritional status on drug disposition.

Rolfes, Sharon Rady, and Linda Kelly DeBruyne. *Life Span Nutrition: Conception Through Life*. St. Paul, MN: West Publishing, 1990. 528p.

This book covers nutrition concepts for all ages and phases of the life span. It is written for both health professionals and lay people. The information is presented in a highly readable and graphic style.

Shils, Maurice E., James A. Olson, and Moshe Shike. *Modern Nutrition in Health and Disease*. 8th ed. Philadelphia: Lea and Febiger, 1994. 2 vols. CORE

A complete and comprehensive classic encompassing all of nutrition: physiologic and metabolic interrelations; adequacy and safety of the food supply, and nutrition in growth, aging and physiologic stress.

Simko, Margaret D., Catherine Cowell, and Judith A. Gilbride. *Nutrition Assessment: A Comprehensive Guide for Planning Intervention*. Rockville, MD: Aspen, 1984. 396p.

The five basic steps (or tools) in the nutritional assessment process (identification, screening, planning, implementation, and evaluation and monitoring) are described in detail. The material illustrates how practical application of nutritional assessment leads to early identification of individuals (or groups) at risk in a community, resulting in health team decisions that can enhance health care quality.

Skipper, Annalynn. *Dietitian's Handbook of Enteral and Parenteral Nutrition*. Rockville, MD: Aspen Publishers, 1989. 452p.

This handbook provides the dietitian with a systems approach to nutritional management.

Spiller, Gene A. *CRC Handbook of Dietary Fiber in Human Nutrition*. 2d ed. Boca Raton, FL: CRC Press, 1992. 483p.

Covers the clinical and nutritional significance of dietary fiber as related to health and nutrition.

Townsend, Carolynn E. *Nutrition and Diet Therapy*. 5th ed. Albany, NY: Delmar, 1989. 457p.

A textbook for beginning students in health care and food service/dietetic programs. This edition emphasizes the relationship between diet and health.

Twin Cities District Dietetic Association. *Manual of Pediatric Nutrition 1990*. 2d ed. St. Paul, MN: The Association, 1990. 595p.

Intended as a single diet manual for health professionals and dietitians to use with pediatric populations. Topics covered include general nutrition, consistency modifications, diabetes, weight control, cholesterol and fat-controlled diets, vitamins and minerals-controlled diets, special pediatric conditions, adolescent health, nutrition for children with special health care needs, and enteral and parenteral nutrition.

Walker, W. Allan and Kristy M. Hendricks. *Manual of Pediatric Nutrition*. Philadelphia: Saunders, 1985. 160p.

This text provides a comprehensive practical guide for dietitians and other health professionals in managing clinical nutritional problems in pediatric patients.

Williams, Sue Rodwell. *Basic Nutrition and Diet Therapy*. 9th ed. St. Louis, MO: Mosby, 1992. 486p.

This concise text covers basic nutrition, community nutrition, and diet therapy. This new edition provides new chapters on weight management, sport and fitness, clinical nutrition and life-cycle nutritional needs.

Williams, Sue Rodwell. *Essentials of Nutrition and Diet Therapy*. 5th ed. St. Louis, MO: Times Mirror/Mosby College Publishing, 1990.

This textbook is designed to meet the needs of beginning students in the allied health professions on the community college level. Major areas covered are introduction to human nutrition, community nutrition and the life cycle, diet therapy, and topics of current relevance. Appendixes include food composition tables, nutritional analysis of foods and brand name products, exchange lists, conversion tables, and a glossary.

Williams, Sue Rodwell et al. *Nutrition Throughout the Life Cycle*. St. Louis, MO: Times Mirror/Mosby College Publishing, 1988. 597p.

This text covers core nutrition concepts throughout the life span and presents such topics as sport/fitness nutrition, alcohol and drug use, and the nutrition for the elderly.

Worthington-Roberts, Bonnie S. *Nutrition in Pregnancy and Lactation*. Edited by

Sue Rodwell Williams. St. Louis, MO: Times Mirror/Mosby College Publishing, 1989. 510p.
Covers nutritional considerations of pregnancy, lactation, and the periods before and between these conditions.

Food Service Management

Kazarian, Edward A. *Foodservice Facilities Planning*. 3d ed. New York: Van Nostrand Reinhold, 1989. 412p.
Covers all aspects of planning a food service facility including the planning process, layout and design, equipment and space requirements, and safety and human design considerations.

Knight, John B. and Lendal H. Kotschevar. *Quantity Food Production, Planning and Management*. 2d ed. New York: Van Nostrand Reinhold, 1989. 445p.
This edition includes the five P's of food service management: people, products, plant/property, profits, and promotions. Also covered are food service planning and quantity food preparation.

Kotschevar, Lendal H. *Standards, Principles, and Techniques in Quantity Food Production*. 4th ed. New York: Van Nostrand Reinhold, 1988. 505p.
This operating guide includes new information on equipment and on the use of computers in foodservice.

Kotschevar, Lendal H. and Charles Levinson. *Quantity Food Purchasing*. 3d ed. New York: Macmillan, 1988. 694p. [F331]
This text emphasizes the management and technical aspects of buying food for a quantity food service operation. Both management and product knowledge are stressed.

Marriott, Norman G. *Principles of Food Sanitation*. 2d ed. New York: Van Nostrand Reinhold, 1989. 387p.
A basic college text on the major aspects and principles of food sanitation.

Pannell, Dorothy VanEgmond. *School Foodservice Management*. 4th ed. New York: Van Nostrand Reinhold, 1990. 275p.
The single-source text that covers all aspects of school food service management.

Puckett, Ruby P. and Bonnie B. Miller. *Food Service Manual for Health Care Institutions*. Rev. ed. Chicago: American Hospital Association, 1988. 404p. [F276]
A comprehensive manual covering the basic principles of management, the process of clinical nutritional management, and the everyday operations of food service departments.

Reed, Lewis. *SPECS: The Comprehensive Foodservice Purchasing and Specification Manual*. 2d ed. New York: Van Nostrand Reinhold, 1992. 1000p. [F361]
A reference manual covering all aspects of food service purchasing along with specifications.

West, Bessie B. and LeVele Wood. *Foodservice in Institutions*. 6th ed. New York: Macmillan Publishing Company, 1988. 662p.
Intended to meet the needs of students preparing to become administrative dieti-

tians or professional food service managers, this book is a ready reference for the planning, production, and service of food in all types of food service operations.

Zaccarelli, Brother Herman E. *Foodservice Management by Checklist.* New York: Wiley and Sons, 1990. 500p.

A reference text that covers basic principles of financial management and control, supervisory techniques, and hospitality operations.

H. Food Tables

Australia Department of Community Services and Health. *Composition of Foods.* Canberra: Australian Government Pub. Service, 1989–.

Bowes and Church's Food Values of Portions Commonly Used. 16th ed. Revised by Jean A. T. Pennington. Philadelphia: Lippincott, 1994. 483p. (Originally titled: *Food Values of Portions Commonly Used.* 1975. 197p.) CORE

This publication contains tables of the food values of commonly consumed foods in the United States. This edition covers 8,500 foods. New features of this edition include information on monounsaturated fat content, references for sources of food data, re-formatting of fat-related nutrients, and two new supplementary tables (Latin names of foods and the caloric and carbohydrate content of chewing gum, mints/candy, and medications).

Food and Agriculture Organization of the United Nations. *Food Composition Tables for the Near East.* Rome: Food and Agriculture Organization of the United Nations, 1982. 275p. *(FAO Food and Nutrition Papers* no. 26.)

This joint publication provides data on the nutrient content of foods consumed in the Near East, defined to include Afghanistan, Bahrein, Cyprus, Egypt, Iran, Iraq, Jordan, Kuwait, Lebanon, Libya, Oman, Pakistan, Qatar, Saudi Arabia, Somalia, Sudan, Syria, and Yemen. Only locally produced foods are considered. Data are presented in three tables: (1) proximate composition, mineral and vitamin content of foods, (2) amino acid content of foods, and (3) fatty acid content of foods.

Hands, Elizabeth S. *Food Finder: Food Sources of Vitamins and Minerals.* 2d ed. Salem, OR: ESHA Research, 1990. 244p.

Instead of looking for food composition data by food, this reference book has the reader look up the nutrient to identify the foods containing that nutrient. The data for each food item include the weight, serving size, calories, and the nutrient density (amount of nutrient per 100 calories).

Human Nutrition Information Service, USDA. *Composition of Foods–Raw, Processed, Prepared.* Washington, DC: Government Printing Office, 1976. (*U.S.D.A. Agriculture Handbook* no. 8. Supplements published in 1989 and 1990.) [F431]

Serves as standard food composition data in the United States. Each volume focuses on a specific food category such as poultry products or fast foods. Titles (and dates of most revisions) include *Dairy and Egg Products* (1976, 158p.), *Spices and Herbs* (1977, 51p.), *Baby Foods* (1978, 255p.), *Fats and Oils* (1979, 142p.), *Poultry Products* (1979, 330p.), *Soups, Sauces, and Gravies* (1980,

228p.), *Sausages and Luncheon Meats* (1980, 92p.), *Breakfast Cereals* (1982, 160p.), *Fruits and Fruit Juices* (1982, 283p.), *Pork Products* (1992, 206p.), *Vegetables and Vegetable Products* (1984, 502p.), *Nut and Seed Products* (1984, 137p.), *Beef Products* (1990, 412p.), *Beverages* (1986, 173p.), *Finfish and Shellfish Products* (1987, 192p.), *Legumes and Legume Products* (1986, 156p.), *Lamb, Veal, and Game Products* (1989, 251p.), *Snacks and Sweets* (1991, 341p.), *Cereal Grains and Pasta* (1989, 137p.), *Fast Foods* (1988, 194p.), *Baked Products* (1992, 467p.).

Human Nutrition Information Service, USDA. *Nutritive Value of Foods*. Washington, DC: U.S. Government Printing Office, 1991. 72p. (*USDA Home and Garden Bulletin* no. 72)
A shorter and simpler version of the preceding reference. Includes 900 of the most commonly consumed foods in the United States.

Kirk, R. S. and R. Sawyer. *Pearson's Composition and Analysis of Foods*. 9th ed. New York: John Wiley & Sons, 1991. (Formerly titled *Chemical Analysis of Foods*.) CORE. [F359]

Klensin, John C. et al. *Identification of Food Components for INFOODS Data Interchange*. Tokyo: United Nations University Press, 1991. 112p.
Contains a comprehensive standardization nomenclature for international nutrient data exchange.

Kraus, Barbara. *Complete Guide to Sodium*. 2d ed. New York: New American Library, 1986. 316p.
The sodium content of thousands of brand name and basic foods are provided.

Kraus, Barbara. *The Dictionary of Sodium, Fats, and Cholesterol*. 5th ed. New York: Putnam, 1992. 382p. [F418]
Over 7,000 brand name and basic food products are listed with their sodium contents.

McCance, R.A. and B. Holland. *McCance and Widdowson's: The Composition of Foods*. 5th ed. Cambridge, U.K.: The Royal Society of Chemistry, 1991. 462p. (Distributed in the United States by CRC Press, Boca Raton, FL.) CORE [F426]
This reference volume covers approximately 1,200 foods. It includes proximates, vitamins, inorganics, dietary fiber, and cholesterol.

Nutritive Value of Convenience and Processed Foods. 4th ed. Schaumburg, IL: West Suburban District of the Illinois Dietetic Association; and Chicago: American Dietetic Association, 1987. 396p.
A comprehensive reference text for food analysts, nutritionists, and dietitians, this work provides extensive tabulations of the macro- and micro-nutrient composition (as provided by food manufacturers) of convenience and processed foods commercially available in the United States.

Scherz, Heimo and Friedrich Senser. *Food Composition and Nutrition Tables, 1989/90: On Behalf of the Bundesministerium fur Ernahrung, Landwirtschaft und Forsten, Bonn*. Edited by Deutsche Forschungsanstalt fur Lebensmittelschemie, Garching b. Munchen. 4th rev. and completed ed. Stuttgart: Wissenschafliche Verlagsgesellschaft, 1989. 1028p. (Also distributed by CRC Press.)
This comprehensive, updated edition consists of a compilation of original publications, monographs, reviews, and unpublished data. The tables introduce new foods in the following food categories: milk and milk products; meat, deer, and

fowl; seafish; oilseed; and wild berries. This fourth edition presents data on meat in a more concise format. Each of the meat portions for animals for slaughter are presented as a comprehensive table in the appendix. New groups of nutritional constituents are purines (e.g., phosphatidylcholine, phosphatidylethanol amine). Salicylic acid is introduced in the group "organic acids." (Former author: S. W. Souci.)

Wenkam, Nao Sekiguchi. *Foods of Hawaii and the Pacific Basin*. V.1,4. Composition, v.2,5. Percentage of U.S. recommended daily allowance. Honolulu: College of Tropical Agriculture and Human Resources, University of Hawaii, 1983–1986. (Hawaii Institute of Tropical Agriculture and Human Resources, Research Extension Series.)

These nutrient tables focus on the foods commonly used in Hawaii and the Pacific Basin. The values have been laboratory analyzed. Raw, processed, and cooked forms of many food items are provided.

I. Dietary Requirements and Recommendations

American Diabetes Association and the American Dietetic Association. *Exchange Lists for Meal Planning*. Chicago: American Dietetic Association, 1986.

An historically significant document that discusses diabetes basics and includes the new exchanges and new symbols flagging foods high in fiber and sodium. Includes the standard U.S. dietary recommendations for diabetics.

Canada. Committee for the Revision of the Dietary Standard for Canada. *Recommended Nutrient Intakes for Canadians*. Ottawa: Health and Welfare Canada, 1983. 181p. CORE.

Food and Agriculture Organization of the United Nations. *Energy and Protein Requirements: Reports of a Joint FAO/WHO/UNU/ Expert Consultation*. Geneva: World Health Organization, 1985. 206p. CORE.

Food and Agriculture Organization of the United Nations. *Requirements of Vitamin A, Iron, Folate and Vitamin B12*. Rome: Food and Agriculture Organization of the United Nations, 1988. 107p. (*FAO Food Nutrition Series* no. 23) CORE.

Institute of Medicine, Committee on Dietary Guidelines Implementation. *Improving America's Diet and Health: From Recommendations to Action*. Edited by Thomas R. Paul. Washington, DC: National Academy Press, 1991. 239p.

This volume provides proposals to facilitate adoption of dietary guidelines by Americans. It contains a set of goals and implementation strategies targeted to various sectors of society: the education community, the health professions, the private sector, and government.

James, W. P. T. and E. C. Schofield. *Human Energy Requirements. A Manual for Planners and Nutritionists*. Oxford: Oxford University Press, 1990. 172p.

This manual contains advice and guidance to planners and nutritionists on how to apply the methodology of the 1985 joint FAO/WHO/UNU report, *Energy and Protein Requirements*. Includes instructions for using ENREQ (Energy Requirements) microcomputer spreadsheet software available from the Food Policy and Nutrition Division of FAO, Rome.

National Research Council. *Recommended Dietary Allowances*. 10th ed. Washington, DC: National Academy Press, 1989. 325p. CORE. [F456]
The accepted source of nutritional requirements for people of all ages in the United States.

Rand, William M., Ricardo Uauy, and Nevin S. Scrimshaw. *Protein-Energy-Requirement Studies in Developing Countries*. Tokyo: United Nations University Press, 1991. 369p.
Focuses on the relevance of research results in resolving the general problem of estimating protein-energy requirements under normal conditions. Based on data from more than fifteen developing countries.

Torun, Benjamin, Vernon R. Young, and William M. Rand. *Protein-Energy Requirements of Developing Countries: Evaluation of New Data*. Tokyo: United Nations University Press, 1991. 268p. CORE.
Based on research data in nineteen countries, this UNU–International Union of Nutritional Sciences report presents dietary requirements for protein/energy.

U.S. Department of Agriculture and U.S. Department of Health and Human Services. *Nutrition and Your Health: Dietary Guidelines for Americans*. 3d ed. Washington, DC: Government Printing Office, 1990. 27p. (*USDA Home and Garden Bulletin* no. 232.)
An historically significant document that states the U.S. dietary guidelines for a healthy population.

U.S. Department of Health and Human Services. *Healthy People 2000: National Health Promotion and Disease Prevention Objectives*. Washington, DC: Government Printing Office, 1991. 154p.
Healthy People is a statement of national opportunities that contains a national strategy for significantly improving the health of the U.S. population by the year 2000. It addresses the prevention of major chronic illnesses, injuries, and infectious diseases.

U.S. Department of Health and Human Services. Public Health, Public Health Service. Office of the Surgeon General. *The Surgeon General's Report on Nutrition and Health*. Washington, DC: U.S. Dept. of Health and Human Services, 1988. 727p.
This report presents a comprehensive discussion of the relationship between diet and chronic disease. The main conclusion is that overconsumption of certain dietary components is now a major concern for Americans. The chief issue is the disproportionately large consumption of foods high in fats and the lack of consumption of foods high in complex carbohydrates and fiber (vegetables, fruits, and whole grain products). The publication includes an examination of the role of diet in major disease groups, a discussion of maternal and child nutrition issues, and a review of common dietary fads and frauds. Extensive citations and supporting documentation are presented to justify conclusions and recommendations. *The Surgeon General's Report on Nutrition and Health: Summary and Recommendations* was also issued (Washington, DC: 1988, 78p.).

J. Legislation, Regulations, Standards, and Inspection

Food Law Facts. Surrey, U.K.: Leatherhead, undated.
This loose-leaf manual explains the EEC's harmonization program and how the Community produces different types of legislation.

Guide to Food Regulations in the U.K. 4th ed. Surrey, U.K.: Leatherhead, undated.
This loose-leaf manual includes explanations of food laws in the United Kingdom, lists of permitted additives, legal aspects of food labeling, composition standards for all foods, and recommendations and references to reports by the Food Advisory Committee. Updated annually.

Hui, Y. H. *United States Regulations for Processed Fruits and Vegetables*. New York: John Wiley and Sons, 1988.
Includes regulations for processed fruits and vegetables covered by several U.S. government agencies.

Institute of Medicine. Committee on the Nutrition Components of Food Labeling. *Nutrition Labeling: Issues and Directions for the 1990's*. Edited by Donna V. Porter and Robert O. Earl. Washington, DC: National Academy Press, 1990. 372p.
Prepared by an independent expert committee, this volume contains a thorough examination of current nutrition labeling practices and recommends ways to make food labeling information consistent with recent dietary recommendations from the U.S. Surgeon General and the National Research Council.

Joint FAO/WHO Expert Consultation on Recommended Allowances of Nutrients for Food Labelling Purposes (Helsinki, Finland). *Recommended Nutrient Reference Values for Food Labelling Purposes*. Rome: Food and Agriculture Organization of the United Nations, 1988. 52p.
This report takes a global look at the presentation of nutrients on food labels. One of the main objectives of nutritional labeling is for it to be easily understood. More consumer research needs to be conducted on the effectiveness of various food label designs and information.

National Archives and Records Administration. *Code of Federal Regulations: Food and Drugs, Parts 100 to 169*. Washington, DC: Office of the Federal Register, 1989.

Overseas Food Legislation (OFL) Manual. 2d ed. Surrey, U.K.: Leatherhead, 1984. [F470]
This loose-leaf manual contains summaries of food legislation of twenty-two major countries. Useful for checking the legality of food and drink products in existing and potential export markets.

U. S. Department of Agriculture. Agricultural Research Service and U.S. Department of Health and Human Services. Public Health Service. Food and Drug Administration. *Insect and Mite Pests in Food*. 2 vol. Washington, D.C.: U.S. Government Printing Office, 1991. (USDA Agricultural Handbook no. 655.)
A comprehensive treatise on the occurrence and identification of food-contaminating insects and their relatives. This work provides the user with a rapid and accurate means of identifying more than 600 species of pests encountered

throughout the food industry. Diagnostic keys and useful illustrations of both adult and immature stages of these pests are presented.

U.S. Department of Agriculture. Animal and Plant Health Inspection Service. Meat and Poultry Inspection Program. *Meat and Poultry Inspection Manual*. Washington DC: U.S. Government Printing Office, latest update 1987. 320p. [F496]
Contains the official procedural guidelines and instructions to aid USDA/FSIS employees in enforcing laws and regulations related to federal meat and poultry inspection. Updated periodically.

U.S. Department of Agriculture. Animal and Plant Health Inspection Service. Meat and Poultry Inspection Program. *Meat and Poultry Inspection Regulations*. Washington, DC: U.S. Department of Agriculture, Animal and Plant Health Inspection Service, 1976–.
Updated periodically, this publication covers the regulations for meat, poultry, and rabbit inspection. Regulations on voluntry inspection and information on the certification service of meat and poultry inspection are provided.

U.S. Department of Agriculture. Food Safety and Inspection Service. *Standards and Labeling Policy Book*. Washington, DC: U.S. Department of Agriculture, Food Safety and Inspection Service, Regulatory Programs, Standards and Labeling Division, 1991. 242p.
Directed toward label reviewers and manufacturers, this policy book sets forth the labeling requirements for meat and poultry products. Updated periodically.

U.S. Department of Health and Human Services. Public Health Service. Food and Drug Administration. *Requirements of Laws and Regulations Enforced by the U.S. Food and Drug Administration*. New York: Macmillan, 1982. 72p.
Directed towards manufacturers and shippers of food, drugs, cosmetics, or medical devices, this publication contains a summary of the principal requirements of laws and regulations enforced by the U.S. Food and Drug Administration.

K. Statistics, Surveys, and Reports

Beasley, Joseph D. and Jerry J. Swift. *The Kellogg Report: The Impact of Nutrition, Environment & Lifestyle on the Health of Americans*. Annandale-on-Hudson, NY: Institute of Health Policy and Practice, The Bard College Center, 1989. 735p.
This report is a result of ten years of research based on government studies, scientific journals, recent books, and news reports about the health of Americans. The report assesses the current health status, suggests how it can be improved, and identifies possible consequences of not taking action.

Cameron, Margaret and Wiji A. van Staveren. *Manual on Methodology for Food Consumption Studies*. Oxford: Oxford University Press, 1988. 259p. CORE
A study supported by the International Union of Nutritional Sciences and EURO-NUT (Concentrated Action Programme on Diet and Health of the Commission of the European Communities). Contains sections on purpose, methods, technical aspects, conversion into nutrients, analysis, validity, economic appraisals of study methods, and practical implementation of food consumption surveys.

Federation of American Societies for Experimental Biology. Life Sciences Research Office. *Nutrition Monitoring in the United States: An Update Report on Nutrition Monitoring*. Hyattsville, MD: U.S. Department of Health and Human Services, Public Health Service, and U.S. Department of Agriculture, Food and Consumer Services, September 1989. (DHHS Publication Series no. (PHS) 89–1255)
Reviews the dietary and nutritional status of the U.S. population as well as the factors determining it, based on the data and information available through the nutrition monitoring activities conducted by the U.S. Departments of Agriculture and Health and Human Services. This report is the second report on the National Nutritional Monitoring System (NNMS) and builds on the framework of the first report, *Nutrition Monitoring in the United States*, submitted in 1986.

Federation of American Societies for Experimental Biology. *Nutrition Monitoring in the United States: A Progress Report from the Joint Nutrition Monitoring Evaluation Committee*. Bethesda, MD: U.S. Department of Health and Human Services, 1986. 356p.
Focuses on the nutritional status of the U.S. population. The U.S. Departments of Agriculture and of Health and Human Services are both responsible for the sampling of the population and the compilation and reporting of the findings.

Food and Agriculture Organization of the United Nations. *Analysis of Food and Nutrition Survey Data for Developing Countries*. Rome: Food and Agriculture Organization of the United Nations, 1980. 146p. (*FAO Food and Nutrition Papers* no. 16.)

Food and Agriculture Organization of the United Nations. *Conducting Small-Scale Nutrition Surveys: A Field Manual*. Rome: Food and Agriculture Organization of the United Nations, 1990. 186p. (*Nutrition in Agriculture* no. 5.)

Food and Agriculture Organization of the United Nations. *Review of Food Consumption Surveys*. Rome: Food and Agriculture Organization of the United Nations, 1989. 197p. (*FAO Food and Nutrition Papers* no. 44.)

Frisancho, A. Roberto. *Anthropometric Standards for the Assessment of Growth and Nutritional Status*. Ann Arbor: University of Michigan Press, 1990. 189p.
Describes the theoretical rationale of the evaluation of nutritional status, techniques for data collection, statistical basis for classifying individuals or populations, standards, reference data for blacks and whites, and graphs that facilitate the interpretation of the data.

Martorell, Reynaldo. *Vitamin A Supplementation: Methodologies for Field Trials*. Washington, DC: National Academy Press; 1987. 91p. (Available from the Food and Nutrition Board.)
An authoritative text for clinical nutritionists, providing guidance on the planning of several longitudinal field trials proposed by the Office of Nutrition of the U.S. Agency for International Development to assess the impact of vitamin A supplementation on child mortality.

O'Mahony, Michael. *Sensory Evaluation of Food: Statistical Methods and Procedures*. New York: Dekker, 1986. 487p.
A reference text for college students, food scientists, and sensory professionals, providing a basic working knowledge of the logic and computation of statistics for the sensory evaluation of foods.

Piggott, J. R. *Statistical Procedures in Food Research.* London: Elsevier Applied Science, 1986. 415p.

An authoritative text with methods and data analysis tools. Topics include: experimental design; one-variable methods; practical approaches to regression analysis; response surface methods; discriminant analysis; methods to aid interpretation of multidimensional data; use of generalized procrustes techniques in sensory analysis; multidimensional scaling and its interpretation; partial least squares regression; and applied cluster analysis.

U.S. Department of Agriculture. Human Nutrition Information Service. *Nationwide Food Consumption Survey, Continuing Survey of Food Intakes of Individuals.* 5 vols. Hyattsville, MD: U.S. Department of Agriculture, Human Nutrition Information Service, 1985–1988.

Presents the data and results of a one-day food and nutrient intake survey for women (ages 19–50 years) and their children (ages 1–5) in the United States.

World Health Organization. *Guidelines for the Study of Dietary Intakes of Chemical Contaminants.* Geneva: World Health Organization, 1985. 104p. (WHO Offset Publication no. 87.)

Guidelines are provided to assist countries in collecting data for dietary intake of contaminant studies. Detailed procedures and methodology are covered as well as suggestions of ways to present the data.

8. Primary Historical Literature, 1850–1950

JENNIE BROGDON
Rockville, Maryland

DAPHNE A. ROE
Nutritional Science, Cornell University

A. Development of Food Science and Human Nutrition in the United States

In 1850, the preparation and processing of food products was based on empirical data and the understanding of the effect of food on the body was based largely on anecdotal observations. By 1950, the scientific foundations of food science and human nutrition were firmly established.

Food Science

Man has always been concerned with a safe, adequate food supply, so the basic techniques of food preservation such as salting, drying, and smoking have been known for thousands of years.[1] While these techniques were improved over time, no major new ones were developed until the invention of canning by Nicholas Appert in the late 1790s. This invention marks the beginning of food science.

During the hundred year period covered in this study, food industries were transformed by the social, cultural, and economic changes in the United States. These included the expansion of the country from the east to the west coast, the change from an agrarian society to an industrial one, the growth of cities, and the ravages of the Civil War. These changes brought about the transport of food products over long distances. Improvements in methods of transportation and the development of refrigeration and freezing

1. (a) George F. Stewart and Maynard A. Amerine, "Evolution of Food Preservation and Preservation," in *Introduction to Food Science and Technology*, 2d ed (New York: Academic Press, 1982). (b) Reay Tannahill, *Food in History* (New York: Stein & Day, 1973). (c) William J. Darby, Paul Ghalioungui, and Louis Grivetti. *Food: The Gift of Osiris*, 2 vols. (New York: Academic Press, 1977).

facilities made this possible. Through technological improvements and inventions, the preparation and processing of food during this period evolved from an "art" (trial and error or procedures based on observation) into a science.[2]

The canning industry in the United States provides an illustration of this evolution. The first description of the canning process, in French by Nicholas Appert in 1810, appeared in an English edition the next year and in an American one soon after.[3] Commercial canning in the United States began within a decade. By 1850 commercial products included seafood, jams, jellies, pickles, various fruits and vegetables, and condensed milk. The need for quantities of food by the armies during the Civil War resulted in a greatly expanded canning industry. However, it wasn't until the 1860s when Louis Pasteur discovered that microbes were the main cause of food spoilage, that there was an explanation of how thermal processing preserved foods. This was the basis for research by S. C. Prescott, W. L. Underwood, and H. L. Russell, which changed the industry into one based on science. One of the first books on food technology and canning, *Commercial Fruit and Vegetable Products* by William J. Cruess, was published in 1924.

The establishment of the United States Department of Agriculture (USDA) in 1862 and of the state agricultural experiment stations in 1887 had an enormous effect on the development of food science and human nutrition. The first chemist appointed by USDA, H. W. Wiley, was concerned with food safety, drugs, and truthful labeling. Under his direction, a series entitled *Foods and Food Adulterants* (*USDA Bulletin No. 13*) were published from 1887 to 1893.[4] Wiley worked for over twenty years for the passage of the first national law regulating the food supply, the Pure Food and Drug Act of 1906. The Meat Inspection Act was also enacted in 1906. Thirty-two years later, the federal Food, Drug and Cosmetic Act of 1938 was enacted along with major amendments to the Meat Inspection Act.

Because of the need for standardization, Wiley joined several state chemists in organizing the Association of Official Agricultural Chemists in 1884, and its *Journal* began publication in 1915.

2. S. A. Goldblith, "Fifty Years of Progress in Food Science and Technology," *Food Technology* 43 (9) (1989): 88–106, 286.

3. Nicholas Appert, *The Art of Preserving all Kinds of Animal and Vegetable Substances for Several Years*, 1st English ed. (London: Black, Perry & Kingsbury, 1811). Translation of *L'Art de Conserver, Pendant Plusieurs Années, Toutes les Substances Animales et Végétales*. (Reprint, St. Louis, Mo.: Mallinckrodt Chemical Works.)

4. (a) Bernard L. Oser, "The Impact of Analytical Chemistry on Food Science," *Food Technology* 29 (1975): 45–47. (b) Peter Barton Hutt, "Development and Growth of the Food and Drug Administration," *Food Technology* 43 (9) (1989): 280–286.

W. O. Atwater, first director of the Connecticut Agricultural Experiment Station and first chief of the USDA Office of Agricultural Experiment Stations, directed studies of food production, composition, digestibility, and metabolism. Along with C. D. Wood in 1896 and later with A. P. Bryant he wrote *The Chemical Composition of American Food Materials (USDA Bulletin No. 28)* which remained the principal source of food composition data for over forty years.

As food companies became technologically more advanced and established laboratories to ensure compliance with food regulations, a need developed for personnel with greater skills than artisans.[5] This need led to the first courses in food technology at the Massachusetts Institute of Technology (MIT) and Oregon State University in 1913. Other institutions developed training courses that reflected the needs of a particular area or industry. Classes were mainly product-oriented and taught in departments of dairy science, horticulture, or animal science. Gradually institutions began offering programs in food technology, and by 1950 courses were available in about thirty institutions.[6] The most rapid growth in university programs in food science occurred after 1950.

In the early 1900s research reports were published mainly in journals with broad subject scope, such as the *Journal of the American Chemical Society*. The journal, *Food Industries*, began in 1928, published by the McGraw-Hill, and *Food Research* began in 1936, published by Garrard Press.

In 1937 a Food Technology Conference was held at MIT with nearly 500 people in attendance.[7] Following this conference, a group of scientists discussed the formation of an organization of food-related scientists. The results of their discussions were presented at the second Food Technology Conference at MIT in 1939, and the group approved the formation of the Institute of Food Technologists (IFT). Established with twenty-two interested individuals, the institute had 839 founding and charter members by the end of the first year. From its beginning, IFT was interested in educational as well as professional advancement. Proceedings of papers presented at the annual conference were published in the early 1940s. The institute introduced *Food Technology* in January 1947. The IFT has been called "the

5. O. Fennema, "Educational Programs in Food Science: A Continuing Struggle for Legitimacy, Respect, and Recognition," *Food Technology* 43 (9) (1989): 170–182.

6. H. W. Schultz, "Educating Our Food Scientists and Technologists," *Food Technology* 18 (1964): 49–52.

7. Neil H Mermelstein, "History of the Institute of Food Technologists: The First Fifty Years," *Food Technology* 29 (1) (1975): 38–42.

single most important vehicle for the development and dissemination of knowledge in food science, technology, and engineering."[8]

In the late 1930s nutritionists, concerned about deficiencies resulting from refining of foods, lobbied for the enrichment of basic foods such as flour. The food industry responded to this concern and the two disciplines began to integrate.[9] This integration was furthered in World War II when research on military feeding demonstrated a need for improved knowledge of food processing and preservation and their effects on nutrition and palatability. Governmental funding of university research in these areas was a major factor in the development of food science as a discipline. The term *food science* was first popularized in 1948, when it was used as the title of a symposium held at the Low Temperature Research Station in Cambridge, Massachusetts.[10]

Human Nutrition

The first active period in the development of knowledge of human nutrition from the biological and social standpoints occurred about 1830, when scientific observation began to replace anecdotal information and dogmas about human nutrition. The years from 1830 to 1950 can be divided into two periods. The first period, 1830 to 1900, was one of emerging knowledge of nutritional physiology and the first realization that specific diseases were clearly linked to diet and poverty. Major advances in the knowledge of gastrointestinal function as well as new understandings of food as a body energy source initiated intense scientific interest in nutrition.

The most important writings which document how new knowledge of physiology was acquired include William Beaumont's description of his own experiments on changes taking place in the stomach in response to food consumption and his observations of changes in intestinal motility in response to dietary change.[11] Indeed, it was his meticulous description of human experiments which stimulated other physiologists in the US to follow this direct approach to the manner in which food was handled in the human body. Later physiologists, working in England and France during the second half of the nineteenth century, contributed to basic knowledge of

8. Goldblith, "Fifty Years of Progress," p. 102.

9. C. O. Chichester and William J. Darby, "The Historical Relationship between Food Science and Nutrition," *Food Technology* 29 (1) (1975): 38–42.

10. J. F. Diehl, "International Cooperation in Food Science and Technology and the Roles of Professional Institutes," *Food Australia* 42 (5) (1990): 286–290.

11. William Beaumont, *Experiments and Observations on the Gastric Juice and the Physiology of Digestion* (Cambridge: Harvard University Press, 1929 [Facsimile of the original 1833 ed.]).

nutrition by defining the need for calories as well as nitrogen during periods of adequate food intake as well as during starvation.

As urbanization increased so did interest in a healthy diet, which began as a vegetarian movement promoted by Sylvester Graham and William Alcott in the 1830s and was later taken up as a business venture by Kellogg and others, who initiated the breakfast cereal industry after the Civil War.[12]

The second period, 1900 to 1950, saw the development of the concept of deficiency diseases, attributable to lack of a specific nutrient. It was also the time of important nutritional interventions, in which nutritional deficiencies in human populations were prevented and also cured by changing diet. Knowledge of nutrition was applied in feeding soldiers, sailors, and airmen in World War I and again in World War II to maintain them in the best health. The feeding of civilian populations in the interest of improving health first became a major concern of the League of Nations after World War I. The League of Nations was the first international organization to develop a nutrition policy.[13]

New knowledge of human nutritional needs and more understanding of the concept of nutritional deficiency diseases initiated development of enriched and fortified food products as a means to prevent deficiencies affecting large subsections of the population. The idea of food fortification, originally applied to the prevention of endemic goiter by addition of iodide to salt, was expanded to other food products. The enrichment of bread and other cereal grains was initiated as a war order in 1943 in response to advice from the Food and Nutrition Board of the National Academy of Sciences. By the simple expedient of adding B vitamins to staple cereal products, it was possible to overcome pellagra, which is caused by a deficiency of the B vitamins, niacin and riboflavin. Similar concerns about childhood rickets, another deficiency disease, led to the addition of vitamin D to milk.

This period may also have been the first period in which was nutritionists cooperated with economists for the purpose of solving the social causes of malnutrition. The best example of this cooperation was the work of Joseph Goldberger and Edgar Sydenstricker, who demonstrated that pellagra was caused not by eating moldy corn, as previously thought, but rather by con-

12. D. A. Roe, "History of Promotion of Vegetable Cereal Diets," *Journal of Nutrition* 116 (1986): 1355–1363.

13. League of Nations, *The Problem of Nutrition*, vol. 3. *Nutrition in Various Countries* (1936. II.B. [Series of League of Nations Publications II], pp. 17–68).

suming a sharecropper's meager rations, which lacked animal protein foods.[14]

Between 1910 and the end of World War I, the infant welfare movement rapidly expanded in cities. In 1915 the National Dairy Council began a program of nutrition education for mothers to inform them of means to provide clean milk for their infants–the first such industry program.[15] The prevalence of diarrheal diseases among infants was reduced due to a better understanding of milk hygiene.

Nutrition literature began to proliferate during this period. One of the first books to present the scientific basis for nutrition was G. Lusk's *The Elements of the Science of Nutrition* in 1906.[16] Advancement of nutrition was greatly stimulated by the publication in 1918 of *The Newer Knowledge of Nutrition*,[17] in which E. V. McCollum presented the current knowledge and the problems still to be solved.[18] Today this book has particular interest because it acknowledges the contributions of women to nutritional science. Many of the early women nutritionists had a home economics background while others had graduate school experience in chemistry and physiology. Women's contributions to nutrition included the development of methods for food analyses and food consumption surveys. Hazel Stiebeling of the Bureau of Home Economics, USDA, was an early director of food consumption surveys among families. The surveys were conducted to examine food expenditures and purchases by families of different economic levels in urban and rural areas. The results were published in 1941 as *Family Food Consumption and Dietary Levels: Five Regions*. Icie Macy Hoobler developed methods to examine the nutrient requirements of children. She wrote *Nutrition and Chemical Growth in Childhood* (1942) and co-authored *The Hidden Hunger* (1945) with Harold Williams.

Early reports were printed in journals whose primary focus was chemistry, medicine, hygiene, or general science. In the 1920s and 1930s, publications specifically on nutrition began: the *Journal of the American Dietetic Association* in 1925, the *Journal of the American Institute of*

14. D. A. Roe, *A Plague of Corn, The Social History of Pellagra* (Ithaca, N.Y.: Cornell University Press, 1973), pp. 99–107.

15. E. Neige Todhunter, "Chronology of Some Events in the Development and Application of the Science of Nutrition," *Nutrition Reviews* 34 (1/2) (1976): 353–365.

16. (a) Graham Lusk, *The Elements of the Science of Nutrition* (Philadelphia: W. B. Saunders, 1906). (b) E. Neige Todhunter, "Some Classics of Nutrition and Dietetics," *Journal of American Dietetic Association* 44 (1964): 100–108.

17. Elmer V. McCollum, *The Newer Knowledge of Nutrition: The Use of Food for the Preservation of Vitality and Health* (New York: Macmillan Company, 1918.)

18. Leonard A. Maynard, " Early Days of Nutrition Research in the United States of America," *Nutrition Abstracts and Reviews* 32 (2) (1962): 345–355.

Nutrition in 1928, the British *Nutrition Abstracts and Reviews* in 1931, *Nutrition Reviews* in 1942, and the *British Journal of Nutrition* in 1947. In 1941 the first tables of recommended dietary allowances for nutrients known to be required by humans were prepared by the National Research Council.[19] This work is now in its tenth edition and ranked first among contemporary core monographs (see Chapter 6).

By 1900, courses in nutrition and dietetics were being taught in many colleges and universities in the United States.[20] The first person appointed with the title Professor of Nutrition was M. S. Rose, at the Teacher's College of Columbia University.

The basic science advances to 1950 included the ability to measure the expenditure of human energy, development of animals models with which to study nutritional physiology deficiencies, the isolation of vitamins and the identification of their biochemical functions, new knowledge of the biochemical cause of diet-related disease such as diabetes, and recognition that pathological states could also be induced by nutrient excess.

Biographical sketches of the nutritionists who were responsible for the major scientific, social, and health-related advances of the period appearing in the *Journal of Nutrition* have been reprinted in *Founders of Nutritional Science*, 1992.[21]

B. Historical Preservation

Since the early literature is physically disintegrating, the historical preservation phase of the Core Agricultural Literature Project, Albert R. Mann Library, Cornell University, is of vital importance. Prior to the 1860s, printing was done on paper with a high rag content which is very stable and remains in good condition. Since then, most paper has been manufactured with ground wood pulp. The resulting paper has a high acid content and, over time, begins to "burn" or turn yellow, becomes brittle, and eventually crumbles to dust. Since it would be prohibitively expensive to preserve all of the literature published during this hundred year period, that which is of most value to future generations must be identified.

In this study, we were primarily interested in English language literature published in the United States and Canada. It is assumed that other coun-

19. National Research Council. Food and Nutrition Board. *Recommended Dietary Allowances; Protein, Calcium, Iron, Vitamin A, Vitamin B (Thiamin), Vitamin C (Ascorbic Acid), Riboflavin, Nicotinic Acid, Vitamin D* (Washington, D.C.: 1941).

20. Jo Anne Cassell, *Carry the Flame: The History of the American Dietetic Association* (Chicago: The American Dietetic Association, 1990).

21. W. J. Darby and T. H. Jukes, eds. *Founders of Nutritional Science: Biographical Articles from the Journal of Nutrition, 1932–1990* (Bethesda, Md.: American Institute of Nutrition, 1992).

tries will preserve the important literature published within their boundaries. It is assumed also that because of their age and historical value that all monographs published before 1850 should have a high priority for preservation. Three types of publications important to food science and human nutrition in the United States have been identified and analyzed in the following categories: monographs, scholarly journals, and trade or popular periodicals.

C. Citation Analysis and Identification of Scholarly Monographic Literature

Methodology

Analysis of citations published in selected source documents were used to identify the scholarly literature. Citation analysis, which involves a count of each monograph, journal, and report series cited in the source documents, is explained in detail in Chapters 4 and 5. The same procedures were used for the historical analysis. The source documents listed here were selected in consultation with professors at Cornell University.

Sources of Citations in Historical Food Science and Human Nutrition

Items marked with an asterisk (*) were not analyzed, but monographs were extracted for evaluation.

Beeuwkes, Adelia, E. Neige Todhunter, and Emma S. Weigley. *Essays on History of Nutrition and Dietetics*. Reprinted. Chicago; American Dietetic Association, 1967. 291p.

Bourne, Geoffrey H. and George W. Kidder, eds. 2 vols. *Biochemistry and Physiology of Nutrition*. New York; Academic Press, 1953.

Cruess, W. V. *Commercial Fruit and Vegetable Products; A Textbook for Student, Investigator, and Manufacturer*. 3d ed. New York; McGraw-Hill, 1948. 906p.

*Falkner, Frank, ed. *Infant and Child Nutrition Worldwide: Issues and Perspectives*. Boca Raton, Fl.; CRC Press, 1991. 297p. (Selected chapters analyzed.)

Goldblith, Samuel A. and Maynard A. Joslyn. *Milestones in Nutrition*. Vol. 2. Westport, Conn.; Avi, 1964. 797p.

Harrow, Benjamin. *Vitamines, Essential Food Factors*. New York; E. P. Dutton & Co., 1921. 219p.

Jacobs, Morris B., ed. *The Chemistry and Technology of Food and Food Products*. 2d ed., rev. and augmented. 3 vols. New York; Interscience, 1951.

Jensen, Lloyd B. *Meat and Meat Foods; Processing and Preservation from Meat Plant to Consumer*. New York; Ronald Press, 1949. 218p.

Kruse, H. D. *Nutrition: Its Meaning, Scope, and Significance*. Springfield, Ill.; Charles C. Thomas, 1969. 195p.

McCollum, Elmer V. *A History of Nutrition: The Sequence of Ideas in Nutrition Investigations*. Boston; Houghton Mifflin, 1957. 451p.
*Powell, Ola. *Successful Canning and Preserving: Practical Hand Book for Schools, Clubs, and Home Use* . . . 4th ed., rev. and reset. Philadelphia; J. B. Lippincott, 1930. 663p.
Prescott, Samuel C. and Bernard E. Proctor. *Food Technology*. New York and London; McGraw-Hill, 1937. 630p.
Pyler, Ernst J. *Baking Science and Technology*. 2 vols. Chicago; Siebel Pub. Co., 1952.
Rogers, Lore A. *Fundamentals of Dairy Science*. 2d ed. New York; Reinhold, 1935. 616p. (Selected chapters analyzed.)
Rose, Mary S. *The Foundations of Nutrition*. New York; Macmillan, 1927. 501p.
*Sharrer, G. Terry, comp. *1001 References for the History of American Food Technology*. Davis; University of California, 1978. 103p. (A Cooperative Project by the Agricultural History Branch, Economic Research Service, U.S. Dept. of Agriculture, and the Agricultural History Center.)
Sherman, Henry C. *Chemistry of Food and Nutrition*. New York; Macmillan, 1911. 355p.
*Storck, John and Walter D. Teague. *Flour for Man's Bread; A History of Milling*. Minneapolis; University of Minnesota Press, 1952. 382p.
von Loesecke, Harry W. *Outlines of Food Technology*. 2d ed. New York; Reinhold, 1949. 585p.

Citation Analysis Results

A total of 11,661 citations were analyzed. Of these, 3,441 (29.6%) were monographs, twenty (0.7%) were dissertations and 133 (1.1%) were patents (Figure 8.1).

Journal literature was the most cited form of literature in both the historical and contemporary periods (69.2% and 75.6%, respectively). The difference was due primarily to the increase in contemporary human nutrition literature. As the percentage of journal literature increased, that of monographic literature decreased.

Nearly all patents cited in the historical literature were in food science (97%), while the majority of cited dissertations were in human nutrition (60%). The percentages of patent and dissertation literature did not differ markedly from the historical to contemporary analysis. When the historical citations were divided into food science and human nutrition fields, the percentages for each literature format differed only slightly. The types of publishers of the monographic literature are shown in Table 8.1. The percentage of commercial publishers was almost three times that of the next highest category, governmental. The high percentage of commercial publishers is especially characteristic of the human nutrition literature. The percentage is less high in food science, where works published by governmental and academic institutions were twice as high as in human nutrition.

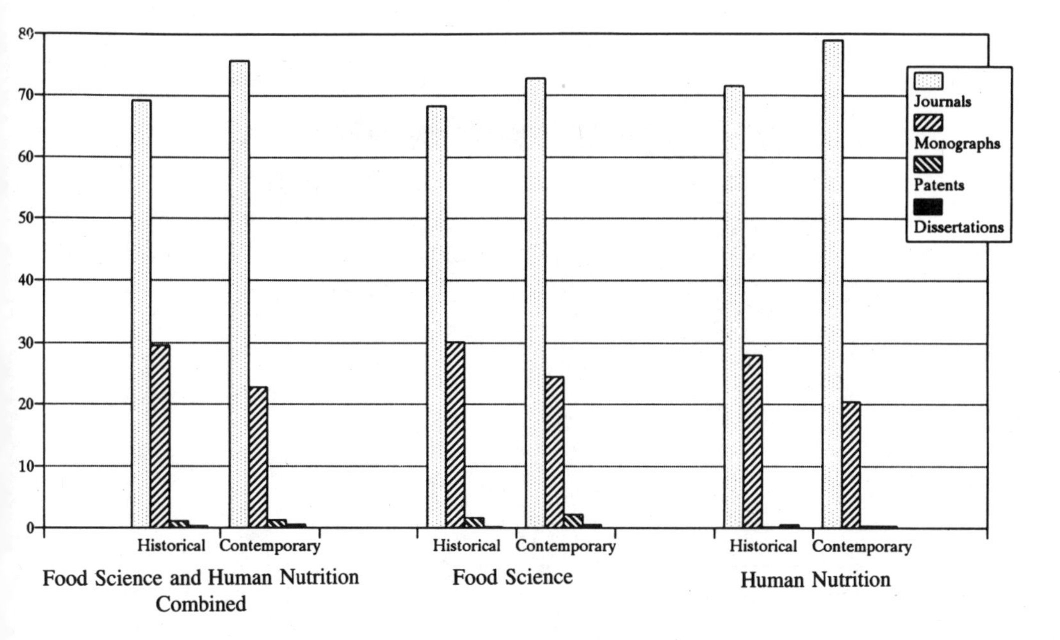

Figure 8.1. Food science and human nutrition literature citation analysis results.

A comparison of publishers in the historical and contemporary periods showed an increase in contemporary commercial publishers and a decrease in publications from universities (Figure 8.2). The top fifteen commercial publishers prior to 1950 are presented in Table 8.2. A comparison of these publishers with those of contemporary monographs shows some consistent carry over of publishers from the older to the more recent. One, Wiley, appears on the top-ranked list of contemporary publishers. McGraw-Hill and W. B. Saunders are on the contemporary list of human nutrition publishers and Interscience on the contemporary food science list (see Chapter 3). Over 79.3% of the monographic titles were published in the United

Table 8.1. Type of publishers of historical monographs

	Combined	Food science	Human nutrition
Commercial	55.1%	50.9%	70.5%
Governmental	19.6	21.8	11.3
University	18.1	20.3	10.1
Organizations	7.2	7.0	8.1

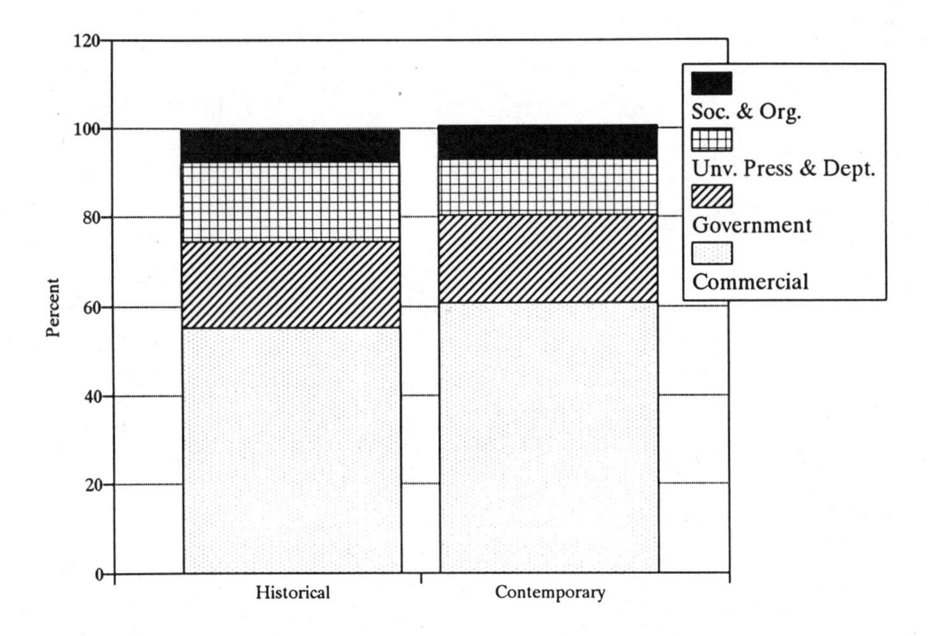

Figure 8.2. Publishers of monographs.

States, followed by the United Kingdom with 12.0%. All other countries accounted for 8.7%.

A total of 1,017 of the monographs were reports in series. These represented 140 different report series of which 40.7% were federal government reports, 37.9% university/agricultural experiment stations reports, and 22.4% organization reports. The United States Department of Agriculture

Table 8.2. Top-ranked commercial publishers before 1950

Rank	Publisher
1	Wiley
2	Macmillan
3	McGraw-Hill
4	Interscience
5	Van Nostrand
6	Reinhold
7	Longman, Green
8	Williams and Wilkins
9	W. B. Saunders
10	Blakiston

report series were the most cited, followed by those of the United States Fish and Wildlife Service. The university/agricultural experiment station publications most cited were from the University of California, Cornell University, and Michigan State University in that order. Organizations with the most cited report series were the National Canners Association and the Carnegie Institute of Washington.

The median half-life for the combined disciplines was 22.3 years. The median half-life for food science was 9.8 years and that for human nutrition was 36.6. The core monographic titles follow.

Core Monographs

In selecting monographs from the cited material, preference was given to English language titles, primarily those published in the United States and Canada. Shorter monographs under fifty pages were excluded as were the majority of land-grant publications in series and federal documents since these are being preserved under established programs. However, select land-grant and federal publications that were clearly of long-lasting historical significance were included. After the monographs were identified, a list of over 800 titles was sent to reviewers for ranking. All reviewers had extensive research and teaching experience. They were:

Hamish Munro
Human Nutrition Research Center on Aging
U.S. Dept. of Agriculture
Boston, Mass.
Helen Guthrie
Dept. of Nutrition
Pennsylvania State University
Samuel A. Goldblith
Massachusett Inst. of Technology
Frank V. Kosikowski
Dept. of Food Science
Cornell University
Daphne Roe
Nutritional Science
Cornell University

Ten additional reviewers were sent lists which were not returned. Reviewers were encouraged to suggest additional titles to incorporate into the list, although no more than fifteen were recommended. Reviewers were asked to rank the titles, keeping in mind the following criteria for important works:

1. The work has had an important influence in the field, either because the author was important, because later authors referred to it frequently, because it was a major compilation or compendium of the time, or because later efforts were built on it.
2. The work was the first of its kind, or one recording major advances in the field.
3. The work embodies an historical record or changes in the field.

4. The title is valuable because it is a superior work of a leader in the food and human nutrition sciences.
5. The work includes unusual or valuable etchings, prints, or illustrations.
6. The title has survived in a very limited number of copies.

A three point scale was used for reviewers' rankings

1. A very important historical title worthy of preservation
2. Worth preserving but of secondary importance
3. A title of marginal historical value

The evaluation list included some major non-English titles as well as large or significant United States government reports, most of which were in a series. Selected foreign language titles were evaluated because they often served as a basis for American work. An effort was made to see if some United States government documents stood out as very important. Of greatest significance in this category is the work of Wilbur O. Atwater and his colleagues with the USDA, who just before 1900 did extensive work concerned with metabolism and the chemical composition of food. Four of his works, all of them in the *Bulletin* series of the USDA Office of Experiment Stations, were rated of top importance. These are not in the final list of core monographs because they are being preserved as part of a USDA series. Atwater, along with Francis G. Benedict, has a non-governmental document in the final historical core listing. Benedict also had four highly rated USDA serial publications and is represented with three non-governmental titles in the historical core monograph list. These are probably the most well-known and highly rated early researchers who worked with the United States government in food science and human nutrition.

The final step was calculating a total score for each title by adding the number of times that the title appeared in the source documents (citations hits) with the cumulative ranks. Each ranking category was weighted; peer rankings of 1 were weighed by a factor of 3; ranks of 2 by a factor of 2, and ranks of 3 by a factor of 1. Thus, the final monograph rankings were calculated using the formula:

$$\text{Final Ranking} = (1 \times \#\ \text{citations hits}) + (3 \times \text{rank 1}) + (2 \times \text{rank 2}) + (1 \times \text{rank 3})$$

The initial 800 monographs identified by the citation analysis was reduced to the following list, which includes 579 monograph titles published after 1850. All monographs earlier than 1850 relating to food science and human nutrition are considered of primary historical value and to be preserved based only on age. The pre-1850 literature most closely allied to this subject area comes primarily from medicine and the chemistry of foods. This literature seems to be the precursor of food science and human nutrition prior to 1900 in United States publications. The removal of the foreign language, pre- 1850, and U.S. federal documents is responsible for the drop to less than 600 final titles. The monographs that remain in the following list are those of greatest value for preservation in United States libraries.

The final rankings were divided into two levels with level one being given the highest priority for preservation.

Primary Historical Monographs Worthy of Preservation

Ranking	
	A
Second	Abderhalden, Emil. Text-Book of Physiological Chemistry in Thirty Lectures . . . transl. by William T. Hall and George Defren. 1st ed. New York; J. Wiley, 1914. 722p.
First	Accum, Friedrich C. A Treatise on Adulterations of Food and Culinary Poisons: Exhibiting the Fraudulent Sophistications of Bread, Beer, Wine, Spiritous Liquors . . . and Methods of Detecting Them. Philadelphia; Printed and published by A. Small, 1820. (Reprinted, St. Louis, Mo.; Mallinckrodt Chemical Works, 1966. 269p.)
Second	Adam, Neil K. The Physics and Chemistry of Surfaces. Oxford; Clarendon, 1930. 332p. (3d ed., London; Oxford University Press, 1941. 436p.)
Second	Adams, Harold S. Milk and Food Sanitation Practice. New York; Commonwealth Fund, 1947. 311p.
First	Adolph, Edward F. Physiology of Man in the Desert. New York; Interscience, 1947. 357p.
Second	Alexander, Jerome. Colloid Chemistry; Principles and Applications. 1st ed. New York; Van Nostrand, 1919. 90p. (4th ed., 1937. 505p.)
Second	Alexander, Jerome, ed. Colloid Chemistry; Theoretical and Applied. New York; Chemical Catalog Co., 1928–1944. 6 vols.
Second	Alexander, Jerome. Glue and Gelatin. New York; Chemical Catalog Co., 1923. 236p.
First	Allen, Alfred H. An Introduction to the Practice of Commercial Organic Analysis. London; J. & A. Churchill; Philadelphia; P. Blakiston, 1879–1882. 2 vols. (5th ed., rev. and edited by Samuel S. Sadler, et al., 1923–1933. 10 vols.)
Second	Allen, Frederick M., Edgar Stillman, and Reginald Fitz. Total Dietary Regulation in the Treatment of Diabetes. New York; Rockefeller Institute for Medical Research, 1919. 646p.

Rank	
Second	Allen, H. Warner. The Romance of Wine. London; E. Benn, 1931. 264p. (Reprinted, New York; Dover, 1971. Also available in Portuguese as Vinho do Porto, O Vinho da Filosofia, 1946.)
First	Alsberg, Carl L., and Alonzo E. Taylor. The Fats and Oils, a General View. Stanford University, Calif.; Food Research Institute, 1928. 103p.
Second	American Association of Cereal Chemists. Cereal Laboratory Methods, with Reference Tables. St. Paul, Minn.; 1935.
First	American Can Company. The Canned Food Reference Manual. New York; American Can Co., 1939. 242p. (3d ed., 1947. 638p.)
Second	American Meat Institute. Pork Operations. 4th ed., rev. Ann Arbor, Mich.; Edwards Brothers, 1936. 197p. (6th ed., rev., Chicago; Institute of Meat Packing, University of Chicago, 1957. 335p.)
Second	American Medical Association. Council on Foods and Nutrition. Handbook of Nutrition; A Symposium . . . Chicago; AMA, 1943. 586p. (2d ed., Philadelphia; Published for AMA by Blakiston, 1951. 717p.)
Second	American Medical Association. The Vitamins; Proceedings of a Symposium . . . arranged by the Council on Pharmacy and Chemistry and the Council on Foods of the AMA. Chicago; AMA, 1939. 637p.
First	American Oil Chemists' Society. Official and Tentative Methods of the AOCS. New York; 1937. 1 vol. (4th ed., Champaign, Ill.; AOCS, 1989)
Second	American Public Health Association. Standard Methods for the Examination of Water and Wastewater. 1st ed. Washington, D.C.; APHA, 1905. 1 vols. (9th ed., 1946. 286p.)
First	Amos, Percy A. Processes of Flour Manufacture. London and New York; Longmans, Green & Co., 1912. 280p. (Later ed., rev. by J. Grant, 1938. 310p.)
Second	Andersen, Aage J. C., and Percy N. Williams. Margarine. New York; Academic Press, 1954. 327p. (2d ed., Oxford and New York; Pergamon Press, 1965. 420p.)
Second	Anderson, J. Ansel, ed. Enzymes and Their Role in Wheat Technology. New York; Published for the American Association of Cereal Chemists by Interscience, 1946. 371p. (AACC Monograph Series no. I)
First	Anonymus Londinensis. The Medical Writings of Anonymus Londinensis . . . by W. H. S. Jones. Cambridge, Eng.; University Press, 1947. 168p. (Reprinted, Amsterdam; Hakkert, 1968.)
First	Anstie, Francis E. On the Uses of Wines in Health and Disease. New York; J.S. Redfield, 1870. 84p. (Later ed., London; Macmillan, 1877. 74p.)
First	Armsby, Henry P. The Conservation of Food Energy. Philadelphia; W. B. Saunders, 1918. 65p.
Second	Armstrong, E. Frankland. The Carbohydrates. London and New York; Longmans, Green, 1934. 252p.
First	Armstrong, E. Frankland. The Simple Carbohydrates and the Glucosides. 1st ed. London; Longmans, Green, 1910. 112p. (4th ed., London and New York; 1924. 293p.)
Second	Ashley, W. J. The Bread of Our Forefathers; An Inquiry in Economic History. Oxford, Eng.; Clarendon Press, 1928. 206p.
First	Association of Official Analytical Chemists. Official and Tentative Methods

Rank

	of Analysis. Washington, D.C.; AOAC, 1920. 417p. (10th ed., 1965. 957p. [Originally publ. as Association of Official Agricülutural Chemists. Committee on Revision of Methods. Official and Provisional Methods of Analysis . . . edited by Harvey W. Wiley. Washington, D.C.; U.S. Govt. Print. Off., 1908. 272p. (USDA Bureau of Chemistry Bulletin No. 107])
Second	Atkinson, Edward. The Application of Science to the Production and Consumption of Food; An Address . . . Meeting of the American Association for the Advancement of Science, Aug. 1885. Salem, Mass.; Salem Press, 1885. 74p.
Second	Atkinson, Edward. The Science of Nutrition. Treatise upon the Science of Nutrition. Springfield; 1892. 179p.
First	Atwater, Wilbur O., and F. G. Benedict. A Respiration Calorimeter with Appliances for the Direct Determination of Oxygen. Washington, D.C.; Carnegie Institution of Washington, 1905. 193p. (CIW Publication no. 42)

B

Second	Badger, Walter L., and G. E. Seavoy. Heat Transfer and Crystallization, a Practical Presentation of the Fundamental Principles Underlying Modern Evaporation and Crystallization Methods and Equipment. Harvey, Ill.; Swenson Evaporator Co., 1945. 52p.
Second	Bailey, Alton E., ed. Cottonseed and Cottonseed Products; Their Chemistry and Chemical Technology. New York; Interscience Publishers, 1948. 936p.
First	Bailey, Alton E. Industrial Oil and Fat Products. New York; Interscience, 1945. 735p. (4th ed., as Bailey's Industrial Oil and Fat Products, edited by Daniel Swern. New York; Wiley, 1979–1985. 3 vols)
First	Bailey, Clyde H. The Chemistry of Wheat Flour. New York; Chemical Catalog Co., 1925. 324p. (American Chemical Society Monograph Series no. 26)
Second	Bailey, Clyde H. The Constituents of Wheat and Wheat Products. New York; Reinhold, 1944. 332p. (Amereican Chemical Society Monograph Series no. 96)
First	Bailey, Edgar H. S. Food Products. 2d ed. Philadelphia; P. Blakiston's, 1921. 551p. (3d ed., rev., by E. H. S. Bailey and Herbert S. Bailey, 1928. 563p.) (1st ed., titled: The Source, Chemistry and Use of Food Products. 1914.)
First	Bailey, Edgar. The Source, Chemistry and Use of Food Products. Philadelphia; P. Blakiston's, 1914. 517p. (Also issued in 1916 & 1918)
First	Ball, Charles O. Mathematical Solution of Problems on Thermal Processing of Canned Foods. Berkeley; University of California Press, 1928. 245p.
Second	Bartlett, Roland W. The Milk Industry; A Comprehensive Survey of Production, Distribution, and Economic Importance. New York; Ronald Press Co., 1946. 282p.
First	Bashforth, Francis, and J. C. Adams. An Attempt to Test the Theories of Capillary Action by Comparing the Theoretical and Measured Forms of Drops of Fluid . . . Cambridge, Eng.; University Press, 1883. 80p.

Rank	
First	Battershall, Jesse P. Food Adulterations and Its Detection. New York and London; E. & F. N. Spon, 1887. 328p.
First	Baumgartner, John G. Canned Foods; An Introduction to Their Microbiology. London; Churchill, 1943. 157p. (7th ed., as Canned Foods: Thermal Processing and Microbiology, by A. C. Hersom and E. D. Hulland. Edinburgh and New York; Churchill Livingstone, 1980. 380p.)
Second	Baylis, John R. Elimination of Taste and Odor in Water. 1st ed. New York and London; McGraw-Hill, 1935. 392p.
First	Bayliss, William M. The Nature of Enzyme Action. London and New York; Longmans, Green, 1908. 90p. (5th ed., 1925. 200p.)
Second	Bayliss, William M. The Physiology of Food and Economy in Diet. London; Longmans, Green, 1917. 107p.
Second	Beaumont, William. Experiments and Observations on the Gastric Juice and the Physiology of Digestion. Facsimile of the original 1833 ed. Cambridge; Harvard University Press, 1929. 280p. (2d ed. as The Physiology of Digestion.)
First	Beeuwkes, Adelia M., E. Neige Todhunter, and Emma S. Weigley, compilers. Essays on History of Nutrition and Dietetics. Chicago; American Dietetic Association, 1967. 291p.
Second	Beilby, George T. Aggregation and Flow of Solids; Being the Records of an Experimental Study of the Micro-Structure and Physical Properties of Solids in Various States of Aggregation, 1900–1921. London; Macmillan, 1921. 256p.
Second	Bell, David J. Introduction to Carbohydrate Biochemistry. London; University Tutorial Press, 1940. 112p. (3d ed., 1952. 100p.)
Second	Ben Meyr, Berl. Sanitation for Food Handlers and Sellers. Los Angeles; American Institute of Sanitary Science, 1948. 126p.
First	Benedict, Francis G. Vital Energetics; A Study in Comparative Basal Metabolism. Washington, D.C.; Carnegie Institution of Washington, 1938. 215p. (Carnegie Institution of Washington, Publication no. 503)
First	Benedict, Francis G., and Thorne M. Carpenter. Food Ingestion and Energy Transformation, with Special Reference to the Stimulating Effect of Nutrients. Washington, D.C.; Carnegie Institution of Washington, 1918. 355p. (Carnegie Institution of Washington, Publication no. 261)
First	Benedict, Francis G., and Thorne M. Carpenter. The Influence of Inanition on Metabolism. Washington, D.C.; Carnegie Institution of Washington, 1907. 542p.
First	Benedict, Francis G., and Thorne M. Carpenter. The Metabolism and Energy Transformations of Healthy Man during Rest. Washington, D.C.; Carnegie Institution of Washington, 1910. 255p.
First	Benedict, Francis G., and Thorne M. Carpenter. Respiration Calorimeters for Studying the Respiratory Exchange and Energy Transformations of Man. Washington, D.C.; Carnegie Institution of Washington, 1910. 102p. (Carnegie Institution of Washington Publication no. 123)
Second	Benedict, Francis G., and Edward P. Cathcart. Muscular Work; A Metabolic Study with Special Reference to the Efficiency of the Human Body as

Rank	
	a Machine. Washington, D.C.; Carnegie Institution of Washington, 1913. 176p. (Carnegie Institution of Washington Publication no. 187)
Second	Benjamin, Earl W. Marketing Poultry Products. New York; J. Wiley & Sons, 1923. 328p. (5th ed., 1960. 327p.)
First	Bennett, Richard, and John Elton. History of Corn Milling. London; Simpkin, Marshall & Co., 1898–1899. 2 vols. (Reissued, New York; B. Franklin, 1964. 4 vols.)
Second	Bennion, Edmund B. Cake Manufacture. London; L. Hill, 1943. 264p. (4th ed., as Cake Making, by E.B. Bennion, James Steward and G.S.T. Bamford, 1966. 347p.)
First	Bergey, D. H. Bergey's Manual of Determinative Bacteriology: A Key for the Identification of Organisms of the Class Schizomycetes. Baltimore; Williams & Wilkins, 1923. 461p. (8th ed., edited by R. E. Buchanan and N. E. Gibbons, 1974. 1246p.)
Second	Berman, Matthew. The How and Why of Candy Making. Chicago; E. Boyles, 1925. 480p.
First	Bevier, Isabel, and Anna R. Van Meter. Selection and Preparation of Food; Laboratory Guide, Department of Household Science, the University of Illinois. Boston; Whitcomb & Barrows, 1907. 86p. (Rev. ed., 1910. 86p.)
Second	Bienfang, Ralph D. The Subtle Sense. 1st ed. Norman; University of Oklahoma Press, 1946. 157p.
First	Bigue, Robert H., ed. The Theory and Application of Colloidal Behavior. New York; McGraw-Hill, 1924. 2 vols.
Second	Bingham, Eugene C. Fluidity and Plasticity. 1st ed. New York; McGraw-Hill, 1922. 440p.
Second	Binsted, Raymond. Pickle and Sauce Making. London; R. H. Binsted, 1939. 128p.
Second	Bisbee, Lewis H., and John C. Simonds. The Board of Trade and the Produce Exchange, Their History, Methods and Law. Chicago; Callaghan & Co., 1884. 435p.
Second	Bitting, Arvill W. Appertizing; or, The Art of Canning; Its History and Development. San Francisco; Trade Pressroom, 1937. 852p.
First	Bitting, Arvill W., and K. G. Bitting. Canning and How to Use Canned Foods. Washington, D.C.; National Canning Association, 1916. 184p.
Second	Bitting, Katherine G. The Effect of Certain Agents on the Development of Some Moulds. Washington, D.C.; National Capital Press, 1920. 176p.
Second	Blakey, Roy G. The United States Beet-Sugar Industry and the Tariff. New York; Columbia University, 1912. 286p.
First	Block, Richard J., and Diana Bolling. The Amino Acid Composition of Proteins and Foods; Analytical Methods and Results. 1st ed. Springfield, Ill.; C. C. Thomas, 1945. 396p. (2d ed., 1951. 576p.)
First	Blum, Harold F. Photodynamic Action and Diseases Caused by Light. New York; Reinhold, 1941. 309p. (ACS Monograph Series no. 85) (Reprinted by Hafner Pub. Co., 1964.)
Second	Blumenthal, Saul. Food Manufacturing; A Compendium of Food Information, with Practical Factory-Tested Commercial Formulae for the Food Man-

Rank

Rank	Entry
	ufacturer, Chemist, Technologist, in the Canning, Flavoring, Beverage, Confectionery, Essence, Condiment, Dairy Products, Meat and Fish, and Allied Industries. Brooklyn, N.Y.; Chemical Pub. Co., 1942. 664p.
First	Blumenthal, Saul. Food Products. Brooklyn, N.Y.; Chemical Pub. Co., 1947. 986p.
First	Blunt, Katharine, and Ruth Cowan. Ultraviolet Light and Vitamin D in Nutrition. Chicago; University of Chicago Press, 1930. 229p.
First	Blyth, Alexander W. Foods: Their Composition and Analysis. London; C. Griffin & Co., 1882. 586p. (7th ed., 1927. 619p.)
First	Bogert, L. Jean. Nutrition and Physical Fitness. Philadelphia and London; W. B. Saunders, 1931. 554p. (Later eds. by George M. Briggs and Doris H. Calloway. 11th ed., New York; Holt, Rinehart & Winston, 1984. 697p.)
First	Boorde, Andrew. The Fyrst Boke of the Introduction of Knowledge . . . A Compendyous Regyment or A Dyetary of Helth Made in Mountpyllier. London; Published for the Early English Text Society by N. Trubner, 1870. 396p. (Early English Text Society, Extra Series no. 10) (Reprinted, edited by F. J. Furnivall, Milwood, N.Y.; Kraus Reprint, 1975.)
First	Borsook, Henry. Vitamins, What They Are and How They Can Benefit You. New York; Viking Press, 1940. 193p.
Second	Bose, Jyoti P. A Handbook on Diabetes Mellitus and Its Modern Treatment. Calcutta and Simla; Thacker, Spink & Co., 1928. 192p. (5th ed., rev., Calcutta; Das Gupta, 1962. 255p.)
Second	Bourne, Geoffrey H., and George W. Kidder, eds. Biochemistry and Physiology of Nutrition. New York; Academic Press, 1953. 2 vols.
First	Braddon, William L. The Cause and Prevention of Beri-Beri. London and New York; Rebman, 1907. 544p.
Second	Bradfield, Edward. Wheat and the Flour Mill; A Handbook for Practical Flour Millers. Liverpool; Northern Pub. Co., 1920. 163p.
First	Braverman, Joseph B. S. Citrus Products: Chemical Composition and Chemical Technology. New York; Interscience, 1949. 424p.
Second	Brayley, Arthur W. Bakers and Baking in Massachusetts: Including the Flour, Baking Supply and Kindred Interests, from 1620 to 1909. Boston; Master Bakers' Association of Massachusetts, 1909. 336p.
Second	Brennemann, Joseph. Practice of Pediatrics. Hagerstown, Md.; Harper & Row, 1933. 4 vols. (Rev. ed., edited by Vincent C. Kelley, Philadelphia; Medical Dept., Harper & Row, 1983. 11 vols.)
First	Brillat-Savarin, Jean A. The Physiology of Tastes: Or, Transcendental Gastronomy . . . transl. from the last Paris ed. by Fayette Robinson. Philadelphia; Lindsay & Blakiston, 1854. 347p. (Translation of Physiologie du Gout.)
Second	Broadhurst, Jean. Home and Community Hygiene; A Text-Book of Personal and Public Health. Philadelphia and London; J. B. Lippincott, 1918. 428p. (4th ed., rev. and enlarged, 1929. 469p.)
First	Brody, Samuel. Bioenergetics and Growth, with Special Reference to the Efficiency Complex in Domestic Animals. New York; Reinhold, 1945. 1023p.
Second	Brooks, Ralph O. Critical Studies in the Legal Chemistry of Foods; For

Rank	
	Chemists, Food Inspection Officials, and Manufacturers and Dealers in Food Products. New York; Chemical Catalog Co., 1927. 280p.
First	Browne, Charles A. A Handbook of Sugar Analysis: A Practical and Descriptive Treatise for Use in Research, Technical and Control Laboratories. 1st ed. New York; J. Wiley & Sons; London; Chapman & Hall, 1912. 787p. (3d ed., rewritten and reset, by C.A. Browne and F.W. Zerban, as Physical and Chemical Methods of Sugar Analysis . . . , 1941. 1353p.)
Second	Browning, Ethel. The Vitamins. London; Bailliere, Tindall & Cox; Baltimore; Williams & Wilkins, 1931. 575p.
Second	Budin, Pierre. The Nursling; The Feeding and Hygiene of Premature and Full-Term Infants. London; Caxton, 1907. 199p.
Second	Buller, A. H. Reginald. Essays on Wheat, Including the Discovery and Introduction of Marquis Wheat, the Early History of Wheat-Growing in Manitoba, Wheat in Western Canada, the Origin of Red Bobs and Kitchener, and the Wild Wheat of Palestine. New York; Macmillan Co., 1919. 339p.
Second	Butt, Hugh R., and Albert M. Snell. Vitamin K. Philadelphia and London; W. B. Saunders, 1941. 172p.
Second	Butterick Publishing Co. The Story of a Pantry Shelf; An Outline History of Grocery Specialties. New York; Butterick, 1925. 224p.
Second	Bywaters, Hubert W. Modern Methods of Cocoa and Chocolate Manufacture. London; Churchill; Philadelphia; P. Blakiston, 1930. 316p.

C

First	Caldwell, G. C. Agricultural Qualitative and Quantitative Chemical Analysis. New York; O. Judd, 1869. 307p.
Second	Cameron, Alexander T. The Taste Sense and the Relative Sweetness of Sugars and Other Sweet Substances. New York; Sugar Research Foundation, 1947. 72p.
First	Cameron, Charles A. The Stock-Feeder's Manual; The Chemistry of Food in Relation to the Breeding and Feeding of Live Stock. London and New York; Cassell, Petter, and Galpin, 1868. 253p.
Second	Cameron, Jenks. The Bureau of Biological Survey: Its History, Activities, and Organization. Baltimore; Johns Hopkins Press, 1929. 339p. (Service Monographs of the U.S. Government no. 54)
First	Campbell, Clyde H. Campbell's Book: A Text Book on Canning, Preserving and Pickling. 1st ed. New York; Canning Age, 1929. 246p. (3d ed., rev., by Rohland A. Isker and Walter A. Maclinn, Chicago; Vance Pub., 1950. 222p.)
Second	Cannon, Paul R. Some Pathologic Consequences of Protein and Amino Acid Deficiencies. Springfield, Ill.; C. C. Thomas, 1948. 49p. (American Lecture Series no. 27)
Second	Cannon, Walter B. The Wisdom of the Body. New York; W. W. Norton & Co., 1932. 312p. (Reissued, Birmingham, Ala.; Classics of Medicine Library, 1989. 333p.)
Second	Carlisle, Anthony. An Essay on the Disorders of Old Age, and on the Means for Prolonging Human Life. London; Printed for Longman, Hurst,

Rank	
	Rees, Orme, & Brown, 1817. 103p. (Reprinted, New York; Arno Press, 1979.)
First	Carlson, Anton J. The Control of Hunger in Health and Disease. Chicago; University of Chicago Press, 1916. 319p.
Second	Carnegie United Kingdom Trust. Report on the Physical Welfare of Mothers and Children. Liverpool; Printed by C. Tinling & Co., 1917. 4 vols.
First	Carter, Herbert W., Paul E. Howe, and Howard H. Mason. Nutrition and Clinical Dietetics. Philadelphia and New York; Lea & Febiger, 1917. 646p. (3d ed., rev., 1923. 731p.)
First	Castle, William B., and George R. Minot. Pathological Physiology and Clinical Description of the Anemias . . . edited by Henry A. Christian. New York; Oxford University Press, 1936. 205p.
First	Cathcart, Edward P. The Physiology of Protein Metabolism. London and New York; Longmans, Green, 1912. 142p. (Later ed., 1921. 176p.)
Second	Charcot, Jean M. Clinical Lectures on Senile and Chronic Diseases. London; New Sydenham Society; New York; W. Wood & Co., 1881. 307p. (New Sydenham Society, Publications no. 95) (Translation of Lecons Cliniques sur les Maladies des Vieillards et les Maladies Chroniques. Reprinted, New York; Arno Press, 1979.)
Second	Charley, Vernon L. S., ed. Recent Advances in Fruit Juice Production. East Malling, Eng.; Commonwealth Bureau of Horticulture and Plantation Crops, 1950. 176p. (Technical Communication no. 21)
Second	Charley, Vernon L., and T. H. J. Harrison. Fruit Juices and Related Products. East Malling, Kent, Eng.; Imperial Bureau of Horticulture and Plantation Crops, 1939. 104p.
Second	Cheadle, Walter B. On the Principles and Exact Conditions to Be Observed in the Artificial Feeding of Infants; The Properties of Artificial Foods; And the Diseases Which Arise from Faults of Diet in Early Life. London; Smith, Elder, 1889. 1 vols. (6th ed., edited and rev. by F. J. Poynton, 1906. 274p.)
Second	Cheever, Lawrence O. The House of Morell. Cedar Rapids, Iowa; Torch Press, 1948. 303p.
Second	Chenoweth, Walter W. Food Preservation; A Textbook for Student, Teacher, Homemaker and Home Factory Operator. New York; J. Wiley; London; Chapman & Hall, 1930. 344p.
Second	Chittenden, Russell H. The Nutrition of Man. New York; F. A. Stokes, 1907. 321p.
Second	Chittenden, Russell H. Physiological Economy in Nutrition, with Special Reference to the Minimal Protein Requirement of the Healthy Man; An Experimental Study. New York; F. A. Stokes, 1904. 478p.
Second	Clarke, A. Flavouring Materials, Natural and Synthetic. London; Frowde, Hodder & Stoughton, 1922. 166p.
Second	Clayton, William. Colloid Aspects of Food Chemistry and Technology. Philadelphia; Blakiston; London; J. & A. Churchill, 1932. 571p.
Second	Clayton, William. The Theory of Emulsions and Emulsification. London; J. & A. Churchill, 1923. 160p. (5th ed., by C.G. Sumner, as The Theory of

Rank

Emulsions and Their Technical Treatment. New York; Blakiston, 1954. 669p.)

First — Cobb, John N. The Canning of Fishery Products; Showing the History of the Art of Canning. Seattle, Wash.; M. Freeman, 1919. 217p.

First — Cocoa and Chocolate. A Short History of Their Production and Use, with Full and Particular Account of Their Properties, and of the Various Methods of Preparing Them for Food. Dorchester, Mass.; Walter Baker & Co., 1886. 165p. (Later ed., 1917. 82p.)

Second — Collins, James H. The Story of Canned Foods. New York; E. P. Dutton & Co., 1924. 251p.

First — A Complete Course in Canning. Being a Thorough Expositon of the Best, Practical Methods of Hermetically Sealing Canned Goods, and Preserving Fruits and Vegetables. 1st ed. Baltimore; Canning Trade Press, 1906. 182p. (12th ed., rev. and enl. by Anthony Lopez, 1987. 3 vols.)

Second — Conn, Herbert W. Agricultural Bacteriology; A Study of the Relation of Germ Life to the Farm, with Laboratory Experiments for Students. Philadelphia; P. Blakiston's Son, 1901. 412p. (3d ed., rev. by Harold J. Conn, 1918. 357p.)

Second — Continental Baking Corporation. The Story of Bread, Its Modern Production under Laboratory Supervision and Sanitary Baking Methods, and a Study of the Importance of Wheat in the World's Health and Nourishment . . . New York; Continental Baking Corp., 1925. 69p.

Second — Cook, Hugh L., and George H. Day. The Dry Milk Industry; An Aid in the Utilization of the Food Constitutents of Milk. Chicago; American Dry Milk Institute, 1947. 169p.

Second — Cornaro, Luigi. The Art of Living Long. Milwaukee, Wis.; W. F. Butler, 1903. 214p. (Translation of Discorsi della Vita sobria. Reprinted, New York; Arno Press, 1979.)

Second — Cory, Lewis. Meat and Man; A Study of Monopoly, Unionism, and Food Policy. New York; Viking Press, 1950. 377p.

Second — Cotter, Oliver. See What You Drink. Read, and Drink No More. Adulteration of Liquors, with a Description of the Poisons Used in Their Manufacture. New York; A. S. Barnes & co., 1874. 45p.

First — Cowgill, George R. The Vitamin B Requirement of Man. New Haven, Conn.; Published for the Institute of Human Relations by Yale University Press; London; H. Milford, Oxford University Press, 1934. 265p.

First — Crichton-Browne, James. Parcimony in Nutrition. London and New York; Funk & Wagnalls, 1909. 111p.

Second — Crissey, Forrest. The Story of Foods. Chicago; Rand, McNally, 1917. 543p.

First — Critchell, James T., and Joseph Raymond. A History of the Frozen Meat Trade; An Account of the Development and Present Day Methods of Preparation, Transport, and Marketing of Frozen and Chilled Meats. London; Constable & Co., 1912. 442p. (Reprinted, London; Dawsons, 1969.)

First — Crocker, Ernest C. Flavor. 1st ed. New York and London; McGraw-Hill, 1945. 172p.

Rank	
Second	Crookshank, Francis G. Epidemiological Essays. London; K. Paul, Trench, Trubner & Co., 1930. 136p. (Also published, New York; Macmillan Co., 1931.)
First	Cruess, William V. Commercial Fruit and Vegetable Products; A Textbook for Student, Investigator and Manufacturer. 1st ed. New York; McGraw-Hill, 1924. 530p. (4th ed., 1958. 884p.)
First	Cruess, William V. The Principles and Practice of Wine Making. New York; AVI, 1934. 212p. (2d ed., 1947. 476p.)
Second	Cummings, Richard O. The American and His Food; A History of Food Habits in the United States. Rev. ed. Chicago; University of Chicago Press, 1941. 291p. (Reprinted, New York; Arno Press and the New York Times, 1970.)
Second	Curwen, E. Cecil. Plough and Pasture. London; Cobbett Press, 1946. 122p. (Later two-part ed., as Plough and Pasture, the Early History of Farming. New York; H. Schuman, 1953. 329p.)

D

First	Dack, Gail M. Food Poisoning. Chicago; University of Chicago Press, 1943. 138p. (3d ed., rev. and enl., 1956. 251p. Reprinted, 1971.)
First	Damon, Samuel R. Food Infections and Food Intoxications. Baltimore; Williams & Wilkins, 1928. 266p.
First	Davies, William L. The Chemistry of Milk. London; Chapman & Hall, 1936. 522p. (2d ed., 1939. 534p.)
Second	Dean, Harry K. Utilization of Fats: A Theoretical and Technical Treatise on the Composition, Extraction, Analysis and Applications of Fats. New York; Chemical Pub. Co., 1938. 292p.
Second	Dedrick, Benjamin W. Practical Milling. 1st ed. Chicago; National Miller, 1924. 576p.
Second	Deerr, Noel. The History of Sugar. London; Chapman & Hall, 1949–1950. 2 vols.
First	DeKruif, Paul. Hunger Fighters. New York; Harcourt, Brace & Co., 1928. 377p.
Second	DeLoach, Daniel B. The Salmon Canning Industry. Corvallis, Oregon; Oregon State College, 1939. 118p.
Second	Depew, Chauncey M., ed. 1795–1895: One Hundred Years of American Commerce . . . A History of American Commerce, by One Hundred Americans. New York; D. O. Haynes, 1895. 2 vols.
Second	Deuel, Harry J. The Lipids; Their Chemistry and Biochemistry. New York; Interscience, 1951–1957. 3 vols.
Second	Deutsch-Renner, Hans. The Origin of Food Habits. London; Faber & Faber, 1944. 261p. (Available in German and Swedish.)
Second	Dewberry, Elliot B. Food Poisoning; Its Nature, History and Causation, Measures for Its Prevention and Control. London; Hill, 1943. 186p. (4th ed., as Food Poisoning; Food-Bourne Infection and Intoxication: Nature, History, and Causation; Measures for Prevention and Control, 1959. 411p.)
Second	Dick, John L. Rickets; A Study of Economic Conditions and Their Effects on the Health of the Nation. New York; E. B. Treat, 1922. 488p.

Rank	
First	Dondlinger, Peter T. The Book of Wheat; An Economic History and Practical Manual of the Wheat Industry. New York; Orange Judd Co., 1908. 369p. (Reprinted, 1919.)
First	Drummond, Jack C., and Anne Wilbraham. The Englishman's Food; A History of Five Centuries of English Diet. London; J. Cape, 1939. 574p. (Rev. ed., 1964. 482p.)
First	Du Bois, Eugene F. Basal Metabolism in Health and Disease. Philadelphia; Lea & Febiger, 1924. 372p. (3d ed., rev., 1936. 494p.)
Second	Dubelle, George H. The "Non Plus Ultra" Soda Fountain Requisites of Modern Times. A Practical Receipt Book . . . New York; Spon & Chamberlain, 1893. 160p. (2d ed., 1901.)
Second	Duddy, Edward A., and David R. Revzan. The Changing Relative Importance of the Central Livestock Market. Chicago; University of Chicago Press, 1938. 122p.
Second	Duncan, Amon O. Food Processing. Atlanta, Ga.; T. E. Smith & Co., 1942. 544p.

E

Second	Earle, Alice M. Home Life in Colonial Days, Written by Alive Morse Earle in the Year MDCCCXCVIII, Illustrated by Photographs, Gathered by the Author, of Real Things, Works, and Happenings of Olden Times. New York and London; Macmillan, 1898. 470p.
Second	Eckey, E. W. Vegetable Fats and Oils. New York; Reinhold, 1954. 836p. (ACS Monograph Series no. 123)
First	Eckles, Clarence H. et al. Milk and Milk Products, Prepared for the Use of Agricultural College Students. 1st ed. New York; McGraw-Hill, 1929. 379p. (4th ed., 1951. 454p.)
First	Edelmann, Richard H. Text-Book of Meat Hygiene, with Special Consideration to Ante-Mortem and Post-Mortem Inspection of Food-Producing Animals . . . transl., with additions, by John R. Mohler and Adolph Eichhorn. Washington, D.C.; G. E. Howard Press, 1908. 402p. (8th ed., rev. Philadelphia; Lea & Febiger, 1943. 468p.)
Second	Edgar, William C. The Story of a Grain of Wheat. New York; 1911. 195p.
Second	Edmund, Carsten. On Deficiency of A Vitamin and Visual Dysaptation. Copenhagen; Levin & Munksgaard; London; H. Milford, Oxford University Press, 1936. 92p.
First	Ehret, George. Twenty-Five Years of Brewing: With an Illustrated History of American Beer . . . New York; Gast Lithograph & Engraving Co., 1891. 120p.
First	Eisen, Gustav. The Raisin Industry: A Practical Treatise on the Raisin Grapes: Their History, Culture and Curing. San Francisco; H. S. Crocker & Co., Stationers & Printers, 1890. 223p.
Second	Ellis, Carleton. The Hydrogenation of Oils; Catalyzers and Catalysis and the Generation of Hydrogen. New York; Van Nostrand, 1914. 340p. (2d ed., rev. and enl., 1919. 767p.)
Second	Ellms, Joseph W. Water Purification. 1st ed. New York; McGraw-Hill, 1917. 485p. (2d ed., 1928. 594p.)

Rank	
First	Emerson, Edward R. Beverages, Past and Present; An Historical Sketch of Their Production, Together with a Study of the Customs Connected with Their Use. New York and London; G. P. Putnam's Sons, 1908. 2 vols.
Second	Emulsol Corporation, Chicago. Mayonnaise and Salad Dressing Products . . . edited by M. H. Joffe. Chicago; Emulsol Corporation, 1942. 169p.
Second	Evans, E. A., ed. The Biological Action of the Vitamins; Proceedings of a Symposium on the Respiratory Enzymes . . . Chicago; University of Chicago Press, 1942. 227p.
First	Evans, Herbert M. Essays in Biology in honor of Herbert M. Evans . . . written by his friends. Berkeley and Los Angeles; University of California Press, 1943. 686p.
Second	Eynon, Lewis. Starch; Its Chemistry, Technology and Uses. Cambridge, Eng.; W. Heffer & Sons, 1928. 256p.

F

Second	Fairrie, Geoffrey. Sugar. 1st ed. Liverpool; Fairrie & Co., 1925. 233p.
Second	Falk, K. George. The Chemistry of Enzyme Actions. New York; Chemical Catalog Co., 1921. 136p. (2d ed., rev., 1924. 249p.)
Second	Falkenhagen, Hans. Electrolytes . . . transl. by R. P. Bell. Oxford; Clarendon Press, 1934. 346p. (Translation of Electrolyte.)
Second	Feer, Emil. The Diagnosis of Children's Diseases, with Special Attention to the Diseases of Infancy . . . transl. by Carl A. Scherer. 2d ed., rev. Philadelphia, London, etc.; J. B. Lippincott Co., 1928. 551p. (Translation of Lehrbuch der Kindeheildunde. Went through 10 German eds.)
First	Fernie, William T. Meals Medicinal: With "Herbal Simples" (of Edible Parts), Curative Foods from the Cook in Place of Drugs from the Chemist. Bristol, Wright and London; Simpkin, Marshall, Hamilton, Kent & Co., 1905. 781p.
Second	Fiene, F., and Saul Blumenthal. Handbook of Food Manufacture; A Handbook of Practical Food Information . . . New York; Chemical Pub. Co., 1938. 603p.
First	Filby, Frederick A. A History of Food Adulteration and Analysis. London; George Allen & Unwin, 1934. 269p.
Second	Finnemore, Horace. The Essential Oils. London; E. Benn, 1926. 880p.
First	Fischer, Martin H. The Physiology of Alimentation. 1st ed. New York; J. Wiley, 1907. 348p.
Second	Fischer, Martin H., and Marian O. Hooder. Fats and Fatty Degeneration; A Physico-Chemical Study of Emulsions and the Normal and Abnormal Distribution of Fat in Protoplasm. New York; Wiley; London; Chapman & Hall, 1917. 155p.
Second	Fisk, Walter W. The Book of Ice-Cream. New ed. New York; Macmillan, 1923. 302p.
First	Fletcher, Horace. The A. B.-Z. of Our Own Nutrition. New York; F. A. Stokes, 1903. 426p. (Reprinted, 1930.)
First	Flosdorf, Earl W. Freeze-Drying; Drying Sublimation. New York; Reinhold Pub., 1949. 280p.

Rank	
First	Folin, Otto K. Preservatives and Other Chemicals in Foods: Their Use and Abuse. Cambridge, Mass.; Harvard University Press, 1914. 60p.
Second	Follis, Richard H. The Pathology of Nutritional Disease; Physiological and Morphological Changes Which Result from Deficiencies of the Essential Elements, Amino Acids, Vitamins, and Fatty Acids. Springfield, Ill.; C. C. Thomas, 1948. 291p.
First	Food and Agriculture Organization. Committee on Calorie Requirements. Calorie Requirements; Report, Sept. 1949. Washington, D.C.; FAO, 1950. 65p. (FAO Nutritional Studies no. 5) (Later ed., 1957. 64p. FAO Nutritional Studies No. 15)
First	Food and Agriculture Organization. Nutrition Division. Rice and Rice Diets; A Survey. Washington, D.C.; FAO, 1948. 72p. (FAO Nutritional Studies no. 1)
Second	Forber, Janet E. Milk and Its Hygienic Relations . . . published under the direction of the Medical Research Committee, National Health Insurance. London and New York; Longmans, Green, 1916. 348p.
Second	Forbes, Robert J. Short History of the Art of Distillation from the Beginnings up to the Death of Celier Blumentahl. Leiden; Brill, 1948. 405p. (2d ed., rev., 1970. 415p.)
Second	Foster, Bertram B. Men, Meat, and Miracles. New York; Messner, 1952. 245p.
First	Francis, Clarence. A History of Food and Its Preservation, a Contribution to Civilization; An Address . . . Princeton, N.J.; Guild of Brackett Lecturers, 1937. 45p.
Second	Franzen, Raymond H. Physical Measures of Growth and Nutrition. New York; American Child Health Association, 1929. 138p. (ACHA School Health Research Monographs no. 2)
Second	Frederiksen, Johan D. The Story of Milk. New York; Macmillan Co., 1919. 188p.
First	Frigidaire Corporation. Food Preservation in Our Daily Life. 2d ed. Dayton, Ohio; Frigidaire Corp., 1929. 84p.
Second	Frozen and Chilled Meat Trade, a Practical Treatise by Specialists in the Meat Trade. London; Gresham Pub. Co., 1929. 2 vols.
First	Funk, Casimir. The Vitamines. Authorized translation from 2d German ed. by Harry E. Dubin. Baltimore; Williams & Wilkins, 1922. 502p. (Translation of Die Vitamine, ihre Bedeutung fur die Physiologie und Pathologie. 1st German ed., Wiesbaden; J.F. Bergmann, 1914. 193p. 3d German ed., Munich; Bergmann, 1924. 522p.)
First	Funk, Casimir, and H. E. Dubin. Vitamin and Mineral Therapy. New York; 1936. 94p.
First	Furnas, Clifford C., and S. M. Furnas. Man, Bread and Destiny. Baltimore; Williams & Wilkins, 1937. 364p. (Reprinted, as The Story of Man and His Food, New York; New Home Library, 1942.)
Second	Furth, Otto ritter von. The Problems of Physiological and Pathological Chemistry of Metabolism, for Students, Physicians, Biologists and Chemists . . . transl. by Allen J. Smith. Philadelphia and London; J. B. Lippincott, 1916. 667p.

Rank	
	G
Second	Gardner, John. Longevity: The Means of Prolonging Life after Middle Age. London; H. S. King & Co., 1874. 168p. (3d ed., Boston; W. F. Gill & Co., 1875. 191p.)
Second	Geiger, Jacob C., E. C. Dickson, and K. F. Meyer. The Epidemiology of Botulism. Washington, D.C.; U.S. Govt. Print. Off., 1922. 119p. (U.S. Public Health Service, Public Health Bulletin no. 127)
First	General Mills, Inc. The Flour Business. Minneapolis; General Mills, 1949. 1 vols.
Second	General Mills, Inc. Products Control Department. The Story of the Cereal Grains. Minneapolis; General Mills, 1944. 30p.
Second	Gephart, Frank C. Analysis and Cost of Ready-to-Serve Foods; A Study in Food Economics. Chicago; Press of American Medical Association, 1915. 71p.
Second	Gerber Products Company. The Story of an Idea and Its Role in the Growth of the Baby Foods Industry. Fremont, Mich.? ; 1953. 95p.
Second	Gerhard, Albert F. Handbook for Bakers. New York and London; Century Co., 1925. 484p.
First	Gibbs, J. Willard. The Collected Works of J. Willard Gibbs . . . edited by W. R. Longley and R. G. Van Name. New York; Longmans, Green & Co., 1928. 2 vols.
Second	Gildemeister, E., and F. Hoffmann. Volatile Oils . . . transl. by Edward Kremers. Milwaukee, Wis.; Pharmaceutical Review Pub. Co., 1900. 733p. (2d ed., by E. Gildemeister. London, etc.; Longmans, Green, 1913–1922. 3 vols.)
Second	Gisvold, Ole, and Charles H. Rogers. The Chemistry of Plant Constituents. Minneapolis; Burgess Pub. Co., Mimeoprint & Offset Pub., 1938. 295p. (Rev. ed., 1943. 484p.)
Second	Gortner, Willis A., Frederick S. Erdman, and Nancy K. Masterman. Principles of Food Freezing. New York; J. Wiley, 1948. 281p.
Second	Grafe, Erich. Metabolic Diseases and Their Treatment . . . transl. by Margaret G. Boise. Philadelphia; Lea & Febiger, 1933. 551p.
First	Great Britain. Committee upon Accessory Food Factors (Vitamines). Report on the Present State of Knowledge Concerning Accessory Food Factors (Vitamines) . . . compiled by the Lister Institute and Medical Research Committee. Oxford; Printed by F. Hall, University Press, 1919. 107p. (Great Britain, National Health Insurance Joint Committee, Medical Research Committee, Special Report Series no. 38) (2d ed., rev. and enl., London; H.M.S.O., 1924. 171p.)
Second	Green, Joseph R. The Soluble Ferments and Fermentation. Cambridge; University Press, 1899. 480p. (2d ed., 1901. 512p.)
Second	Greenberg, David M. Amino Acids and Proteins; Theory, Methods, Application. Springfield, Ill.; Thomas, 1951. 950p.
Second	Greenwood, Major. Epidemiology: Historical and Experimental. Baltimore; Johns Hopkins Press; London; H. Milford, Oxford University Press, 1932. 80p.
Second	Grimshaw, Robert. Modern Milling: Being the Substance of Two Addresses

Rank

Rank	Entry
	Delivered by Request, at the Franklin Institute, Philadelphia, January 19 and January 27, 1881. Philadelphia; H. Baird & Co., 1881. 51p.
First	Grindley, Harry S. Studies in Nutrition; An Investigation of the Influence of Saltpeter on the Nutrition and Health of Man with Reference to Its Occurence in Cured Meats. Champaign, Ill.; University of Illinois, 1911–1929. 5 vols.
First	Grossman, Harold J. Grossman's Guide to Wines, Beers, and Spirits. New York; Sherman & Spoerer, 1940. 404p. (7th ed., rev. by Harriet Lembeck, New York; Scribner, 1983. 638p.)
Second	Guenther, Ernest et al. The Essential Oils. New York; Van Nostrand, 1948–1952. 6 vols.
First	Guilliermond, Alexandre. The Yeasts . . . transl. and rev. by Fred W. Tanner. New York; J. Wiley, 1920. 424p.

H

Rank	Entry
Second	Haas, Paul, and T. G. Hill. An Introduction to the Chemistry of Plant Products. London and New York; Longmans, Green, 1913. 401p. (3d ed., 1921. 2 vols.)
First	Haldane, John B. S. Enzymes. London and New York; Longmans, Green, 1930. 235p. (Reprinted, Cambridge; M.I.T. Press, 1965.)
Second	Hall, Constant J. J. van. Cocoa. 1st ed. London; Macmillan, 1914. 515p. (2nd ed., Titled Cacao. 1932. 514p.)
Second	Halliday, Evelyn G. Hows and Whys of Cooking. Chicago; University of Chicago Press, 1928. 179p. (Later ed., 1946. 328p.)
First	Halliday, Evelyn G., and Isabel T. Nobel. Food Chemistry and Cookery. Chicago; University of Chicago Press, 1943. 346p.
First	Hammarsten, Olof. A Text-Book of Physiological Chemistry . . . transl. from 2d Swedish ed. and enl. and rev. German ed. by John A. Mandel. 1st ed. New York; J. Wiley, 1893. 511p. (7th ed., transl. from author's enl. and rev. 8th German ed., 1914. 1026p.)
Second	Harden, Arthur. Alcoholic Fermentation. London, etc.; Longmans, Green, 1911. 128p. (4th ed., 1932. 243p.)
First	Harris, Henry F. Pellagra. New York; Macmillan, 1919. 421p.
First	Harris, James A., and Francis G. Benedict. A Biometric Study of Basal Metabolism in Man. Washington, D.C.; Carnegie Institution of Washington, 1919. 266p. (Carnegie Institution of Washington Publication no. 279)
Second	Harrow, Benjamin. Vitamines, Essential Food Factors. New York; E. P. Dutton & Co., 1921. 219p. (New and enl. ed., 1922. 261p.)
Second	Hartley, Robert M. An Historical, Scientific and Practical Essay on Milk as an Article of Human Sustenance. New York; Arno Press, 1942. 358p. (Reprinted, 1977.)
Second	Harvey, William C., and Harry Hill. Milk Products. London; H. K. Kewis, 1937. 387p. (2d ed., 1948. 343p.)
First	Hausbrand, Eugen. Evaporating, Condensing and Cooling Apparatus; Explanations, Formulae, and Tables for Use in Practice . . . transl. from 2d rev. German ed. by A. C. Wright. London; Scott, Greenwood & Co., 1908.

Rank

400p. (5th English ed., rev. and enl. by Basil Heastie, London; E. Benn, 1933. 503p.)

Second Hausner, A. The Manufacture of Preserved Foods and Sweetmeats; A Handbook of All the Processes for the Preservation of Flesh, Fruit, and Vegetables, and for the Preparation of Dried Fruit, Dried Vegetables, Marmalades, Fruit-Syrups, and Fermented Beverages, and of All Kinds of Candies, Candied Fruit, Sweetmeats, Rocks, Drops, Dragees, Pralines, etc. . . . transl. from the 3d enlarged German ed. by Arthur Morris and Herbert Robson. London; Scott, Greenwood & Co., 1902. 223p. (2d English ed., 1912. 238p.)

First Hawk, Philip B. Practical Physiological Chemistry: A Book Designed for Use in Courses in Practical Physiological Chemistry in Schools of Medicine and of Science. Philadelphia; Blakiston, 1907. 416p. (14th ed., edited by Bernard L. Oser, New York; McGraw-Hill, 1965. 1472p.)

First Haworth, Walter N. The Constitution of Sugars. London; E. Arnold, 1929. 100p. (Available in German as Die Konstitution der Kohlenhydrate, 1932)

First Helmholtz, Hermann L. F. von. Helmholtz's Treatise on Physiological Optics . . . transl. from the 3d German ed., edited by James P. C. Southall. Rochester, N.Y.; Optical Society of America, 1924–1925. 3 vols. (Translation of Handbuch der Physiologischen Optik.)

First Henderson, Lawrence J. The Fitness of the Environment; An Inquiry into the Biological Significance of the Properties of Matter. New York; Macmillan Co., 1913. 317p. (Reprinted, Boston; Beacon Press, 1958.)

First Henrici, Arthur T. Molds, Yeasts, and Actinomycetes; A Handbook for Students of Bacteriology. Minneapolis; Burgess-Roseberry Co., 1929. 159p. (2d ed., as Henrici's Molds Yeasts, and Actinomycetes . . . by Charles E. Skinner, Chester W. Emmons and Henry M. Tsuchiya. New York; J. Wiley & Sons; London; Chapman & Hall, 1947. 409p.)

Second Henry, Thomas A. The Plant Alkaloids. Philadelphia; P. Blakiston's Son & Co., 1913. 466p. (4th ed., London; Churchill, 1949. 804p.)

Second Hernstein, Karl M., and Thomas C. Gregory. Chemistry and Technology of Wines and Liquors. New York; Van Nostrand, 1935. 360p. (2d ed., by K. M. Herstein and Morris B. Jacobs, 1948. 436p.)

Second Herrington, Barbour L. Milk and Milk Processing. 1st ed. New York; McGraw-Hill, 1948. 343p.

Second Hess, Alfred F. Scurvy, Past and Present. Philadelphia and London; J. P. Lippincott, 1920. 279p.

Second Hier, Wayland G. The Manufacture of Tomato Products. Denver, Colo.; W. G. Hier, 1919. 132p.

Second Hilditch, Thomas P. The Chemical Constitution of Natural Fats. New York; Wiley, 1940. 437p. (4th ed., by T. P. Hilditch and P. N. Williams, 1964. 745p.)

Second Hilditch, Thomas P. The Industrial Chemistry of the Fats and Waxes. New York; Van Nostrand, 1927. 461p. (3d ed., London; Bailliere, Tindall & Cox, 1949. 604p.)

Second Hill, H. Pasteurization. London; Lewis, 1943. 152p.

Rank	
Second	Hill, Janet M. Canning, Preserving and Jelly Making. Boston; Little, Brown & Co., 1915. 189p. (Later ed., rev. by Sally Larkin, 1943. 143p.)
Second	Himsworth, Harold. Lectures on the Liver and Its Diseases, Comprising the Lowell Lectures Delivered at Boston, Massachusetts, in March 1947. 2d ed. Cambridge, Mass.; Harvard University Press, 1950. 222p.
Second	Hind, H. Lloyd. Brewing: Science and Practice. New York; J. Wiley & Sons, 1938. 2 vols.
Second	Hiss, Philip H., and Zinsser. A Text-Book of Bacteriology, a Practical Treatise for Students and Practitioners of Medicine. New York and London; D. Appleton & Co., 1910. 745p. (5th–15th eds., by H. Zinsser, later eds. as Microbiology. 15th ed., edited by Wolfgang K. Joklik and David T. Smith, 1972. 1120p.)
Second	Historic Tinned Foods. 2d ed. Greenford, Middlesex, Eng.; International Tin Research and Development Council, 1939. 70p.
Second	History of Rice Country. Minneapolis; Minnesota Historical Co., 1882. 603p.
Second	Hoffman, Frederick L. Cancer and Diet, with Facts and Observations on Related Subjects. Baltimore; Williams & Wilkins, 1937. 767p.
First	Hopkins, Frederick G. Newer Aspects of the Nutrition Problem. New York; Columbia University Press, 1922. 19p.
Second	Hopkins, Reginald H., and Civilingenior B. Krause. Biochemistry Applied to Malting and Brewing. New York; Van Nostrand, 1937. 342p. (2d ed., London; Allen & Unwin, 1948. 342p. Reprinted, 1951.)
Second	Hoskins, Thomas H. What We Eat: An Account of the Most Common Adulterations of Food and Drink. Boston; T. O. H. P. Burnham, 1861. 218p.
Second	Howell, William H., ed. An American Text-Book of Physiology, by Henry P. Bowditch, et al. Philadelphia; Saunders, 1896. 1052p. (21st ed., edited by Harry D. Patton, et al., 1989. 2 vols.)
Second	Howes, Frank N. Nuts: Their Production and Everyday Uses. London; Faber & Faber, 1948. 264p.
Second	Hufeland, Christoph W. The Art of Prolonging Life . . . transl. from German. London; J. Bell, 1797. 2 vols. (Translation of Die Kunst das Menschlishe Leben zu Verlangern. Reprinted, New York; Arno Press, 1979.)
Second	Hughes, Osee G. Introductory Foods. New York; Macmillan, 1940. 522p.
Second	Hurd, Louis M. Modern Poultry Farming. New York; Macmillan, 1944. 599p. (4th ed., 1956. 575p.)
Second	Hutchison, Robert. Food and the Principles of Dietetics. 1st ed. New York; W. Wood, 1905. 548p. (12th ed., by Hugh M. Sinclair and Dorothy F. Hollingsworth, as Food and the Principles of Nutrition. London; E. Arnold, 1969. 644p.)

I

Rank	
Second	Institute of American Meat Packers. Sausage and Ready to Serve Meats. Chicago; Institute of Meat Packing, 1938. 361p. (Rev. ed., 1953. 335p.)

Rank

J

Second	Jackson, Clarence M. The Effects of Inanition and Malnutrition upon Growth and Structure. Philadelphia; P. Blakiston's Son & Co., 1925. 616p.
Second	Jacob, Heinrich E. The Saga of Coffee. London; G. Allen & Unwin, 1935. 384p.
First	Jacobs, Morris B. The Chemical Analysis of Foods and Food Products. 1st ed. New York; Van Nostrand, 1938. 537p. (3d ed., Princeton, N.J.; 1958. 970p.)
First	Jacobs, Morris B., ed. The Chemistry and Technology of Food and Food Products. 1st ed. New York; Interscience, 1944. 2 vols. (2d ed., rev. and augmented, 1951. 3 vols.)
Second	Jacobs, Morris B. Synthetic Food Adjuncts: Synthetic Food Colors, Flavors, Essences, Sweetening Agents, Preservatives, Stabilizers, Vitamins and Similar Food Adjuncts. New York; Van Nostrand, 1947. 335p.
Second	Jago, William, and William C. Jago. The Technology of Bread-Making, Including the Chemistry and Analytical and Practical Testing of Wheat, Flour, and Other Materials Employed in Bread-Making and Confectionery. London; Simpkin, Marshall, Hamilton, Kent & Co., 1911. 908p. (A development of the writer's former works on the same subject, which appeared in 1886 and 1895. Later ed., Liverpool; Northern Pub. Co., 1921. 630p.)
Second	Jamieson, George S. Vegetable Fats and Oils; the Chemistry, Production and Utilization of Vegetable Fats and Oils for Edible, Medicinal and Technical Purposes. New York; Chemical Catalog Co., 1932. 444p. (American Chemical Society, Monograph Series no. 58) (2d ed., New York; Reinhold, 1943. 508p.)
Second	Jensen, Harold R. The Chemistry, Flavouring and Manufacture of Chocolate Confectionery and Cocoa. Philadelphia; P. Balkiston's Son, 1931. 406p.
First	Jensen, Lloyd B. Meat and Meat Foods. New York; Ronald Press Co., 1949. 218p.
First	Jensen, Lloyd B. Microbiology of Meats. Champaign, Ill.; Garrard Press, 1942. 252p. (3d ed., 1954. 422p.)
Second	Johnston, J. F. W. Chemistry of Common LIfe. New ed., rev. New York; D. Appleton & Co., 1880. 592p.
Second	Johnston, James F. W. Elements of Agricultural Chemistry and Geology. New York; Wiley & Putnam, 1842. 249p. (17th ed., by Charles A. Cameron, rev. and rewritten by C. M. Aikman. London; W. Blackwood & Sons, 1894. 482p.)
First	Johnston, James F. W. Lectures on Agricultural Chemistry and Geology. New York; Wiley & Putnam, 1842. 255p. (Later ed., New York; A. O. Moore & Co., 1859. 619p.)
Second	Jones, Osman. Canning Practice and Control. New York; Chemical Pub. Co., 1937. 254p. (3d ed., London; Chapman & Hall, 1949. 322p.)
First	Jordan, Edwin O. Food Poisoning. Chicago; University of Chicago Press, 1917. 115p. (2d ed., as Food Poisoning and Food-Borne Infection, 1931.)
First	Jordan, Edwin O. A Text-Book of General Bacteriology. Philadelphia; Saunders, 1908. 557p. (13th ed., rev., 1941. 731p.)

Rank

Second Jordan, Stroud. Chocolate Evaluation. New York; Applied Sugar Laboratories, 1934. 225p. (Confectionery Studies no. 3)

Second Jordan, Stroud. Confectionery Problems. Chicago; National Confectioner's Association, 1930. 347p. (Confectionery Studies no. 1)

Second Jordan, Stroud. Confectionery Standards. New York; Applied Sugar Laboratories, 1933. 370p. (Confectionery Studies no. 2)

Second Jordan, Stroud, and Katheryn E. Langwill. Confectionery Analysis and Composition. Chicago; Manufacturing Confectioner, 1946. 116p.

Second Jorgensen, Alfred P. C. Micro-Organisms and Fermentation. New ed., transl. from 3d ed. in German by Alex K. Miller and E. A. Lennholm. London; F. W. Lyon, 1893. 257p. (7th English ed., rewritten by Albert Hansen, London; C. Friddin, 1948. 550p.)

First Joslin, Elliott P. Treatment of Diabetes Mellitus. 4th ed. Philadelphia; Lea & Febiger, 1928. 998p. (12th ed., 1985. 1007p.)

First Judge, Arthur I. History of the Canning Industry by Its Most Prominent Men. Baltimore; Canning Trade, 1914. 161p.

K

First Kansas. State College of Agriculture and Applied Science, Manhattan. Department of Food Economics and Nutrition. Practical Cookery and the Etiquette and Service of the Table, a Compilation of Principles of Cookery and Recipes with Suggestions for Etiquette for Various Occasions. 20th ed. Manhattan, Kans.; Dept. of Printing, Kansas State College of Agriculture and Applied Science, 1941. 506p. (Later ed., New York; Wiley, 1956. 364p.)

First Karo, Joseph ben Ephraim. The Kosher Code of the Orthodox Jew. Minneapolis; University of Minnesota Press, 1940. 243p. (Reprinted, New York; Hermon Press, 1975.)

Second Kellogg, Ella E. Science in the Kitchen: A Scientific Treatise on Food Substances and Their Dietetic Properties. Rev. ed. Battle Creek, Mich.; Health Pub. Co., 1898.

First Kellogg, John H. The New Dietetics, What to Eat and How; A Guide to Scientific Feeding in Health and Disease. Battle Creek, Mich.; Modern Medicine Pub. Co., 1921. 933p. (Rev. ed., 1927. 1031p.)

Second Kellogg, Vernon L., and Alonzo E. Taylor. The Food Problem. New York; Macmillan Co., 1917. 213p.

Second Kenneth, John H. An Experimental Study of Affects and Associations Due to Certain Odors. Princeton, N.J., and Albany, N.Y.; The Psychological Review Co., 1927. 64p.

First Kent-Jones, Douglas W. Modern Cereal Chemistry. Liverpool, Eng.; Northern Pub. Co., 1924. 324p. (6th ed., by D. W. Kent-Jones and A. J. Amos, London; Food Trade Press, 1967. 730p.)

First Kent-Jones, Douglas W., and J. Price. The Practice and Science of Bread-Making. 2d ed. Liverpool; Northern Pub., 1951. 278p.

Second Kerr, Ralph W. E., ed. Chemistry and Industry of Starch; Starch Sugars and Related Compounds. New York; Academic Press, 1944. 472p. (2d ed., rev. and enl., 1950. 719p.)

Rank	
Second	Kick, Freidrich. Flour Manufacture: With Supplement, Recent Progress in Flour Manufacture . . . transl. by H. H. P. Powles. London; C. Lockwood, 1888. 291p.
Second	King, Frederic T. Feeding and Care of Baby. 1st ed. London; Macmillan, 1917. 162p. (Later ed., rev. and enlarged, Christchurch, N.Z.; Whitcombe & Tombs, 1940. 257p.)
Second	Kirschenbauer, H. G. Fats and Oils, and Outline of Their Chemistry and Technology. New York; Reinhold Pub., 1944. 154p. (2d ed., 1960. 240p.)
Second	Klocker, Albert. Fermentation Organisms; A Laboratory Handbook . . . transl. from German by G. E. Allan and J. H. Millar. London, etc.; Longmans, Green, 1903. 392p.
Second	Knapp, Arthur W. Cacao Fermentation: A Critical Survey of Its Scientific Aspects. London; J. Bale, Sons & Curnow, 1937. 171p.
First	Kohman, Edward F. Vitamins in Canned Foods. Washington, D.C.; 1929. 117p. (National Canners Association, Research Laboratory Bulletin no. 19–L, rev.) (4th ed., 1937. 95p.)
Second	Kozmin, Peter Q. Flour Milling; A Theoretical and Practical Handbook of Flour Manufacture for Millers, Millwrights, Flour-Milling Engineers, and Others Engaged in the Flour-Milling Industry . . . transl. from Russian by M. Falkner and Theodor Fjelstrup. New York; Van Nostrand, 1917. 584p.
Second	Kuehn, Henry E. Wheat to Flour: A Brief Story of Wheat Production, Wheat Marketing and Wheat Milling. Minneapolis; King Midas Mill Co., 1927. 33p.
Second	Kuhlmann, Charles B. The Development of the Flour Milling Industry in the United States. Boston; Houghton Mifflin Co., 1942. 349p.
Second	Kyrk, Hazel. The American Baking Industry, 1849–1923. Stanford University, Calif.; Stanford University Press, 1925. 108p.

L

Second	Lafar, Franz. Technical Mycology: The Utilization of Micro-Organisms in the Arts and Manufactures. A Practical Handbook on Fermentation and Fermentative Processes, for the Use of Brewers and Distillers, Analysts, Technical and Agricultural Fermentation . . . transl. by Charles T. C. Salter. London; C. Griffin & Co., 1898–1910. 2 vols.
Second	Lampert, Lincoln M. Milk and Dairy Products; Their Composition, Food Value, Chemistry, Bacteriology and Processing. Brooklyn, N.Y.; Chemical Pub. Co., 1947. 291p. (3d ed., rev. and enlarged, as Modern Dairy Products: Composition, Food Value, Processing, Chemistry, Bacteriology, Testing, Imitation Dairy Products, 1975. 437p.)
Second	Lang, Otto W. Thermal Processes for Canned Marine Products. Berkeley; University of California Press, 1935. 182p. (UC Publications in Public Health, Vol. 2 no. 1)
Second	Leach, Albert E. Food Inspection and Analysis. For the Use of Public Analysts, Health Officers, Sanitary Chemists, and Food Economists. 1st ed. New York; J. Wiley, 1904. 787p. (4th ed., 1936. 1000p.)
First	League of Nations. The Problem of Nutrition. Geneva, Switzerland; League of Nations, 1936. 4 vols.

Rank

Second Lewkowitsch, J. Chemical Analysis of Oils, Fats, Waxes and of the Commercial Products Derived Therefrom, Founded on Benedikt's 2d ed. of Analyse der Fette. 2d ed., rev. and enl. London and New York; Macmillan, 1898. 834p. (6th ed., rewritten and enl. as Chemical Technology and Analysis of Oils, Fats and Waxes, 1921–1923. 3 vols.)

First Lind, James. Treatise on Scurvy; A Bicentenary Volume Containing a Reprint of the First Edition, with Additional Notes . . . edited by C. P. Stewart and Douglas Guthrie. Edinburgh; University Press, 1953. 440p.

Second Ling, Edgar R. A Text Book of Dairy Chemistry, Theoretical and Practical, for Students of Agriculture and Dairying. London; Chapman & Hall, 1930. 213p. (3d ed., reprinted with revisions, 1963. 2 vols.)

Second Lloyd, Dorothy J. Chemistry of the Proteins and Its Economic Applications. London; J. & A. Churchill, 1926. 279p. (2d ed., 1938. 532p.)

Second Lockwood, J. F. Flour Milling. Liverpool, Eng.; Northern Pub. Co., 1945. 511p. (4th ed., Stockport, Cheshire, Eng.; H. Simon, 1960. 526)

Second Lodder, Johannes. The Anascosporogenous Yeasts . . . transl. by Adolf Kadner. Berkeley, Calif.; 1936. 394p. (Translation of Die Anaskosporogenen Hefen.)

Second Loeb, Jacques. Proteins and the Theory of Colloidal Behavior. 1st ed. New York; McGraw-Hill, 1922. 292p. (2d ed., 1924. 380p.)

Second Long, George. The Mills of Man. London; H. Joseph, 1931. 224p.

Second Loomis, Henry M. The Canning of Foods, and Some Tested Recipes. Washington, D.C.; National Canners Association, 1925. 106p.

First Lowe, Belle. Experimental Cookery from the Chemical and Physical Standpoint. New York; Wiley, 1932. 498p. (4th ed., 1955. 573p.)

First Lusk, Graham. The Elements of the Science of Nutrition. Philadelphia and London; W. B. Saunders, 1906. 326p. (4th ed., reset, 1928. 844p.)

First Lusk, Graham. Food in War Time. Philadelphia; Saunders, 1918. 46p.

First Lusk, Graham. The Fundamental Basis of Nutrition. New Haven; Yale University Press, 1914. 62p. (2d ed., 1923. 55p.)

First Lusk, Graham. Nutrition. New York; P. B. Hoeber, 1933. 142p.

Second Lyle, Oliver. Technology for Sugar Refinery Workers. 2d ed. London; Chapman & Hall, 1950. 525p.

M

First M'Gonigle, George C. M, and J. Kirby. Poverty and Public Health. London; V. Gollancz, 1936. 278p. (Reprinted, New York; Garland, 1985.)

Second MacDonald, Aeneas. Whisky. Garden City; Henry & Longwell, 1930. 24p.

Second Maclean, Hugh. Lecithin and Allied Substances: The Lipins. London and New York; Longmans, Green, 1918. 206p. (Later ed., 1927. 230p.)

Second Malin, James C. Winter Wheat in the Golden Belt of Kansas; A Study in Adaption to Subhumid Geographical Environment. Lawrence; University of Kansas Press, 1944. 290p.

Second Mann, Gustav. Chemistry of the Proteids . . . based on Professor Otto Cohnheim's Chemie der Eiweisskorper. London and New York; Macmillan, 1906. 606p.

Rank	
Second	Markley, Klare S., ed. Soybeans and Soybean Products. New York; Intersicence, 1950. 2 vols.
Second	Markley, Klare S., and Warren H. Goss. Soybean Chemistry and Technology. Brooklyn, N.Y.; Chemical Pub. Co., 1944. 261p.
Second	Marshall, Charles R. Microbiology, a Text-Book of Microoraganisms, General and Applied. Philadelphia; P. Blakiston, 1912. 724p. (3rd ed., rev. and enl., 1921. 1043p.)
Second	Martin, Charles R. A. Practical Food Inspection. London; H. K. Lewis & Co., 1932. 1 vol. (9th ed., 1978. 827p.)
Second	Martin, Geoffrey. Animal and Vegetable Oils, Fats, and Waxes; Their Manufacture. London; C. Lockwood & Son, 1920.
Second	Mathews, Albert P. Physiological Chemistry; A Text-Book and Manual for Students. New York; Wood, 1915. 1040p. (6th ed., Baltimore; Williams & Wilkins, 1939. 1488p.)
First	Mayer, Oscar G. America's Meat Packing Industry: A Brief Survey of Its Development and Economics. Princeton, N.J.; Newcomen Society, American Branch, 1939. 35p.
First	Mayo Clinic. Lectures on Nutrition; A Series of Lectures given at the Mayo Foundation and the Universities of Wisconsin, Minnesota, Nebraska, Iowa, and Washington (St. Louis), 1924–1925. Philadelphia and London; W. B. Saunders, 1925. 283p.
First	McCance, R. A., and E. M. Widdowson. The Chemical Composition of Foods. London; H.M.S.O., 1940. 150p. (4th ed., rev. and extended, Royal Society of Chemistry and Ministry of Agriculture, Fisheries and Food, 1991. 163p.)
Second	McCann, Alfred W. This Famishing World; Food Follies That Maim and Kill the Rich and the Poor, That Cheat the Growing Child and Rob the Prospective Mother of Health, That Burn up Millions in Treasure and Fill Untimely Graves, and the Remedy. New York; George H. Doran Co., 1918. 387p. (Later ed. as The Science of Eating.)
First	McCarrison, Robert. Nutrition and Health; Being the Cantor Lectures Delivered before the Royal Society of Arts, 1936, Together with Two Earlier Essays. New ed., rev. and enl. London; Faber & Faber, 1953. 125p.
Second	McCarrison, Robert. Studies in Deficiency Disease. London; H. Frowde and Hodder & Stoughton, 1921. 270p.
First	McCay, David. The Protein Element in Nutrition. London; E. Arnold; New York; Longmans, Green & Co., 1912. 216p.
Second	McCleary, George F. Infantile Mortality and Infants Milk Depots. London; P. S. King & Son, 1905. 135p.
Second	McClendon, Jesse F. Iodine and the Incidence of Goiter. Minneapolis; University of Minnesota Press; London; H. Milford, Oxford University Press, 1939. 126p.
First	McCollum, Elmer V. A History of Nutrition; The Sequence of Ideas in Nutrition Investigations. Boston; Houghton Mifflin, 1957. 451p.
First	McCollum, Elmer V. The Newer Knowledge of Nutrition; The Use of Food for the Preservation of Vitality and Health. New York; The Macmillan

Rank	
	Company, 1918. 199p. (5th ed., entirely rewritten by E.V. McCollum, Elsa Orent-Keiles and Harry G. Day, 1939. 701p.)
First	McCollum, Elmer V., and Nina Simmonds. The American Home Diet; An Answer to the Ever Present Question What Shall We Have For Dinner. Detroit, Mich.; Frederick C. Mathews Co., 1920. 237p.
First	McCulloch, Ernest C. Disinfection and Sterilization . . . illustrated with 53 engravings. Philadelphia; Lea & Febiger, 1936. 525p. (2d ed., rev., 1945. 472p.)
First	McLester, James S. Nutrition and Diet in Health and Disease. Philadelphia and London; W. B. Saunders, 1927. 783p. (6th ed., 1952. 710p.)
Second	McNair, James B. Citrus Products. Chicago; 1926–1927. 2 vols. (Field Museum of Natural History, Publication no. 238, 245)
Second	Medical Research Council (Great Britain). Vitamins: A Survey of Present Knowledge . . . compiled by a Committee appointed jointly by the Lister Institute and Medical Research Council. London; H.M.S.O., 1932. 332p. (MRC Special Report Series no. 167)
First	Mellanby, Edward. Nutrition and Disease; The Interaction of Clinical and Experimental Work. Edinburgh; Oliver & Boyd, 1934. 171p.
Second	Mellanby, Edward. A Story of Nutritional Research; The Effect of Some Dietary Factors on Bones and the Nervous System. Baltimore; Williams & Wilkins, 1950. 454p. (The Abraham Flexner Lectures, Series no. 9)
First	Mendel, Lafayette B. Nutrition: The Chemistry of Life. New Haven, Conn.; Yale University Press, 1923. 150p. (Hitchcock Lectures delivered at the University of California, 1923.)
Second	Mendelsohn, Simon. Baking Powders, Including Chemical Leavening Agents, Their Development, Chemistry and Valuation. New York; Chemical Pub. Co., 1939. 178p.
Second	Meyer, Ernst C. Infant Mortality in New York City; A Study of the Results Accomplished by Infant-Life Saving Agencies 1885–1920. New York; Rockefeller Foundation, International Health Board, 1921. 135p. (RF International Health Board, Publication no. 10)
Second	Michaelis, Leonor. The Effects of Ions in Colloidal Systems. Baltimore; Williams & Wilkins, 1925. 108p.
Second	Michaelis, Leonor. Hydrogen Ion Concentration, Its Significance in the Biological Sciences and Methods for Its Determinations . . . transl. from the 2d rev. and enlarged German ed. by William A. Perlzweig. Baltimore; Williams & Wilkins, 1926. 2 vols.
Second	Miller, Edgar S. Observations on Milling. 1st ed. Chicago; National Miller, 1923. 128p. (Originally puglished in National Miller in serial form, August 1921 through August 1922.)
Second	Miller, Edgar S. Studies in Practical Milling. Minneapolis; Miller Pub. Co., 1941. 618p.
Second	Mitchell, C. Ainsworth. Vinegar: Its Manufacture and Examination. London; C. Griffin & Co.; Philadelphia; J. B. Lippincott, 1916. 201p. (2d ed., rev., 1926. 211p.)
Second	Mojonnier, Timothy, and Hugh C. Troy. The Technical Control of Dairy

Rank	
	Products; A Treatise on the Testing, Analyzing, Standardizing and the Manufacture of Dairy Products. 1st ed. Chicago; Mojonnier Bros. Co., 1922. 909p. (2d ed., 1925. 936p.)
First	Moncrieff, R. W. The Chemical Senses. New York; J. Wiley, 1946. 424p. (3d ed., London; L. Hill, 1967. 760p.)
Second	Monier-Williams, Gordon W. Chemistry in Relation to Food. London; E. Benn, 1924. 20p.
Second	Monroe, Day, and Lenore M. Stratton. Food Buying and Our Markets. Boston; M. Barrows & Co., 1925. 321p. (Later ed., New York; M. Barrows & Co., 1940. 430p.)
Second	Moore, C. Ulysses. Nutrition of Mother and Child. 1st ed. Philadelphia and London; J. B. Lippincott, 1923. 230p. (2d ed., rev., 1924. 234.)
Second	Morgan, R. Harold. Beverage Manufacture (Non-Alcoholic) . . . edited by Arthur T. E. Binsted. New York; Chemical Pub. Co., 1939. 240p.
First	Morgulis, Sergius. Fasting and Undernutrition; A Biological and Sociological Study of Inanition. New York; Dutton, 1923. 407p.
Second	Morris, Thomas N. The Dehydration of Food. Toronto and New York; Van Nostrand, 1946. 174p.
Second	Morris, Thomas N. Principles of Fruit Preservation, Jam Making, Canning and Drying. London; Chapman & Hall, 1933. 239p. (2d ed., New York; Van Nostrand, 1947. 198p.)
Second	Morrison, Abraham C. The Baking Powder Controversy. New York; American Baking Powder Association, 1907. 2 vols.
Second	Morse, John L., and Fritz B. Talbot. Diseases of Nutrition and Infant Feeding. New York; Macmillan Co., 1915. 345p. (2d ed., rev., 1920. 384p.)
Second	Moulton, C. Robert. Meat through the Microscope; Applications of Chemistry and the Biological Sciences to Some Problems of the Meat Packing Industry. Chicago; University of Chicago Press, 1929. 528p. (2d ed., 1940. 592p.)
Second	Muir, M. M. Pattison. Heroes of Science: Chemists. London; Society for Promoting Christian Knowledge; New York; E. & J. B. Young & Co., 1883. 332p.
Second	Mullendore, William C. History of the United States Food Administration, 1917–1919. Stanford University, Calif.; Stanford University Press, 1941. 389p.
Second	Munsell, Albert H. Atlas of the Munsell Color System. Malden, Mass.; Wadsworth, Howland & Co., 1915. 15p.

N

Second	Nachod, Frederick C. Ion Exchange: Theory and Application. New York; Academic Press, 1949. 411p.
Second	Nascher, Ignatz L. Geriatrics; The Diseases of Old Age and Their Treatment, Including Physiological Old Age, Home and Institutional Care, and Medico-Legal Relations. Philadelphia; P. Blakiston, 1914. 517p. (2d ed., rev., 1916. 527p.)
First	National Canners Association. Research Laboratories. Processes for Low-

Rank	
	Acid Canned Foods in Metal Containers. 11th ed. Washington, D.C.; NCA, 1976. 61p. (NCA Bulletin no. 26–L)
Second	National Institutes of Health (U.S.). Manual of Industrial Hygiene and Medical Service in War Industries. Philadelphia and London; W. B. Saunders, 1943. 508p.
First	National Research Council (U.S.). Committee on Maternal and Child Feeding. Maternal Nutrition and Child Health; An Interpretative Review . . . by Kirsten U. Toverud, Genevieve Stearns and Icie G. Macy Hoobler. Washington, D.C.; National Academy of Sciences, 1950. 174p. (NRC Bulletin no. 123)
First	National Research Council (U.S.). Committee on Nutrition Surveys. Nutrition Surveys: Their Techniques and Value. Washington, D.C.; National Academy of Sciences, 1949. 144p. (NRC Bulletin no. 117)
First	National Research Council (U.S.). Food and Nutrition Board. Recommended Dietary Allowances; Protein, Calcium, Iron, Vitamin A, Vitamin B (Thiamin), Vitamin C (Ascorbic Acid), Riboflavin, Nicotinic Acid, Vitamin D. Washington, D.C.; 1941. 5p. (Issued by the Board under its earlier name, Committee on Food and Nutrition. 10th ed., rev., 1989. 284p.)
Second	Nettleton, John A. The Manufacture of Spirit: As Conducted at the Various Distilleries of the United Kingdom. London and New York; M. Ward, 1893. 431p.
Second	Neuberg, Carl, and Irene S. Roberts. Invertase. New York; Sugar Research Foundation, 1946. 62p.
Second	Newlands, John A. R., and Benjamin E. R. Newlands. Sugar: A Handbook for Planters and Refiners, Being a Comprehensive Treatise on the Culture of Sugar-Yielding Plants, and the Manufacture, Refining, and Analysis of Cane, Beet, Palm, Maple, Melon, Sorghum, and Starch Sugars: With Copious Statistics of Their Production and Commerce, and a Chapter on the Distillation of Rum. London; E. & F. Spon; New York; Spon & Chamberlain, 1909. 876p.
Second	Newman, George. Infant Mortality; A Social Problem. New York; E. P. Dutton & Co., 1907. 356p. (Earlier ed., London; Methuen, 1906.)
Second	Newsholme, Arthur. Fifty Years in Public Health: A Personal Narrative with Comments. London; G. Allen & Unwin, 1935. 415p.
Second	Nickerson, Dorothy. Application of Color Measurement in the Grading of Agricultural Products. Washington, D.C.; 1932. 36p. (Later ed., as Color Measurement and Its Application to the Grading of Agricultural Products; A Handbook on the Method of Disk Colorimetry, 1946. 62p. USDA Miscellaneous Publication No. 580.)
Second	Nierenstein, Maximilian. The Natural Organic Tannins; History, Chemistry, Distribution. London; J. & A. Churchill, 1934. 319p. (American ed., Cleveland, Ohio; Sherwood Press, 1935.)
Second	Noorden, Karl H. von. Metabolism and Practical Medicine. Chicago; W. T. Keener & Co., 1987. (Anglo- American issue under the editorship of I. Walker Hall.)
First	Northrop, John H. Crystalline Enzymes. New York; Columbia University Press, 1939. 176p. (2d ed., 1948. 352p.)

Rank

O

Second	Onslow, Muriel W. The Anthocyanin Pigments of Plants. Cambridge; University Press, 1916. 318p. (2d ed., 1925. 314p.)
Second	Onslow, Muriel W. The Principles of Plant Biochemistry. Cambridge; University Press, 1931. 1 vols.
Second	Oppenheimer, Karl. Ferments and Their Actions . . . transl. from German by C. Ainsworth Mitchell. London; C. Griffin & Co., 1901. 343p.
First	Orr, John B. Food, Health and Income; Report on a Survey of Adequacy of Diet in Relation to Income. London; Macmillan & Co., 1936. 71p. (Reprinted, along with Feeding the People in War-Time, by J. b. Orr and David Lubbock, New York; Garland, 1985. 88p.)
First	Orr, John B., and I. Leitch. Iodine in Nutrition, a Review of Existing Information. London; H.M.S.O., Printed by J. Johnson, University Press, Oxford, 1929. 108p. (Medical Research Council, Special Report Series no. 123)
Second	Osborne, Thomas B. The Proteins of the Wheat Kernel. Washington, D.C.; Carnegie Institution, 1907. 119p. (Carnegie Institution of Washington, Publication no. 84)
Second	Osborne, Thomas B. The Vegetable Proteins. London and New York; Longmans, Green & Co., 1909. 125p. (2d ed., 1924. 154p.)
Second	Osborne, Thomas B., and Lafayette B. Mendel. Food Experiments with Isolated Food-Substances. Washington, D.C.; Carnegie Institution of Washington, 1911. 1 vol. (Carnegie Institution of Washington Publication no. 156) (From the laboratories of the Connecticut Agricultural Experiment Station and the Sheffield Laboratory of Physiological Chemistry of Yale University.)
Second	Ostertag, Robert von. Handbook of Meat Inspection . . . transl. by Earley V. Wilcox. New York; W. R. Jenkins, 1904. 884p. (New English ed., as Textbook of Meat Inspection, edited by T. Dunlop Young. London; Bailliere, Tindall & Cox, 1934. 744p.)

P

Second	Palmer, Leroy S. Carotinoids and Related Pigments: The Chromolipoids. New York; Chemical Catalog Co., 1922. 316p. (American Chemical Society Monograph Series no. 38)
Second	Parker, George H. Smell, Taste, and Allied Senses in the Vertebrates. Philadelphia and London; J. B. Lippincott Co., 1922. 192p.
Second	Parker, Milton E. Food-Plant Sanitation. 1st ed. New York; McGraw-Hill, 1948. 447p.
Second	Parry, Ernest J. The Chemistry of Essential Oils and Artificial Perfumes. London; Scott, Greenwood & Co., 1899. 411p. (4th ed., rev. and enlarged, 1921–1922. 2 vols.)
Second	Parry, John W. The Spice Handbook. Brooklyn, N.Y.; Chemical Pub. Co., 1945. 254p.
Second	Pattee, Alida F. Practical Dietetics, with Reference to Diet in Disease. 6th ed., rev. and enl. Mount Vernon, N.Y.; A. F. Pattee, 1910. 527p. (22d ed., 1940. 880p.)

Ranking	
Second	Pavy, Frederick W. A Treatise on Food and Dietetics, Physiologically, and Therapeutically Considered. London; J. & A. Churchill, 1874. 559p. (2d ed., New York; William Wood & Co., 1881. 402p.)
Second	Pearl, Raymond. The Nation's Food; A Statistical Study of a Physiological and Social Problem. Philadelphia and London; W. B. Saunders, 1920. 274p.
Second	Perkin, Arthur G., and Arthur E. Everest. The Natural Organic Colouring Matters. London and New York; Longmans, Green, 1918. 655p.
Second	Perla, David, and Jessie Marmorston. Natural Resistance and Clinical Medicine. Boston; Little, Brown, 1941. 1344p.
Second	Peterson, Marjorie W. Baking Flour Mixtures at High Altitudes. Fort Collins; Colorado Agricultural College, Colorado Experiment Station, 1930. 180p.
Second	Pieron, Henri. The Sensations: Their Functions, Processes, and Mechanisms . . . transl. by M. H. Pirenne and B. C. Abbott. New Haven; Yale University Press, 1952. 468p. (Translation of Aux Sources del la Connaissance.)
Second	Pigman, William W., and Rudolph M. Goepp. Chemistry of the Carbohydrates. New York; Academic Press, 1948. 748p.
Second	Plimmer, Robert H. The Chemical Constitution of the Proteins. 1st ed. London; Longmans, Green, 1908. 2 vols. (3d ed., 1917. 1 vol.)
First	Plimmer, Violet G. S., and R. H. A. Plimmer. Vitamins and the Choice of Food. London and New York; Longmans, Green, 1922. 164p.
Second	Pollock, Ivan L. The Food Administration in Iowa. Iowa City; Iowa State Historical Society, 1923. 2 vols.
Second	Powell, Ola. Successful Canning and Preserving; Practical Hand Book for Schools, Clubs, and Home Use. Philadelphia and London; J. B. Lippincott Co., 1917. 371p. (4th ed., rev. and entirely reset, by Ola Powell Malcolm, 1930. 663p.)
Second	Prescott, A. B. Chemical Examination of Alcoholic Liquors; A Manual of the Constituents of the Distilled Spirits and Fermented Liquors of Commerce, and Their Qualitative and Quantitative Determination. New York; D. Van Nostrand, 1875. 108p. (Later printing, 1880.)
First	Prescott, Samuel C., and Cecil G. Dunn, eds. Industrial Microbiology. 1st ed. New York and London; McGraw-Hill, 1940. 541p. (4th ed., as Prescott and Dunn's Industrial Microbiology, edited by Gerald Reed. Westport, Conn.; Avi, 1982. 883p.)
First	Prescott, Samuel C., and Bernard E. Proctor. Food Technology. 1st ed. New York; McGraw-Hill, 1937. 630p.
Second	Price, Weston A. Nutrition and Physical Degeneration; A Comparison of Primitive and Modern Diets and Their Effects. New York and London; P. B. Hoeber, 1939. 431p. (50th anniversary ed., New Canaan, Conn.; Keats, 1989. 526p.)
Second	Pringsheim, Hans. The Chemistry of the Monosaccharides and the Polysaccharides. New York and London; McGraw-Hill, 1932. 413p.
First	Prinson Geerligs, H. C. Cane Sugar and Its Manufacture. Altrincham, Manchester; N. Rodger, 1909. 350p. (2d ed., rev., 1924. 342p.)

Ranking	
	R
Second	Race, Joseph. The Examination of Milk for the Public Health Purposes. 1st ed. New York; J. Wiley, 1918. 224p.
Second	Radley, Jack A. Starch and Its Derivatives. New York; Van Nostrand, 1940. 346p. (4th ed., London; Chapman & Hall, 1968. 558p.)
Second	Ralston, Anderson W. Fatty Acids and Their Derivatives. New York; Wiley, 1948. 986p.
First	Rector, Thomas M. Scientific Preservation of Food. New York; J. Wiley, 1925. 213p.
First	Richards, Ellen H. Food Materials and Their Adulterations. Boston; Estes & Laurial, 1886. 183p. (Later ed., 1906.)
Second	Richards, Lenore. Quantity Cookery; Menu Planning and Cooking for Large Numbers . . . Boston; Little, Brown, 1922. 200p. (4th ed., by Nola Treat and L. Richards, 1966. 660p.)
First	Richmond, Henry D. Dairy Chemistry: A Handbook for Dairy Chemists and Others Having Control of Dairies. London; Charles Griffin & Co., 1899. 384p. (5th ed., rev. by J. G. Davis and F. J. Macdonald, as Richmond's Dairy Chemistry, 1953. 603p.)
First	Richmond, Walter L. Candy Production: Methods and Formulas. Chicago; Manufacturing Confectioner Pub., 1948. 622p.
Second	Rideal, Samuel. The Carbohydrates and Alcohol. London; Bailliere, Tindall & Cox, 1920. 219p.
Second	Rideal, Samuel. Disinfection and the Preservation of Food, Together with an Account of the Chemical Substances Used as Antiseptics and Preservatives. London; Sanitary Pub. Co.; New York; J. Wiley, 1903. 494p.
Second	Rigby, Will O., and Fred Rigby. Rigby's Reliable Candy Teacher, with Complete and Modern Soda, Ice Cream and Sherbet Sections. 13th ed. Topeka, Kans.; Rigby Pub. Co., 1920. 271p. (14th ed., 1923. 268p.)
First	Roberts, Lydia Jane. Nutrition Work with Children. Chicago; University of Chicago Press, 1927. 394p. (Rev. and enl. ed., 1935. 639p.)
Second	Roberts, Stewart R. Pellagra; History, Distribution, Diagnosis, Prognosis, Treatment, Etiology. St. Louis; Mosby, 1912. 272p.
Second	Robertson, T. Brailsford. The Chemical Basis of Growth and Senescence. Philadelphia and London; J. B. Lippincott, 1923. 389p.
First	Robertson, T. Brailsford. The Physical Chemistry of the Proteins. New York; Longmans, Green, 1918. 483p.
Second	Rooker, William A. Fruit Pectin. New York; Avi, 1928. 170p.
First	Rose, Mary S. Feeding the Family. New York; Macmillan Co., 1917. 449p. (4th ed., 1940. 421p.)
First	Rose, Mary S. The Foundations of Nutrition. New York; Macmillan Co., 1927. 501p. (6th ed., by Clara Mae Taylor and Orrea F. Pye, 1966. 564p.)
First	Rose, Mary S. A Laboratory Handbook for Dietetics. 4th ed. New York; Macmillan Co., 1937. 322p. (5th ed., rev. and rewritten by Clara Mae Taylor and Grace MacLeod, 1949. 358p.)
First	Rosenberg, Hans R. Chemistry and Physiology of the Vitamins. New York; Interscience, 1945. 676p.
Second	Rutgers University. Bureau of Biological Research. Cooperative Determina-

Ranking	
	tions of the Amino Acid Content, and of the Nutritive Value of Six Selected Protein Food Sources, 1946–1950. New Brunswick; 1950. 114p.

S

Ranking	
Second	Sahyun, Melville. Proteins and Amino Acids in Nutrition. New York; Reinhold, 1948. 566p.
Second	Salter, William T. The Endocrine Function of Iodine. Cambridge, Mass.; Harvard University Press, 1940. 351p. (Harvard University Monographs in Medicine and Public Health no. 1)
Second	Savage, William G. Canned Foods in Relation to Health. Cambridge, Eng.; University Press, 1923. 146p. (Milroy Lectures, 1923.)
Second	Savage, William G. Food Poisoning and Food Infections. Cambridge; University Press, 1920. 247p.
Second	Scarborough, N. F. Sweets Manufacture. London; Leonard Hill, 1937. n.p.
Second	Scheele, Carl W. The Collected Papers of Carl Wilhelm Scheele . . . transl. from Swedish and German originals by Leonard Dobbin. London; G. Bell & Sons, 1931. 367p.
Second	Scherer, Robert. Casein: Its Preparation and Technical Utilisation . . . transl. from German by Chas. Salter. London; Scott, Greenwood & Son; New York; Van Nostrand, 1906. 163p. (Translation of Kassein, dessen Zusammensetzung, Eigenschaften, Herstellung und Berwertung. 3d English ed., rev. and enl. by H. B. Stocks, 1921. 216p.)
Second	Schmidt, Carl L. A., ed. The Chemistry of the Amino Acids and Proteins. Springfield, Ill., and Baltimore; C. C. Thomas, 1938. 1031p. (2d ed., 1945. 1290p.)
Second	Schneider, Albert. The Microanalysis of Powdered Vegetable Drugs. 2d ed. Philadelphia; P. Blakiston, 1921. 548p.
First	Schoenheimer, Rudolf. The Dynamic State of Body Constituents. Cambridge, Mass.; Harvard University Press, 1942. 78p. (Harvard University Monographs in Medicine and Public Health no. 3) (2d ed., 1946.)
Second	Schoonmaker, Frank, and Tom Marvel. The Complete Wine Book. New York; Simon & Schuster, 1934. 315p. (Rev. ed., London; G. Routledge & Sons, 1938. 262p.)
Second	Schryver, Samuel B. The General Characters of the Proteins. London and New York; Longmans, Green, 1909. 86p.
Second	Schulerud, Arne. Das Roggenmehl. 2d ed. Detmold; Schafer, 1957. 200p. (Translation from original Norwegian.)
Second	Schwartz, Anthony M., and James W. Perry. Surfact Active Agents, Their Chemistry and Technology. New York; Interscience, 1949–1958. 2 vols. (Vol. 2 reprinted, 1977. 869p.)
Second	Scott, James H. Flour Milling Processes. New York; Van Nostrand, 1936. 416p. (2d ed., rev. London; Chapman & Hall, 1951. 670p.)
Second	Scott Blair, George W. Foodstuffs, Their Plasticity, Fluidity, and Consistency. Amsterdam; North-Holland; New York; Interscience, 1953. 264p.
First	Sedgwick, William T. Principles of Sanitary Science and the Public Health: With Special Reference to the Causation and Prevention of Infectious Dis-

Ranking	
	eases. New York; Macmillan, 1902. 368p. (Later ed., as Sedgwick's Principles of Sanitary Science and Public Health, rewritten and enlarged by Samuel C. Prescott and Murray P. Horwood, 1935. 654p.)
Second	Semichon, Lucien. Traite des Maladies des Vins, Description, Etude, Traitement. Montpellier; Coulet et Fils, 1905. 654p.
Second	Shand, Philip M. A Book of Other Wines—Than French. New York; A. A. Knopf, 1929. 185p.
First	Sherman, Henry C. Chemistry of Food and Nutrition. New York; Macmillan Co., 1911. 355p. (8th ed., 1952. 721p.)
First	Sherman, Henry C. Food Products. New York; Macmillan, 1914. 594p. (4th ed., 1948. 428p.)
Second	Sherman, Henry C. The Nutritional Improvement of Life. New York; Columbia University Press, 1950. 270p.
First	Sherman, Henry C. The Science of Nutrition. New York; Columbia University Press, 1943. 253p.
Second	Sherman, Henry C., and S. L. Smith. The Vitamins. New York; Chemical Catalogue Co., 1922. 273p.
Second	Shinkle, Charles A. American Commercial Methods of Manufacturing Preserves, Pickles, Canned Foods, etc. Rev. ed. Menominee, Mich.; C. A. Shinkle, 1912. 212p.
Second	Shohl, Alfred T. Mineral Metabolism. New York; Reinhold, 1939. 384p. (American Chemical Society, Monograph Series no. 82)
Second	Shrader, James H. Food Control, Its Public Health Aspects; A Manual for Regulatory Officers, Food Technologists, and Students of the Food Industry. New York; J. Wiley; London; Chapman & Hall, 1939. 513p.
Second	Sickson, Ernest C. Botulism; A Clinical and Experimental Study. New York; Rockefeller Institute for Medical Research, 1918. 117p. (Monographs of the Rockefeller Institute for Medical Research no. 8)
Second	Simon, Ernest D. The Physical Science of Flour Milling. Liverpool, Eng.; Northern Pub. Co., 1930. 222p.
Second	Smallzreid, K. A. The Everlasting Pleasure: Influences on American Kitchens, Cooks and Cookery from 1565 to the Year 2000. Appleton-Century-Crofts Co., 1956.
Second	Smith, Edward. Practical Dietary for Families, Schools, and the Labouring Classes. London; Walton & Maberly, 1864. 265p.
Second	Smith, J. Russell. The World's Food Resources. New York; H. Holt & Co., 1919. 634p.
Second	Smith, Leslie. Flour Milling Technology. 3d ed., rev. Liverpool, Eng.; Northern Pub. Co., 1944. 571p.
Second	Smyth, Henry F., and Walter L. Obold. Industrial Microbiology; The Utilization of Bacteria, Yeasts and Molds in Industrial Processes. Baltimore; Williams & Wilkins, 1930. 313p.
Second	Society of Chemical Industry Food Group. Vitamin E; Proceedings of a Symposium . . . School of Hygiene and Tropical Medicine, London, April 1939. London; Chemical Pub. Co., 1940. 88p.
Second	Sorensen, S. P. L. Proteins; Lectures Given in the United States of America in 1924. New York; Fleischmann Laboratories, 1925. 142p.

Ranking	
Second	Soskin, Samuel, and Rachmiel Levine. Carbohydrate Metabolism, Correlation of Physiological, Biochemical and Clinical Aspects. Chicago; University of Chicago Press, 1946. 316p. (2d ed., rev., 1952. 346p.)
Second	Spencer, Guilford L. A Hand-Book for Sugar Manufacturers and Their Chemists. New York; J. Wiley, 1889. 221p. (8th ed., rev., rewritten and enlarged, 1945, as Cane Sugar Handbook. 834p. 11th ed., by George P. Meade and James C. P. Chen.)
Second	Squibb, Edward R. Proposed Legislation on the Adulteration of Food and Medicine. New York; G. P. Putnam's Sons, 1879. 57p.
Second	Stanley, Louis, and Jessie A. Cline. Foods, Their Selection and Preparation. Boston and New York; Ginn & Co., 1935. (Rev. ed., 1950. 388p.)
Second	Starling, Ernest H. Mercers' Company Lectures on Recent Advances in the Physiology of Digestion, Delivered in the Michaelmas Term, 1905, in the Physiological Department of University College, London. Chicago; W. T. Keener, 1907. 156p.
Second	Starling, Ernest H. The Oliver-Sharpey Lectures on the Feedings of Nations, a Study in Applied Physiology, given at the Royal College of Physicians, London, June 3 and 5, 1919. London and New York; Longmans, Green, 1919. 146p.
First	Stephenson, Marjory. Bacterial Metabolism. London and New York; Longmans, Green, 1930. 320p. (3d ed., Cambridge, Mass.; M.I.T. Press, 1949. 398p. Reprinted, 1966.)
Second	Stewart, George N. A Manual of Physiology, with Practical Exercises. Philadelphia; W. B. Saunders, 1897. 796p. (8th ed., London; Bailliere, Tindall & Cox, 1921. 1245p.)
Second	Stewart, Jean J. Foods: Production, Marketing, Consumption. New York; Prentice-Hall, 1938. 737p. (2d ed., by J. J. Stewart and Alice L. Edwards, 1948. 490p.)
Second	Stiles, Percy G. Nutritional Physiology. Philadelphia and London; W. B. Saunders, 1912. 271p. (7th ed., 1931. 313p.)
First	Straus, Lina G. Disease in Milk; The Remedy, Pasteurization: The Life Work of Nathan Straus. New York; E. P. Dutton & Co., 1917. 383p.
Second	Sulz, Charles H. A Treatise on Beverages, or, The Complete Practical Bottler: Full Instructions for Laboratory Work with Original Practical Recipes for All Kinds of Carbonated Drinks, Mineral Waters, Flavorings, Extracts, Syrups, etc. New York; Dick & Fitzgerald Pub., 1888. 818p.
Second	Sumner, James B., and G. Fred Somers. Chemistry and Methods of Enzymes. New York; Academic Press, 1943. 365p. (3d ed., 1953. 462p.)
First	Sunkist Growers, Inc. Exchange Citrus Pectin; Preservers Handbook. New York and Ontario, Calif.; California Fruit Growers Exchange, 1941. 117p. (7th ed., Ontario, Calif.; Sunkist Growers, 1964. 146p.)
Second	Sutermeister, Edwin. Casein and Its Industrial Applications. New York; Chemical Catalog Co., 1927. 296p. (American Chemical Society, Monograph Series no. 30) (2d ed., by E. Sutermeister and Frederick L. Browne. New York; Reinhold Pub., 1939. 433p.)
Second	Swank, Edith E. The Story of Food Preservation. Pittsburgh, Penn.; H. J. Heinz Co., 1942. 101p.

Ranking

Second Swanson, Charles O. Physical Properties of Dough. Minneapolis; Burgess Pub. Co., 1943. 258p.

Second Swanson, Charles O. Wheat and Flour Quality. Minneapolis; Burgess Pub. Co., 1938. 227p.

Second Swanson, Charles O. Wheat Flour and Diet. New York; Macmillan Co., 1928. 203p.

Second Sweetman, Marion D. Food Preparation; A Textbook for Colleges on the Science of Food Processing. New York; J. Wiley; London; Chapman & Hall, 1932. 344p. (4th ed., 1954. 645p.)

T

First Tanner, Fred W. Bacteriology and Mycology of Foods. 1st ed. New York; J. Wiley & Sons, 1919. 592p.

First Tanner, Fred W. Food-Borne Infections and Intoxications. 1st ed. Champaign, Ill.; Twin City Printing Co., 1933. 439p. (2d ed., by F. W. Tanner and Louise P. Tanner, published by Garrard Press, 1953. 769p.)

First Tanner, Fred W. The Microbiology of Foods. 1st ed. Champaign, Ill.; Twin City Print. Co., 1932. 768p. (2d ed., Champaign, Ill.; Garrard Press, 1944. 1196p.)

Second Tauber, Henry. The Chemistry and Technology of Enzymes. New York; Wiley, 1949. 550p.

Second Tauber, Henry. Enzyme Technology. New York; J. Wiley; London; Chapman & Hall, 1943. 275p.

Second Tauber, Henry. Experimental Enzyme Chemistry. Minneapolis; Burgess Pub. Co., 1936. 118p.

First Thom, Charles, and Margaret B. Church. The Aspergilli. Baltimore; Williams & Wilkins, 1926. 272p. (Later ed., by C. Thom and Kenneth B. Raper, 1945. 373p.)

Second Thom, Charles, and Walter W. Fish. The Book of Cheese. New York; Macmillan, 1918. 392p. (rev. ed., 1938. 415p.)

Second Thom, Charles, and Albert C. Hunter. Hygienic Fundamentals of Food Handling. Baltimore; Williams & Wilkins, 1924. 228p.

Second Thornton, M. K. Cottonseed Products. 1st ed. Wharton, Tex.; Oil Mill Gasetteer, 1932. 268p.

Second Thresh, John C., and Arthur E. Porter. Preservatives in Food and Food Examination. Philadelphia; P. Blakiston, 1906. 484p.

First Thudichum, John L. W. A Treatise on the Origin, Nature, and Varieties of Wine; Being a Complete Manual of Viticulture an Oenology. London and New York; Macmillan, 1872. 760p.

Second Tibbles, William. Foods; Their Origin, Composition, and Manufacture. London; Bailliere, Tindall & Cox, 1912. 950p.

Second Tomhave, William H. Meats and Meat Products. Philadelphia and Chicago; J. B. Lippincott, 1925. 418p.

Second Topley, William W. C., and G. S. Wilson. The Principles of Bacteriology and Immunity. New York; W. Wood, 1929. 2 vols. (6th ed., by G. S. Wilson and A. Miles, Baltimore; Williams & Wilkins, 1975.)

First Tressler, Donald K. Marine Products of Commerce; Their Acquisition,

Ranking

Handling, Biological Aspects, and the Science and Technology of Their Preparation and Preservation. New York; Chemical Catalog Co., 1923. 762p. (2d ed., rev. and enlarged. New York; Reinhold, 1951. 782p.)

First — Tressler, Donald K., and Clifford F. Evers. The Freezing Preservation of Foods. New York; Avi, 1943. 763p. (4th ed., edited by D. K. Tressler, Wallace B. Van Arsdel and Michael J. Copley. Westport, Conn.; Avi, 1968.)

First — Tressler, Donald K., Maynard A. Joslyn, and George L. March. Fruit and Vegetable Juices. New York; Avi, 1939. 549p.

Second — Tucker, J. H., A Manual of Sugar Analysis, Including the Applications in General of Analytical Methods to the Sugar industry. With an Introduction on th Chemistry of Cane-Sugar, Dextrose, Levulose, and Milk-Sugar. New York; D. Van Norstrand, 1881. 353p.

U

First — Ukers, William H. All About Coffee. New York; Tea and Coffee Trade Journal, 1935. 2 vols.

First — Ukers, William H. All About Tea. New York; Tea and Coffee Trade Journal, 1935. 2 vols.

Second — Ukers, William H. Coffee Merchandising. New York; Tea and Coffee Trade Journal Co., 1924. 245p. (Later ed., 1930. 245p.)

First — Ukers, William H. The Romance of Coffee; An Outline History of Coffee and Coffee-Drinking through a Thousand Years. New York; Tea and Coffee Trade Journal Co., 1948. 280p.

Second — Underhill, Frank P. The Physiology of the Amino Acids. New Haven, Conn.; Yale University Press, 1915. 169p.

Second — United States Army. Surgeon General's Office. Military Meat and Dairy Hygiene . . . compiled by Horace S. Eakins. Baltimore; Williams & Wilkins, 1924. 647p.

V

First — Van Slyke, Lucius L. Modern Methods of Testing Milk and Milk Products; A Handbook Prepared for the Use of Dairy Students, Butter Makers, Cheese Makers, Producers of Milk, Operators in Condenseries, Managers of Milk-Shipping Stations, Milk-Inspectors, Physicians . . . New York; O. Judd, 1906. 214p. (3d ed., rev., 1940. 344p.)

Second — Van Slyke, Lucius L., and Walter V. Price. Cheese; A Treatise on the Manufacture of American Cheddar Cheese and Some Other Varieties . . . Rev. and enlarged ed. New York; O. Judd, 1952. 522p.

First — Van Slyke, Lucius L., and Charles H. Publow. The Science and Practice of Cheese-Making; A Treatise on the Manufacture of American Cheddar Cheese and Other Varieties, Intended as a Text-Book for the Use of Dairy Teachers and Students in Classroom and Workroom. New York; O. Judd, 1909. 483p.

Second — Vaughan, Victor C., and J. Walter Vaughan. Protein Split Products in Relation to Immunity and Disease. Philadelphia and New York; Lea & Febiger, 1913. 476p.

Rank	
Second	Vedder, Edward B. Beriberi . . . illustrated by numerous engravings and by five colored plates. New York; W. Wood, 1913. 427p.
Second	Vernon, Horace M. Intracellular Enzymes; A Course of Lectures Given in the Physiological Laboratory, University of London. London; J. Murray, 1908. 240p.
Second	Verwey, Evert J. W., and J. T. G. Overbeek, with the collaboration of K. van Nes. Theory of the Stability of Lyophobic Colloids; The Interaction of Sol Particles Having an Electric Double Layer. New York; Elsevier, 1948. 205p.
Second	Verworn, Max. General Physiology; An Outline of the Science of Life . . . transl. from 2d German ed. and edited by Frederic S. Lee. London; Macmillan, 1899. 615p.
Second	Vincent, Ralph H. The Nutrition of the Infant. New York; Wood, 1904. 295p. (2d ed., rev. and enlarged. London; Bailliere, Tindall & Cox, 1904. 321p.)
First	von Loesecke, Harry W. Drying and Dehydration of Foods. New York; Reinhold Pub., 1943. 302p. (2d ed., 1955. 300p.)
First	von Loesecke, Harry W. Outlines of Food Technology. New York; Reinhold Pub. Corp., 1942. 505p. (2d ed., 1949. 585p.)
Second	Vulte, Hermann T. Food Industries. Easton, Penn.; Chemical Pub. Co., 1914. 309p.

W

Rank	
Second	Wagner, Philip M. American Wines and How to Make Them. New York; Alfred A. Knopf, 1933. 295p. (Later ed., 1956. 264p.)
First	Waksman, Selman A., and Wilburt C. Davison. Enzymes; Properties, Distribution, Methods and Applications. Baltimore; Williams & Wilkins Co., 1926. 364p.
Second	Waldschmidt-Leitz, Ernst. Enzyme Actions and Properties . . . transl. by Robert P. Walton. New York; J. Wiley; London; Chapman & Hall, 1929. 255p.
First	Walker, William H. Principles of Chemical Engineering. 1st ed. New York; McGraw-Hill, 1923. 637p. (3d ed., 1937. 749p.)
Second	Walton, Robert P. A Comprehensive Survey of Starch Chemistry. New York; Chemical Catalog Co., 1928. 1 vols.
Second	Wanklyn, James A. Milk-Analysis. A Practical Treatise on the Examination of Milk and its Derivatives, Cream, Butter, and Cheese. New York; D. Van Nostrand, 1874. 73p.
Second	Warcollier, Georges. The Principles and Practice of Cider-Making . . . transl. by Vernon L. S. Charley and Pamela M. Mumford. London; L. Hill, 1949. 367p. (Translation of La Cidrerie, 1928.)
Second	Ward, Alan G. Colloids: Their Properties and Applications. New York; Interscience, 1946. 133p.
Second	Ware, Lewis S. Beet-Sugar Manufacture and Refining. 1st ed. New York; J. Wiley, 1905–1907. 2 vols.
Second	Warren, Shields. The Pathology of Diabetes Mellitus. Philadelphia; Lea & Febiger, 1930. 212p. (4th ed., 1966. 528p.)

Rank	
Second	Warth, Albin H. The Chemistry and Technology of Waxes. New York; Reinhold, 1947. 519p. (2d ed., 1956. 940p.)
Second	Weber, G. M., and C. L. Alsberg. The American Vegetable-Shortening Industry: Its Origin and Development. Stanford University, 1934. (Stanford University Food Research Institute, Fats and Oils Studies no. 5)
Second	Weinmann, J. Manual of the Industry of Sparkling Wines; Description of the Chemical and Practical Processes Customarily Used in Champagne . . . transl. by Charles A. Wetmore. Piedmont, Calif.; 1917. 105p.
Second	Whipple, George C. The Microscopy of Drinking Water. 1st ed. New York and London; Wiley & Sons, 1899. 300p. (4th ed., rewritten and enlarged, rev. by Gordon M. Fair and Melville C. Whipple, 1927. 586p.)
Second	Whymper, Robert. Cocoa and Chocolate, Their Chemistry and Manufacture. Philadelphia; P. Blakiston, 1912. 327p. (2d ed., rev. and enlarged, 1921. 568p.)
Second	Wihlfahrt, Julius E. Treatise on Baking. 3d ed. New York; Standard Brandt, 1935. 468p.
First	Wilder, Russell M., and Robert R. Williams. Enrichment of Flour and Bread: A History of the Movement. Washington, D.C.; National Research Council, 1944. 130p.
First	Wiley, Harvey W. Beverages and Their Adulteration. Philadelphia; P. Balkiston's & Co., 1919. 421p.
First	Wiley, Harvey W. Foods and Their Adulteration: Origin, Manufacture and Composition of. Food Products; Description of Common Adulterations; Food Standards and National Food Laws and Regulation. Philadelphia; P. Blakiston's Son & Co., 1907. 625p.
First	Wiley, Harvey W. The History of a Crime Against the Food Law. Washington, D.C.; The author, 1929. 413p.
Second	Willard, Florence, and Lucy H. Gillett. Dietetics for High Schools. New York; Macmillan, 1920. 201p. (Rev. ed., 1930. 290p.)
Second	Williams, Robert R., and Tom D. Spies. Vitamin B1 (Thiamin) and Its Use in Medicine. New York; Macmillan, 1938. 411p.
Second	Willows, Richard S., and E. Hatschek. Surface Tension and Surface Energy and Their Influence on Chemical Phenomena. London; J. & A. Churchill, 1915. 80p. (3d ed., 1923. 134p.)
Second	Willstatter, Richard M. Problems and Methods in Enzyme Research. Ithaca, N.Y.; Cornell University, 1927. 62p.
Second	Wilson, Graham S. The Pasteurization of Milk. London; E. Arnold, 1942. 212p.
First	Winton, Andrew L. The Microscopy of Vegetable Foods, with Special Reference to the Detection of Adulteration and the Diagnosis of Mixtures. 1st ed. New York; J. Wiley, 1906. 701p. (2d ed., 1916. 701p.)
First	Winton, Andrew L., and Kate B. Winton. The Structure and Composition of Foods. New York; J. Wiley & Sons; London; Chapman & Hall, 1932–1939. 4 vols.
Second	Wolf, Stewart, and Harold G. Wolff. Human Gastric Function; An Experimental Study of a Man and His Stomach. London; Oxford University Press, 1943. 195p. (Later ed., 1947. 262p.)

Rank	
First	Woodman, Alpheus G. Food Analysis, Typical Methods and Interpretation of Results. 1st ed. New York; McGraw-Hill, 1915. 510p. (4th ed., 1941. 607p.)
	Z
Second	Zavalla, Justo P. The Canning of Fruits and Vegetables, Based on the Methods in Use in California, with Notes on the Control of the Microorganisms Effecting Spoilage. 1st ed. New York; J. Wiley & Sons, 1916. 214p.
First	Ziegler, P. Thomas. The Meat We Eat. Danville, Ill.; Interstate, 1948. 497p. (12th ed., by John R. Romans, et al., 1985. 850p.)

Non-English Monographs Cited in Source Documents

As the citation analysis continued through the nineteen source documents, foreign language titles were extracted. They were later removed from the primary monograph list, since they are not being recommended for preservation by United States libraries. These monographs, however, represent the background and scientific basis for much of the work in the United States, and in the review process they were rated of historical value. Although the list is brief, the titles are provided here for information and preservation consideration. A more comprehensive list would include all similar documents mentioned in the beginning of this chapter and in Chapters 1 and 2.

Primary Historical Non-English Monographs

Albu, Albert, and Carl Neuberg. Physiologie und Pathologie des Mineralstoffwechsels; Nebst Tabellen uber die Mineralstoffzusammensetzung der menschlichen Nahrungs- und Genussmittel sowie der Mineralbrunned und -Bader. Berlin; Springer, 1906. 255p.

Ammon, Robert, and Wilhelm Dirscherl. Fermente, Hormone, Vitamine, und die Beziehungen Dieser Wirkstoffe Zueinander. Leipzig, Germany; Thieme, 1938. 451p. (2d ed., 1948. 1051p.)

Andrade, J. L. Estudios sobre la Leche. Caracas, Venezuela; n.p., 1940. 159p.

Antonini, Giuseppe. La Pellagra; Storia, Eziologia, Patogenesi, Profilassi. Milan; Hoepli, 1902. 166p.

Arlt, Ferdinand Ritter von. Die Krankheiten des Auges, fur Praktische Arzte. Prague; Credner & Kleinbub, 1851–1956. 3 vols.

Aschoff, Ludwig, ed. Pathologische Anatomie: Eine Lehrbuch fur Studierende und Aerzte. Jena; Fischer, 1923. 2 vols. Auervain, Fritz de, and C. Wegelin. Der Endemische Kretinismus. Berlin; Springer, 1936. 206p.

Babo, August W. von. Handbuch des Weinbaues und der Kellerwirthschaft. Berlin; P. Parey, 1881–1883. 2 vols. (Later ed., 1910–1923. 2 vols. in 4.)

Barthel, Christian. Die Methoden zur untersuchung von Milch und Molkereiprodukten. Leipzig; M. Heinsius, 1907. 271p. (2d ed., 1911. 309p.)
Beccari, Jacopo B. Prolegomena Institutionum Medicarum. Introduzione, Traduzione e Note a Cura di Giuseppe Alberti. Gologna; Cappelli, 1955. 229p. (Classici Italiani della Medicina no. 3) (Report of 1750 ed.)
Beer, August. Einleitung in die Hohere Optik. Braunschweig; F. Vieweg, 1853. 430p. (2d ed., 1882. 423p.)
Berg, Ragnar. Die Vitamine, Kritische Ubersicht der Lehre von den Erganzungsstoffen. Leipzig; Hirzel, 1922. 336p. (2d ed., 1927. 714p.)
Bernard, Claude. Lecons sur le Diabete et la Glycogenese Animale. Paris; J.-B. Bailliere & Fils, 1877. 576p. (Reissued, Cercle du Livre Precieux, 1966. 390p.)
Bernard, Claude. Lecons sur les Phenomenes de la Vie Communs aux Animaux et aux Vegetaux. 2d ed. Paris; J.-B. Bailliere, 1879–1885. 2 vols. (Reprinted, Paris; Vrin, 1966.)
Berthelot, Marcellin. Chimie organique fondee sur la Synthese. Paris; Mallet-Bachelier, 1860. 2 vols. (Reprinted, Brussels; Culture et Civilisation, 1966.)
Berzelius, Jons J. Forelasningar i Djurkemien. Stockholm; Delen, 1806–1808. 2 vols.
Bibra, Ernst von. Chemische untersuchungen uber die Knochen und Zahne des Menschen und der Wirbelthiere. Wshweinfurt; Kunstverlag, 1844. 435p.
Bidder, Friedrich H., and C. Schmidt. Die Verdauungssaefte und der Stoffwechsel; Eien Physiologisch-Chemische Untersuchung. Mitau; Beyer, 1852. 413p.
Bindoni, Mario. Trattato di Enologia ad uso Degli Industriali, dei Commerciante e Degli Agricoltori. Albano Laziale; Fratelli Strini, 1930. 394p.
Bischoff, Theodor L. W. von, and Carl Voit. Die Gesetze der Ernahrung des Fleischfressers durch neue Untersuchungen festgestellt. Leipzig; n.p., 1860. 304p.
Blondlot, Nicolas. Traite analytique de la Digestion consideree particulierement dans l'Homme et dans les Animaux vertebres. Nancy; Grimblot, Raybois, 1843. 471p.
Bunge, Gustav von. Lehrbuch der physiologischen und pathologischen Chemie. 2d ed. Leipzig; Verlag von F. C. W. Vogel, 1889. 404p. (4th ed., 1898. 510p.)
Bunge, Gustav von. Lehrbuch der Physiologie des Menchen. Leipzig; Vogel, 1901. 2 vols. (2d ed., 1905.)
Le Canu, Louis R. Etudes Chimiques sur le Sang Humain: These Presentee et Soutenue a la Faculte de Medecine de Paris, Nov. 1837. Paris; Imprimerie et Fonderie de Rignoux et Cie, 1837. 128p.
Cuvier, Georges. Lecons d'Anatomie Comparee de Georges Cuvier, Recueillies et Publiees par M. Dumeril. 3d ed. Brussels; H. Dumont; London; Dulau, 1836–1840. 3 vols.
Dugast, J. Vinification dans les Pays Chauds, Algerie et Tunisie. Paris; G. Carre et C. Naud, 1900. 281p. (3d ed., Alger, Aumeran, 1930. 396p.)
Eberle, J. N. Physiologie der Verdauung, nach Versuchen auf naturlichem und kunstlichem Wege. Wruzburg; Etlinger, 1834. 408p.
Euler-Chelpin, Hans K. Chemie der Enzyme. 2d ed. Munich; Bergmann, 1920–1934. 2 vols.
Fabre, Jean-Henri. Traite Encyclopedique des Vins. 4th ed. Algiers; Biblioteque du Colon de l'Afrique du Nord, 1929. 3 vols.
Fincke, Heinrich. Handbuch der Kakaoerzeugnisse; Ihre geschichte, rohstoffe, herstellung, beschaffenheit, zusammensetzung, anwendung, wirkung, gesetzliche regelung und zahlberichte, dargestellt fur gewerbe handel und wessenschaft. Berlin; J. Springer, 1936. 568p. (2d ed., 1965. 570p.)

Fischer, Emil. Untersuchungen uber Aminosauren, Polypeptide und Proteine (1899–1906). Berlin; J. Springer, 1906–1923. 2 vols.

Fleischmann, Wilhelm. Lehrbuch der Milchwirtschaft. Bremen; M Heinsius Nachfolger, 1870. 483p. (5th ed., Berlin; P. Parey, 1915. 597p.)

Fracastoro, Girolamo. De Contagione et Contagiosis Morbis et Eorum Curatione, Libri III. New York and London; G. P. Putman's Sons, 1930. 356p. (In English and Latin.)

Freudenberg, Kove. Tannin, Cellulose, Lignin. 2d ed of Chemie der Naturlichen Gerbstoffe. Berlin; J. Springer, 1933. 165p.

Freundlich, Herbert. Kapillarchemie; Eine Darstellung der Chemie der Kololoide und Verwandter Gebiete. 1st ed. Leipzig; Akademische Verlagsgessellschaft, 1909. 591p. (4th ed., rev. by J. Bikerman, 1930–1932. 2 vols.)

Gamgee, Arthur. Die Physiologische Chemie der Verdauung mit Einschluss der Pathologischen Chemie. Leipzig; F. Deuticke, 1897. 524p.

Goldschmidt, Fritz. Der Wein von der Rebe bis zum Konsum. Mainz am Rhein; J. Diemer, 1900. 408p. (6th ed., 1925. 928p.)

Gorup-Besanez, E. F. von. Lehrbuch der Physiologischen Chemie. Braunschweig; F. Viewig, 1878. 902p.

Haldane, J. B. S., and Kurt G. Stern. Allgemeine Chemie der Enzyme. Dresden; T. Steinkipff, 1932. 367p.

Haller, Albrecht von. Auctarium ad Alberti Halleri Elementa Physiologiae Corporis Humani. Lausanne, Switzerland; Sumptibus Julii Henrici Pott et Socior, 1782.

Hefter, Gustav, ed. Chemie und Technologie der Fette und Fettprodukte. 2d ed. Vienna; Springer, 1936. 3 vols.

Henle, Jakob. Von den Miasmen und Kontagien und von den Miasmatisch-Kontagiosen Krankheiten (1840) Einleitung von Felix Marchand. Leipzig; J. A. Barth, 1910. 88p. (Klassiker der Medizin no. 3)

Henneberg, Wilhelm, and F. Stohmann. Beitrag zur Begrundung einer Rationellen Futterung der Weiderkauer: Praktisch-Landwirthschaftliche und Chemischphysiologische Untersuchungen. Braunschweig; C. A. Schwetschke & Sohn, 1860–1864. 2 vols.

Henning, Hans. Der Geruch. Leipzig; Barth, 1916. 533p. (2d ed., 1924. 434p.)

Hoesch, Kurt. Emil Fischer, sein Leben und sein Werk. Berlin; Verlag Chemie, 1921. 480p.

Hoppe-Seyler, Felix. Physiologische Chemie. Berlin; A. Hirschwald, 1877–1881. 4 vols.

Hutinel, Victor H. Les Maladies des Enfants. Paris; Asselin et Houzeau, 1909. 5 vols.

Jayle, Gaetan E., and Albert G. Ourgaud. La Vision Nocturne et Ses Troubles. Paris; Masson, 1950. 863p. (Eng. ed., transl. by L.F. Baisinger and W.J. Holmes, 1959. 408p.)

John, Johann F. Chemische Tabellen der Pflanzenanalysen, oder, Versuch eines systematischen Verzeichnisses der bis jezt zerlegten Fegetabilien nach den vorwaltenden naheren Bestandtheilen. Nurnberg; Johan L. Schrag, 1814. 94p.

Koller, Raphael. Salz, Rauch und Fleisch. Salzburg; Kiesel, 1941. 388p.

Konig, Franz J. Chemie der menschlichen Nahrungs- und Genussmittel. Berlin; Springer, 1882–1883. 2 vols. (Later ed., 1919–1923.)

Kroemer, Karl, and Gottfried Krumbholz. Obst- und Beerenweine; Fachbuch der Gewerbsmassigen Obst- und Beerenweinbereitung. Braunschweig; Serger & Hempel, 1932. 292p.

Lederer, Edgar. Les Carotenoides des Plantes. Paris; Hermann, 1934. 82p.

Lippmann, Edmund O. von. Die Chemie der Zuckerarten. 2d ed. Braunschweig; F. Vieweg, 1895. 1174p. (3d ed., 1904. 2 vols.)
Lombroso, Cesare. Trattato Profilattico e Clinico della Pellagra. Torino; Bocca, 1892. 410p.
Micheel, Fritz. Chemie der Zucker und Polysaccharide. Leipzig; Akademische Verlagsgesellschaft, 1939. 399p. (2d ed., 1956. 512p.)
Moleschott, Jacob. Physiologie des Stoffwechsels in Pflanzen und Thieren. Ein Handbuch fur Naturforscher, Landwrithe und Aerzte. Erlangen; F. Enke, 1851. 592p.
Monvoisin, Alexandre. Le Traitement frigorifique des Fruits et des Legumes. Paris; Dunod, 1947. 95p.
Morelli, Carlo. La Pellagra nei suoi Rapporti Medici i Sociali; Studi. Florence; Murate, 1855. 279p.
Nageli, Carl. Pflanzenphysiologische Untersuchungen. Zurich; F. Schulthess, 1855–1858. 4 vols.
Naunyn, Bernhard. Der Diabetes melitus. Vienna; Holder, 1898. 526p. (Specielle Pathologie und Therapie no. 7) (2d ed., 1910. 3 pts. in 1 vol.)
Neumeister, Richard. Lehrbuch der physiologischen Chemie, mit Berucksichtigugn der pathologischen Verhaltnisse; fur Studierende und Aerzte. Jena; Fischer, 1893. 2 vols. (Later ed., 1897. 927p.)
Noorden, Carl von. Die Zuckerkrankheit und ihre Behandlung. Berlin; A. Hirschwald, 1895. 212p.
Nothnagel, Hermann. Specielle Pathologie und Therapie. XXIV Band, II Halfte, II Abtheilung Victor Babes' Die Lepra. Vienna; Alfred Holder, 1901. 338p.
Ostwald, Carl W. W. Die Welt der vernachlassigten Dimensionen: Eine Einfuhrung in die Kolloidchemie, mit besonderer Berucksichtigung ihrer Anwendungen. Dresden and Leipzig; T. Steinkopff, 1915. 219p.
Ottavi, Ottavio. Enologia Teorico—Pratica. 12th ed. Casale Monferrato, Italy; Casa Editrice Fratelli Ottavi, 1931. 741p.
Pacottet, Paul. Vinification; Vin, Eau-de-Vie, Vinaigre. Paris; J.-B. Bailliere et Fils, 1904. 447p. (5th ed., 1926. 463p.)
Pasqualini, Rodolfo O. Stress: Enfermedades de Adaptacion; ACTH y Cortisona. Buenos Aires; El Ateneo, 1952. 618p.
Pasteur, Louis. Etudes sur le Vinaigre et sur le Vin. Paris; Masson et Cie, 1924. 519p.
Pauli, Wolfgang. Kolloidchemie der Eiweisskorper. Dresden; Steinkopff, 1920. 111p. (2d ed., 1933. 353p.)
Petren, Karl A. Uber Eiweissbeschrankung in der Behandlung des Diabetes gravis. Halle; C. Marhold, 1927. 72p.
Pfaundler, M., and A. Schlossmann. Handbuch der Kinderheilkunde: Ein Buch fur den praktischen Arzt. Leipzig; Vogel, 1906. 2 vols. (4th ed., 1931.)
Pfeffer, W. Osmotische untersuchungen. Studien zur Zellmechanik. Leipzig; W. Engelmann, 1877. 236p. (2d ed., 1921.)
Pfeffer, Wilhelm F. P. Pflanzenphysiologie. Ein Handbuch des Stoffwechsels und Draftwechsels in der Pflanze. Leipzig; W. Engelmann, 1881. 2 vols. (2d ed., 1897–1904.)
Phisalix, Marie. Animaux Venimeux et Venins: La Fonction Venimeuse chez Tous les Animaux; Les Appareils Venimeux; Les Venins et Leurs Proprietes; Les Fonctions et Usages des Venins; L'Envenimation et Son Traitement. Paris; Masson & Cie, 1922. 2 vols.

Pommer, Gustav. Untersuchungen uber Osteomalacie und Rachitis, nebst Beitragen zur Kenntniss der Knochenresorption und -Apposition in verschiedenen altersperioden und der durchbohrneden Gefasse. Leipzig; Vogel, 1885. 506p.

Porcher, Charles. La Methode Synthetique dans l'Etude du Lait: Le Lait au Point de Vue colloidal; Recherches sur le Mecanisme de l'Action de la Presure. Lyon; Le Lait, 1929. 530p.

Regnard, Paul. Recherches Experimentales sur les Variations Pathologiques des Combustions Respiratoires. Paris; Delahaye, 1879. 394p.

Ritthausen, Heinrich. Die Eiweisskorper der Getreidearten, Helsenfruchte und Olsamen: Beitrage zur Physiologie der Samen der Culturgewachse, der Nahrungs- und Futtermittel. Bonn; M. Cohen, 1872. 252p.

Roll, M. F. Lehrbuch der Pathologie und Therapie der nutzbaren Hausthiere. Vienna: L. W. Seidel, 1856. 680p.

Rolle, M. F. Lehrbuch der Pathologie und Therapie der Hausthiere. 3d ed. Vienna; W. Braumuller, 1867. 2 vols.

Roussel, Theophile. Traite de la Pellagre et des Pseudo-Pellagres. Paris; J. B. Bailliere, 1866. 656p.

Rubner, Max. Die Gesetze des Energieverbrauchs bei der Ernahrung. Leipzig; F. Deuticke, 1902. 426p. (Nutrition Foundations' reprint of The Laws of Energy Consumption in Nutrition . . . transl. by Allan Markoff and Alex Sandri- White, edited by Robert J. T. Joy. New York; Academic Press, 1982. 371p.)

Salm-Horstmar, Wilhelm F. K. A. Versuche und Resultate uber die Nahrung der Pflanzen . . . Braunschweig; F. Vieweg, 1856. 39p.

Sannino, F. Antonio. Tratado de Enologia. Barcelona; G. Gili, 1925. 920p. (2d ed., Buenos Aires; G. Gili, 1948.)

Scheunert, Arthur. Der Vitamingehalt der deutschen Nahrungsmittel. Berlin; J. Springer, 1929–1930. 2 vols.

Schmidt, Karl S. Charakteristik der Epidemischen Cholera Gegenuber Verwandten Transsudationsanomalieen. Leipzig; Reyher, 1850. 168p.

Speck, Carl. Physiologie des Menschlichen Athmens nach eigenen Untersuchungen dargestellt. Leipzig; Vogel, 1892. 262p.

Stelling-Dekker, Nellie M. Die Sporogenen Hefen. Amsterdam; Drukkerig Holland, 1931. 546p.

Stepp, Wilhelm O. et al. Die Vitamine und ihre klinische Anwendung. 2d ed. Stuttgart; Enke, 1937. 189p. (6th ed., 1944. 480p.)

Stohmann, Friedrich C. A. Die Milch- und Molkereiproducte: Ein Handbuch fur Milchtechniker und Nahrungsmitelchemiker. Braunschweig; Friedrich Vieweg und Sohn, 1898. 1031p.

Sucharipa, Rudolf. Die Pektinstoffe; Eine Leicht Fassliche Darstellung der Bisherigen Wissenschaftlichen Arbeiten und der Such Daraus fur den Praktiker Ergebenden Winke. Braunschweig; Serger & Hempel, 1925. 188p. (2d ed., 1937. 404p.)

Tiedemann, Friedrich. Physiologie des Menschen. Darmstadt; Leske, 1830–1836. 2 vols.

Tollens, Bernhard C. Kurzes Handbuch der Kohlenhydrate. Breslau; Tresendt, 1895–1898. 2 vols. (4th ed., Leipzig; J. A. Barth, 1935. 627p.)

Tuczek, Franz. Klinische und anatomische Studien uber die Pellagra. Berlin; Fischer, 1893. 113p.

Ulzer, Ferdinand. Allgemeine und Physiologische Chemie der Fette fur Chemiker, Mediziner und Industrielle. Berlin; J. Springer, 1906. 317p.

Ventre, Jules. Traite de Vinificaiton Pratique et Rationnelle. Montpellier; Coulet, 1930–1932. 3 vols. (3d ed., 1946.)

Willstatter, Richard M., and Arthur Stoll. Untersuchungen uber Chlorophyll; Methoden und Ergebnisse. Berlin; J. Springer, 1913. 424p.

Ziemssen, Hugo von. Handbuch der speciellen Pathologie und Therapie. Leipzig; Vogel, 1882. 9 vols. Zwaardemaker, Hendrik. Die Physiologie des Geruchs. Leipzig; W. Engelmann, 1895. 324p. (Translated into French, 1925.)

D. Identification of Scholarly Journals

A list of scholarly journal titles was developed from the citation analysis of the source documents previously described. Each time a journal title was cited a tally was made and the year of publication noted. These titles denote the primary scholarly journals prior to 1950 and are potential candidates for preservation. Average and median half-lives were also determined.

A total of 990 titles were represented in the 8,067 journal citations analyzed. Of these 990 titles, 632 or 63.8% were cited only once or twice, and another 15.9% were cited three to five times, illustrating the scattering of the literature (Table 8.3).

Table 8.3. Cited scholarly journal titles

Times cited	Number of titles	Percentage
1	506	51.1
2	126	12.7
3–5	157	15.9
6–20	136	13.7
21–50	38	3.8
51–100	11	1.1
Over 100	16	1.6
Total	990	99.9

Only half of these titles were published in the United States; foreign language titles made a heavy showing of 37.9% of all titles. Titles from Germany accounted for 17% of all titles in the list, demonstrating early reliance on German food chemistry. Abstracting publications were often cited and counted for 0.2% of all titles. Only English-language titles are included in the list of scholarly journals that have top priority for preservation (Table 8.4). Eight additional European titles ranked equally high and are worthly of preservation, given here in order of importance:

Table 8.4. Core scholarly journals

Journal	Microfilmed[a]
American Journal of Physiology	UMI
American Journal of Public Health	UMI
American Miller	—
American Society of Bakery Engineers, Proceeding & Annual Meeting	—
American Society of Horticultural Science, Proceeding	—
Archives of Internal Medicine	UMI
Baker's Digest	—
Biochemical Journal	UMI
Canner	UMI
Canning Age	UMI
Cereal Chemistry	UMI
Food Industry	—
Food Technology (Chicago)	UMI
Fruit Products Journal	—
Industrial and Engineering Chemistry	—
Institute of Food Technologist, Proceeding	—
JAMA; Journal of the American Medical Association	UMI
Journal of Agricultural Research	UMI
Journal of Bacteriology	UMI
Journal of Biological Chemistry	UMI
Journal of Dairy Science	UMI
Journal of Experimental Medicine	UMI
Journal of Infectious Diseases	UMI
Journal of Nutrition	UMI
Journal of Physiology	UMI
Journal of the American Chemical Society	UMI
Journal of the Association of Official Agricultural Chemists	DATAMATICS
Journal of the Society of Chemical Industry	PR
Lancet	UMI
Nature	UMI
Oil and Soap	UMI
Philosophical Magazine	UMI
Plant Physiology	UMI
Proceedings of the Society of Experimental Biology and Medicine	—
Science	UMI
Soap	UMI
U S Public Health Report	—
Western Canner and Packer	—

[a]UMI = University Microfilm, Inc.; PR = Princeton Microfilm.

Zeitschrift fur Physiologische Chemie and Hopp-Seyler's Zeitschrift fur Physiologische Chemie. Strassburg: Verlag von Karl J. Trubner, 1877–1984.

Biochemische Zeitschrift (superseded by *European Journal of Biochemistry*). Berlin: J. Springer, 1906–1967.

Comptes Rendus Hebdomadaires des Seances de l'Academie des Sciences. Paris: Academie des Sciences, 1835–1965.
Berichte. Koniglich Preussische Akademie der Wissenschaften zu Berlin. Berlin: Akademie der Wissenschaften, 1836–1855.
Annales de Chimie et de Physique. Paris: Masson, 1789–1913.
Zeitschrift fur Untersuchung der Lebensmittel. Berlin: J. Springer, 1926–1943.
Zeitschrift fur Biologie. Munich: J. F. Lehmann, 1865–1971.

All of these titles have been preserved in microfilm.

Thirty-eight titles were found statistically valid to constitute the core scholarly journals in Table 8.4. Each is important for historical preservation.

The top-ranked journals were also ranked within food science and human nutrition as determined by the subject of the source documents. Their rankings are given in Table 8.5. Three titles appear on both lists: the *Journal of Biological Chemistry*, *Biochemical Journal*, and the *Journal of the American Chemical Society*.

Table 8.5. Top-ranked scholarly journals

Food science	Rank	Human nutrition
Journal of Biological Chemistry	1	Journal of Biological Chemistry
Cereal Chemistry	2	Biochemical Journal
Industrial and Engineering Chemistry	3	JAMA; Journal of the American Medical Association
Food Industry	4	Journal of Nutrition
Journal of the American Chemical Society	5	Journal of the American Chemical Society
Biochemical Journal	6	American Journal of Physiology
Food Research	7	Journal of Physiology
Fruit Products Journal	8	Lancet
Journal of Agricultural Research	9	Proceedings of the Society of Experimental Biological Medicine
Journal of Dairy Science	10	Nature

An analysis of 2,732 articles published in the *Journal of Nutrition* in 1945 and 1946 showed that only forty-eight different serial titles were cited more than five times.[22] Of these, twenty-one were classified in the field of medicine, six in agriculture, five in biochemistry, and four in nutrition, although the greatest number of citations per title were in nutrition. The top five titles accounted for 50.5% of the citations. These titles were: *Journal of Nutrition*, *Journal of Biological Chemistry*, *Proceedings of the Society*

22. James G. Hodgson, "The Use of Periodicals in a Special Field: Nutrition," *Library Bulletin* 19 (1948); mimeographed, 6p..

for Experimental Biology and Medicine, *Biochemical Journal*, and *American Journal of Physiology*, all of which are in the top ten human nutrition titles in the present study (see Table 8.5).

The median half-life for journals was 14.8 years for the combined subjects. For works that concerned food science, the half-life was 8.9, while for human nutrition it was 22.5. There was a considerable range in the half-life for the publications. In food science the range was from 3.7 to 13.2, and in human nutrition from 2.5 to 37.6.

E. Identification of Trade or Popular Periodicals

The citation analysis method does not identify non-scientific publications used by practitioners or commercial firms, the "popular" periodicals. Other means had to be used to identify these titles and establish their relative merit for preservation. The journal lists, library catalogs and historical catalogs, and writings which served as sources for popular titles are listed below. Criteria were established with the highest preference for preservation: early age of a title, length of a run, and national or international influence. Selected titles were omitted from the final list, such as those for hotel or restaurant service, works written for union workers, and those for the liquor industry. The list of selected titles was ranked. A rank of one was given to periodicals with primary preservation priority, which included periodicals published for more than twenty years, those of national and international importance, and those beginning before 1900. A rank of two was given to periodicals worthy of preservation but of lesser importance.

The list was reviewed by N. N. Potter of Cornell University and by Z. Holmes of Oregon State University, each of whom has extensive knowledge of the history of their disciplines.

Historically Important Popular and Trade Periodicals in Food Science and Human Nutrition, 1850–1950 (N=356)

Not all changes of names and cessations have been noted, particularly those after 1950.

Rank

1 American Baker. Minneapolis; v.1– 1942–.
1 American Bakers' Association, Bulletin. Chicago; no.1– 1928–.
2 American Bakers' Association, Bulletin . . . Cake and Retail. Chicago; no.1–23, 1929–1932//.

Rank

1 American Bakers' Association, Monthly Bulletin. Chicago; v.1– 1936/37–.

2 American Beverage and Food Journal. Cincinnati, Ohio; v.1–9, 1906–1910//. Began as Bar and Buffet. (1906–1909).

1 American Brewer. New York; 1868–1969//. Also German edition with title "Amerikanische bierbrauher".

2 American Brewers' Gazette and Malt and Hop Trades' Review. New York; U.S. Brewers' Association, v.1– 4, 1871–1874//? Merged with Brewers' Journal and Barley, Malt and Hops Trades' Reports.

1 American Brewers' Review. Chicago; v.1–53, no.1, 1884–1939//. Began as American Brewers Review and Beverage Bulletin (1887–1918).

1 American Brewing Institute, Transactions. New York; v.1–5, 1901–1910//.

1 American Cookery. Boston, etc.; v.1–52, no.9, 1896–1947//. Began as Boston Cooking School Magazine (1896–1913). Merged with Practical Home Economics.

1 American Food Journal. Chicago; v.1–23, no.2, 1906–1928//. Merged with the Home Economist.

2 American Ginner and Cotton Oil Miller. Little Rock, Ark.; v.1–15, no.6, 1924–1938//. Began as Arkansas Ginner (1924–1925), 1925–1927 as American Cotton Ginner. Merged with Cotton and Cotton Oil Press.

1 American Home Economics Association, Bulletin. Baltimore. Md.; v.1–24, 1912–1942//. Suspended 1917– 1918; 1921–1925. Continued in Journal of Home Economics.

1 American Independent Baker and the Retail Baker. New York; 1909–. Began as Retail Baker.

2 American Institute of Food Distribution, Inc. Washington Food Report. New York; v.1– 1933–. Began as Washington Service Letter (1933–1941).

1 American Institute of Food Distribution, Inc. Weekly Digest. no.500, 1941, v.27, no.12– 1941–.

2 American Kosher Butcher Weekly. New York; American Federation of Retail Kosher Butchers, Inc., v.1–3, 1938–1941//.

2 American Meat Institute, Bulletin. Chicago; Dept. of Nutrition, v.1–3, 1922–1928//.

1 American Meat Trade and Retail Butchers' Journal. New York; v.1–23, 1898?-1920//. Merged with Butchers' Advocate.

1 American Miller. Prospect Heights, Ill.; v.1– 1873–1968//. Also known as American Miller and Processor. Began as American Miller (1873–1930, 1935–1943), 1930–1931 National Miller and American Miller, 1931–1934 as National and American Miller. Continued as American Miller and Processor.

2 American Pure Food and Health Journal. v.1–3, 1909–1911//. Began as American Pure Food and Drug Journal.

2 American Society of Bakery Engineers Bakery Engineers Information Service, E.I.S. no.1– 1936–.

2 American Society of Bakery Engineers, Bulletin. v.1– 1924–.

2 American Society of Bakery Engineers, Proceedings. v.2– 1925–. Vol. 1 never published.

1 American Society of Brewing Chemists, Proceedings, Annual Meeting. Madison,

Ranking

	Wis.; v.3– 1940–1975//. Vols. 1–2 never published. Continued as the Journal of the American Society of Brewing Chemists.
2	American Society of Brewing Technology, Journal. Chicago; v.1–8, 1910–1918//.
1	American Soft Drink Journal. Atlanta, Ga.; v.1– 1905–. Began as Southern Carbonator and Bottler (1905–1925), 1925–1930 as Carbonator and Bottler, 1930–1945 as National Carbonator and Bottler, 1945–1949 as American Carbonator and Bottler, 1950–1955 as American Bottler.
2	American Sugar Bulletin. New York; v.1–9, 1916–1924//. Began as Willett's Sugar Bulletin.
1	American Wine Press (and Mineral Water News). New York; v.1–42, 1897–1918//.
2	Anti-Adulteration Journal. Williamsport, Penn.; American Society for Prevention of Adulteration of Food, v.1–7, 1885–1891//. Began as Universal Benefactor (1885–1886), continued as Anti-Adulteration Journal, Universal Benefactor (1886–1891).
2	Armour Magazine. Chicago.
1	Associated Food Dealer. Chicago Ill.; Associated Food Retailers of Illinois, v.1– 1937–. Began as Associated Food Dealer (1937–1953). Continued as Associated Food Retailer (1954–1962). Continues as Illinois Food Retailer.
1	Bakers' and Confectioners' Journal. Chicago; Bakery and Confectionery Workers' International Union of America, v.1– 1888–. Also known as Bakers' Journal.
1	Bakers Digest. Chicago; Siebel Institute of Technology, v.1– 1926–. Began as Siebel Technical Review (1926–1936); 1936–1939 as Bakers Technical Digest.
1	Bakers' Journal. Toronto; v.1– 1938–.
1	Bakers Letter. Chicago; no.1– 1942–.
1	Bakers Review. New York; v.1– 1898–.
1	Bakers Weekly. New York; v.1– 1904–1969//. Merged with Bakery Production and Marketing.
1	Bakery Management. Chicago; v.1– 1922–.
2	Bakery Sales Association, Proceedings. v.1–?, 1932–?. Began as Bakery Sales Promotion Association.
1	Barrel and Box and Packages. Louisville, Kent. and Chicago; v.1– 1895–. Began as Barrel and Box (1895–1929).
1	Bakers' Helper. Chicago; v.1– 1887–. Continues as Baking Industry, 1952–.
2	Baking Technology. Chicago; American Bakers' Association, v.1–6, 1922–1927//. Superseded by American Bakers' Association, Journal.
1	Better Nutrition. v.1– 1938–.
2	Beverage Industry News. San Francisco; v.1– 1935–. Began as Liquor Industry News.
1	Beverage News. New York; v.1–34, 1918–1935//. Supersedes American Wine Press and Mineral Water News. Merged with Beverage Retailer and Wholesaler.
1	Biscuit and Cracker Baker. New York; 1912–. Began as Cracker Baker (1912–1949).
1	Bonfort's Circular. New York; v.1–89, 1871–1919//.
1	Borden Review of Nutrition Research. New York;[Columbus, Ohio?], v.1–31, 1940–1971//.

Ranking

1 Bottling Industry. New York; v.1– 1946–.
2 Bread and Butter. New York; v.1–7, 1941–1947//. Merged with Consumer Reports.
1 Brewer and Maltster and Beverageur. Chicago; v.1–9, 1882–1937//. Merged with Brewers Journal.
1 Brewers Bulletin. Chicago; v.1– 1907–.
1 Brewers Digest. Chicago and Beloit, Wis.; v.9– 1934–. Continues in part Siebel Technical Review. 1934–1937 as Brewers Technical Review.
1 Brewers Journal. Chicago and Philadelphia; v.1–116, 1876–1960//. Began as Western Brewer (1876–1920), 1920–1932 as Beverage Journal.
1 Brewers' Journal and Barley, Malt and Hop Trades' Reporter, and American Brewers' Gazette, Consolidated. New York; v.1–47, 1876–1922//. Began as German and American Brewers' Journal (1876–1921).
2 Brewers News. New York; v.1–11, 1932–1938//. Merged with Brewers Journal.
2 Brewery Age. Chicago; v.1–8, 1933–1940//. Merged with Modern Brewer to form Modern Brewery Age.
1 Brewery, Flour, Cereal, Malt, Yeast, Soft Drink and Distillery Worker. Cincinnati, Ohio, etc.; International Union of United Brewery, Flour, Cereal, Soft Drink and Distillery Workers of America, v.1– 1886–. Began as Brauer-zeitung (1886–1910), 1910–1917 as Brauerei-arbeiter-zeitung, 1918–1934 as Brewery, Flour, Cereal and Soft Drink Workers' Journal, 1934–1949 as Brewery Worker.
2 Brewing Chemists' News Letter. New York; American Society of Brewing Chemists, v.1– , 1940–1966. Continued as American Society of Brewing Chemists Newsletter.
1 California Citrograph: the Magazine of the Citrus Industry. Los Angeles; v.1–54, 1915–1969//. Continued as Citrograph.
1 California Fruit and Trucker's Journal. 1896–.
1 Canadian Baker. Toronto, etc.; v.1– 1888–. Began as Canadian Baker and Confectioner (1888–1922), 1922–1942? as Canadian Baker and Soda Fountain Dispenser.
1 Canadian Beverage Review. Toronto; v.1– 1930–.
1 Canadian Food Industries. Gardenvale, Quebec; v.1–42, 1930–1971?. Began as Canadian Canner and Preserver (1930–1931), 1932–1936 as Canadian Canner and Food Manufacturer, 1937–1947 as Canadian Food Packer. Merged with Food in Canada.
1 Canadian Grain Journal, Miller and Processor. Winnipeg, Canada; v.1– 1945–.
2 Canadian Home Economics Newsletter. Winnipeg, Canada; v.1– 1943–. Supersedes the Associations News Letter.
2 Canadian Miller and Cerealist. Montreal, Canada; v.1–8, 1909–1916//.
2 Candy. Chicago; v.1–8, 1921–1928//. Began as Candy Factory (1921–1925). Merged with Confectioners' Weekly Gazette, later Candy (N.Y.).
1 Candy. New York; v.1–50, 1881–1930//?. Began as Confectioners' and Bakers' Gazette (1881–1913), 1913–1926 as Confectioners' Gazette. Also known as Confectioners' Weekly Gazette, Candy Gazette, and Candy Weekly.
2 Candy. Toronto; v.1–5, 1922–1926//?.
1 Candy and Ice Cream Retailer. Chicago; v.1–38, 1889–1927//. Merged with Candy Factory-jobber, later Candy.

Ranking

2 Candy Industry. New York. N.Y.; v.1–25, 1944–1956//. Merged with Confectioners Journal to form Candy Industry and Confectioner's Journal.
2 Candy Jobber. Chicago; v.1–5, 1921–1925//. Merged with Candy Factory to form Candy Factory-Jobber, later Candy (Chicago).
1 Candy Merchandising. Chicago; v.1– 1937–.
1 Canner/Packer. Louisville, Kent., etc.; v.1– 1895–. Began as Canner and Dried Fruit Packer (1895–1915), 1916–1955 as Canner, 1955–1958 as Canner and Freezer.
1 Canning Trade, the Canned Food Authority of the World. Baltimore; v.1– 1878–. Also known as Trade in 1904 and Canned Goods Trade, 1904–1912.
2 Canners' Market Report. New York; American Institute of Food Distribution.
2 Carolina Fruit and Truckers' Journal. Wilmington, N.C.; v.1– 1886–. Began as Carolina Fruit and Truck Grower's Journal.
1 Chain Store Age. New York; v.1– 1925–.
2 Chain Store Management. Los Angeles; v.1–13, 1925–1937//. Began as Chain Store Manager (1925–1930).
2 Chain Store Merchandise. New York; v.1–6, 1928–1932//. Began as Food Chain Store Merchandising (1928–1929).
2 Chain Store Progress. New York; National Chain Store Association, v.1–3, 1929–1931//.
2 Chef and Steward. Chicago; v.1–29, 1891–1920//?.
1 Citrus Industry. Florida; 1920–.
2 Citrus Leaves. Redlands and Los Angeles; Mutual Orange Distributors, v.1– 1921–.
1 Coffee and Tea Digest. New York; v.1– 1930–.
1 Coffee and Tea Industries and the Flavor Field. New York; v.1– 1878–. Also known as Spice Mill, 1921– 1949 and Simmons Spice Mill, 1913–1920.
2 Colhecon (AHEA). Washington, D.C.; v.1–6, 1945–1951//.
1 Commercial Review. Portland, Ore.; v.1– 1889–.
2 Confectioner. Milwaukee, Wis.; v.1– 1916–. Began as Northwestern Confectioner (1916–1940).
1 Confectioner and Baker. Chicago; v.1–39, 1879–1913//. Began as Western Confectioner and Baker (1879–1880?).
1 Confectioners Journal for Candy Manufacturers. Philadelphia; v.1–82, 1874–1956//. Merged with Candy Industry to form Candy Industry and Confectioner's Journal.
2 Confectioners News. Philadelphia; v.1– 1935–.
2 Confectioners' Review. Cincinnati, Ohio; v.1– 1902–.
1 Confectionery, Biscuit and Chocolate Journal. Toronto; v.1– 1927–.
1 Confectionery and Ice Cream World. New York; v.1– 1929–.
2 Confectionery Studies. Chicago; National Confectioners' Association, v.1–3, 1930–1934//?.
1 Consumer Packaging. Chicago; v.1– 1938–. Supersedes Packaging Digest. Began as Packaging Parade (1938–1959).
2 Cooking for Profit. Madison, Wis.
2 Cooking Club Magazine. Goshen, Ind.; v.1–19, 1895–1917//?.

Ranking

1 Corn Miller; Devoted to Corn, Rye, Oat Milling, etc. Indianapolis, Ind.; v.1–9, 1885–1892//?.
1 Culinary Review. New York; American Culinary Federation, v.1– 1932–.
1 Detaillant, Le; en Produits Alimentaires. Montreal, Canada; v.1– 1927–.
1 Diet; Rejuvenation. Chicago; v.1– 1934–.
2 Diet and Health Digest. San Francisco; v.1– 1937–. Began as Diet Digest.
2 Diet for Health and Happiness. Tujunga, Calif.; v.1– 1934–.
1 Dietetic and Hygienic Gazette. New York; v.1–30, 1886–1914//. Began as Journal of Reconstructives, Dietetics and Alimentation. 1888–1891 as Dietetic Gazette. Merged with Medicopharmaceutical Critic and Guide.
2 Dietary Administration and Therapy. Cleveland, Ohio; v.1–5; 1923–1927//.
1 Distributor. New York; Associated Grocery Manufacturers of America, v.1– 1928–.
1 Dixie Miller; A Monthly Journal Devoted to Milling, Flour and Grain. Atlanta, Ga., etc.; v.1–62, 1892–1924//. Merged with Miller's Review to form Miller's Review and Dixie Miller.
1 Epicure. Boston; v.1– 1887–.
1 Evaporator (Dried Fruits). Webster, N.Y.; N.Y. State Evap. Association, v.1– 1908–.
1 Everyday Housekeeping, A Magazine for Practical Housekeepers and Mothers. Boston; v.1–24, 1894–1908//. Began as New England Kitchen Magazine (1894–1895), 1895–1903 as American Kitchen Magazine, 1903–1905 as Home Science Magazine, 1905–1906 as Modern Housekeeping.
2 Executive Service on Food Distribution. New York; American Institute of Food Distribution, v.1–5, 1928– 1932; no.117–301, 1932–1941//. Began as Facts in Food Distribution (1928–1934), 1934–1935 as Food Distribution.
2 Executive Service on Food Markets. New York; American Institute of Food Distribution, v.1–5, 1928–1932; no.117–302, 1932–1941//. Began as Facts in the Food Markets (1928–1934), 1934–1935 as Food Markets.
2 Facts and Figures; An Authoritative Food Trade Magazine. Jacksonville, Fla., Washington, D.C.; National American Wholesale Grocers Association, v.1–21, 1915–1935//. Began as Association Bulletin.
2 Family Grocer Meat Dealer Magazine.
1 Fast Food. New York; v.1– 1902–. Began as Soda Fountain (1902–1932), 1933–1940 as Soda Fountain Magazine, 1941–43 as Soda Fountain Service, 1945–1951 as Fountain Service, 1951–1956 as Fountain and Fast Food.
2 Flavoring Extract Journal. New York; v.1–4, 1929–1931//. Continues Flavoring Extracts section in Spice Mill 1910–1930. Continued as Flavors section in Spice Mill.
1 Flour and Feed; Devoted to the Interests of Flour and Feed Stores. Milwaukee, Wis.; v.1–57 1900–1956. Continues as Feed Bag.
2 Flour and Grain World. Seattle. v.1–11, 1916–1926//. Began as Flour and Grain, then Flour and Grain Critic.
2 Flour Trade News; Hay, Grain and Feed. New York; v.1–10, 1902–1907//. Merged with American Hay, Four and Food Journal, later Feedingstuffs.
1 Food Engineering. Randor, Pa.; v. 1–49, 1928–1977//. Began as Food Industries,

Ranking

v. 1–23, 1928–1951. Continued by Chilton's Food Engineering.

1 Food Facts. Chicago; Wheat Flour Institute, v.1– 1930–.

2 Food Facts. Los Angeles; v.1–4, 1926–1928//. Began as Western Dietitian. Merged with Western Hospital and Nurses Review.

1 Food Field Reporter. New York; v.1– 1932–19652.

2 Food Forum. Chicago; v.1– 1944–.

2 Food Freezing. New York; v.1–3, 1945–1948//. Merged with Quick Frozen Foods and the Locker Plant.

1 Food, Home and Garden. Philadelphia; Vegetarian Society of America, v.1–7, 1889–1895; nsv.1–4, 1896–1900//. Merged with Vegetarian Magazine.

2 Food in Canada. Toronto; v.1– 1941–.

2 Food Law Bulletin. Chicago; v.1–13, 1906–1918//. Merged with American Food Journal.

2 Food Materials and Equipment. New York; v.1–8, 1941–1948//.

1 Food Merchants' Advocate. New York; v.1–61, 1877–1930; no.2617–3017, 1930–1935; nsv.55– 1940–. Began as Retail Grocers' Advocate (1877–1935).

2 Food News and Food Magazine.

2 Food Packer. Pontiac, Ill.; v.1–39, 1920–1958//. 1922–1943 as Canning Age, 1943 as Food Packer and Canning Age. Merged with Canner/Packer.

2 Food Processing. Chicago; v.1– 1940/1941–. Began as Food Equipment Preview (1940/1941–1943), 1943– 1947 as Food Preview, 1947–1949 as Food Processing Preview.

1 Food and Drink; The Pure Food Advocate. New York; v.1–12, 1899–1907//.

1 Food and Nutrition News. Chicago; Chicago National Livestock and Meat Board, v.1– 1930–.

1 Food Retailing Magazine. Chicago; v.1– 1808–. Began as Butchers' and Packers Gazette (1808–1935), 1935–1939 as Meat Dealer and Butchers' and Packers' Gazette, 1939–1941 as Meat Dealer and Butchers Gazette, 1941–1945 as Food Retailing and Butchers' Gazette.

2 Food Service News. Madison, Wis.; v.1– 1939–.

2 Food Topics; A Monthly Magazine for the Housekeeper. Milwaukee, Wis.; v.1–3, 1903–1905//?.

2 Foods for Health and Enjoyment. New York; v.1– 1941—.

1 Forecast for Home Economists. New York and Philadelphia; v.1– 1910–. Began as Forecast; America's Pure Food Champion (1910–1939).

2 Freezing and Cold Storage. Toronto and Gardenvale, Quebec, Canada; v.1–12, 1946–1957//. Began as Locker Plants and Frosted Foods (1946–1953).

2 Fresh Fruit and Vegetable Merchandising. Los Angeles; National League of Wholesale Fresh Fruit and Vegetable Distributors, v.1–4, 1947–1951//?.

2 Frozen Food Industry and Locker Plant Journal. New York; v.1–4, 1945–1948//. Merged with Quick Frozen Foods and the Locker Plant.

2 Frozen Food Merchandiser. San Francisco; v.1– 1941–.

1 Fruit Products Journal and American Food Manufacturer. New York; v.1–29, 1921–1950//?. Began as American Vinegar Industry (1921–1922), 1922–1923 as American Vinegar Industry and Fruit Products Journal, 1923–1943 as Fruit Products Journal and American Vinegar Industry.

Ranking

1 Fruit Trade Journal and Produce Record. New York; National League of Wholesale Fresh Fruit and Vegetable Distributors, v.1–87, 1888–1933//.

2 Glass Packer. New York; v.1–4, 1928–1931; v.10, 1931–. Merged with Glass Container and continued its numbering.

1 Good Food Magazine. New York; v.1– 1937–. Began as Home and Food (1937–1944).

1 Good Health. Battle Creek, Mich.; v.1– 1866–. Began as Health Reformer (1866–1878), 1879–1912 as Good Health, 1912–1914 as Good Health Magazine.

2 Good Health. Chicago; v.1–8 1910–1917//?.

1 Good Health. Boston; v.1–4, 1869–1872//.

1 Grocer-Graphic. New York; v.1– 1937–.

2 Groceries; Chain Store Review. New York; v.1–13, 1926–1939//?. Began as Groceries, A National Publication for the Wholesale Grocer (1926–1932).

2 Grocers' Association News. Columbus, Ohio; v.1–29, 1910–1939//.

1 Grocers' Criterion; A Journal of Trade for the Wholesaler and Retailer. Chicago; Retail Grocers' and Butchers' Association, v.1–39, 1873–1912//.

1 Grocers' Magazine. Boston; v.1–49, 1900–1935; yr.36–38, 1936–1938//?.

2 Grocers' Register. Seattle; v.1–47, 1892–1917//. Began as Trade Register (1892–1916).

1 Grocers' Regulator. Chicago; v.1–12, 1886–1898//?.

1 Grocers' Review. Philadelphia; Retail Grocers' Association, v.1–36, 1891–1927//.

2 Grocers' Spotlight. Detroit, Mich.; v.1– 1933–.

2 Health Bulletin. Guthrie, Okla.

2 Homemaker Combined with Better Cooking. New York; Institute for Better Cooking, v.1–9, 1941–1946//. Began as Better Cooking and Homemaking (1941–1943).

2 Ideal Grocer. New York; v.1–9, 1910–1918//?.

1 Independent Grocergram. Chicago; v.1– 1926–. Continued as IGA Grocergram, 1950–.

2 Inland Grocer and Butcher. Cleveland, Ohio; v.1–33, 1901–1914//. Began as Inland Grocer (1901–1910).

2 Inland Merchant. Chicago and New York; v.1–35, 1910–1928//?. Began as Inland Storekeeper (1910–1920). Merged with Notion and Novelty Review.

2 Inland Miller. Louisville, Kent.; v.1–8, 1923–1927//?.

1 International Confectioner. New York; v.1– 1892–.

2 Interstate Merchant. St. Louis; v.1– 1889–. Vol. 1–47 as Interstate Grocer.

2 Iowa Food Dealer. Cedar Rapids; Iowa Retail Grocers and Meat Dealer Association, v.1– 1932–.

1 Jewish Food Merchant. Chicago; v.1– 1933–. Yiddish Title: Idisher Shpeiz Soher.

1 Journal of Home Economics. Baltimore; American Home Economics Association, 1909–. Supersedes Lake Placid Conference on Home Economics, Quarterly Bulletin.

2 Journal of Living. New York; v.1– 1935–. Continued as Journal of Lifetime Living, 1955–.

Ranking

1 Journal of Practical Medicine. Lowell, Mass. and New York; v.1–11, 1892–1900//. Began as Food, A Journal of Hygiene and Nutrition (1892–?).
1 Kansas City Packer. 1883–1899.
1 Kosher Butcher News. New York; Federation of Kosher Butchers of Greater New York, v.1– 1914–.
1 Lake Placid Conference on Home Economics, Lake Placid, N.Y., Proceedings. Lake Placid, N.Y.; v.1–10, 1899–1908//.
1 Macaroni Journal. Minneapolis; National Macaroni Manufacturers Association, v.1– 1919–. Supersedes Macaroni and Noodle Manufacturers Journal. Began as New Macaroni Journal (1919–1923).
2 Macaroni and Noodle Manufacturers Journal. Cleveland, Ohio; National Macaroni Manufacturers Association, 1903–1919//. Superseded by New Macaroni Journal.
2 Machinery and Supply Bulletin for Millers and Grain Dealers. Olathe, Kans.; v.1–18, 1902–1919; nsv.4– 1920–. Also know as: Southwestern Grain and Flour Journal; Southwestern Journal of Grain, Flour and Coal; Southwestern Journal of Grain-Flour; 1919–1922 as Western Grain Journal.
2 Martha Logan's Food News and Views, Bulletin.
2 Master Brewers' Association of America, Annual Convention, Technical Proceedings. Technical Proceedings prior to 1944 as Proceedings.
2 Master Brewers' Association of America, Communications.
1 Meat Merchandising. St. Louis, Mo.; v.1– 1925–. 1952–1953 as Meat, Fresh and Frozen Food Merchandising, 1953–1958 as Meat and Food Merchandising. Continues as Food Merchandising.
1 Meat; The Idea Magazine for Meat Packers and Related Manufacturers. Chicago; v.1– 1934–.
2 Merchant's Journal, Topeka, Kans.; v.1–38, 1891–1935//. Merged with Interstate Grocer (St. Louis).
2 Merchant's Journal and Commerce. Richmond and Raleigh, Va.; v.1–36, 1904–1928//?.
1 Merchants' Review. New York; v.1–58, 1879–1908//?.
1 Mida's Criterion. Chicago; v.1–52, 1885–1941//. Merged with American Wine and Liquor Journal.
2 Mid Continent Bottler. Kansas City, Mo.
2 Milk and Food Sanitation. Albany, N.Y.; International Association of Milk and Food Sanitarians, v.1– 1948–.
1 Milk Industry Foundation, Proceedings.; v.1– 1909–. Also known as Association Bulletin, 1938–1946.
2 Milk Market Bulletin. Indianapolis, Ind.; 1936–.
2 Milk Market News. Hampshire, Ill.; Chicago Milk Producers Council, v.1– 1941–.
1 Millers' Journal and Flour and Grain Reporter. New York; v.1–24, ?-1886//.
1 Millers' Journal and Hydraulic Engineer. New York; v.1–9, ?-1876//?.
2 Millers' National Federation, Report.
1 Millers' Review and Feed Forum. Philadelphia; New York; v.1–43, 1882–1924; v.86–98, 1924–1934//. Absorbed Dixie Miller and assumed its numbering. Merged with National and American Miller.
1 Milling. Indianapolis, Ind.; Chicago; nsv.1–8, 1892–1896//?.

Ranking

1 Milling and Feed. Montreal, Canada; v.1– 1920–. Began as Canadian Milling and Feed Journal (1920–1944).

1 Milling and Grain News. Omaha, Nebr.; v.1–42, 1902–1923//?. Began as Spring Wheat Milling News (1920–?).

1 Milling Engineer. Milwaukee, Wis.; v.1–2, nsv.1–4, v.6, 1884–1889//. Began as Millwright and Engineer (1884–1885). Absorbed Miller and Manufacturer, 1885, and adopted its numbering 1889. Merged with United States Miller.

1 Milling Journal and Corn Exchange Review. New York; v.1–3, 1869–1871//?.

2 Milling Production; Issued Monthly by the Publishers of the Northwestern Miller. Minneapolis; v.4– 1939–. Volumes 1–3 as Production Number of Northwestern Miller.

1 Milling World and Chronicle of the Grain and Flour Trade. Buffalo, N.Y.; v.1–38, 1879–1898//.

1 Millstone. Indianapolis, Ind.; v.1–17, 1875–1892//.

2 Minnesota Food Guide. Minneapolis; v.1– 1928–. Began as Grocers Commercial Bulletin and Meat Dealers News (1928–1950). Formerly issued as part of Northwest Commercial Bulletin.

1 Modern Brewery Age. St. Louis, Mo.; New York; Chicago; v.1– 1923–. Began as Brewer's Art (1923–1932), 1933–1935 as Modern Brewery, 1936–1940 as Modern Brewer.

1 Modern Grocer. Chicago; v.1– 1898–.

2 Modern Grocer. New York; v.1– 1921–. Also known as Independent Grocer.

2 Modern Grocer's Merchandiser. New York; v.1–9, 1935–1945//.

1 Modern Housekeeping and Food News. New York; v.1–13, 1899–1911//. Began as Food News (1899–1902).

1 Modern Merchant and Grocery World. Philadelphia; v.1–1113, 1887–1942//. Began as Grocery World (1887–1914).

1 Modern Miller and Bakers News. Moline and Chicago; v.1–. 1878–. Began as Grain Cleaner (1878–1883), 1899–1901 as Weekly Modern Miller; 1946 as Modern Miller.

2 Modern Nutrition. Los Angeles; American Academy of Nutrition, v.1– 1948–. Began as the Academy's Monthly Newsletter Journal. Academy also known as the American Academy of Applied Nutrition.

2 Modern Packaging. nsv.1– 1927–.

1 NARGUS Bulletin. Chicago; National Association of Retail Grocers of U.S., v.1– 1912–. Began as National Grocers Bulletin (1912–1953).

2 NEGM; The New England Grocery and Market Magazine. v.1– 1932–. Supersedes the New England Grocer and Tradesman. Began as New England Grocery and Market Magazine (1932–1952).

2 Naborhood Grocer. Roanoke, Va.; v.1– 1932–. Absorbed the Virginian in Foods 1942.

2 National Association of Food Chains, Washington, D.C., Agricultural Bulletin.

2 National Association of Food Chains, Washington D.C., Proceedings of Annual Meeting. v.1 1934?—

1 National Baker, Devoted Solely to the Baking Interests. Philadelphia; v.1–27, 1896–1922//. Merged with Baker's Weekly.

1 National Bottlers' Gazette. New York; 1882–.

Ranking

1 National Butter, Cheese, and Egg Association, Proceedings. Davenport, Iowa; v.1–14, 1874–1887//?.

1 National Canners Association Annual Convention. v.1– 1908–. Volumes 1–4 in Canner.

2 National Coffee Association, Bulletin. New York; no.1– 1940–.

2 National Coffee Association, News-Comment. New York; v.1–7, 1930–1937//?.

2 National Coffee Association, New York, Proceedings of Convention . . .

2 National Coffee Association, Scientific Bulletin. New York; v.1– 1939--.

1 National Food Magazine. Minneapolis; Chicago; v.1–45, 1896–1920//. Began as What to Eat; the National Food Magazine (1896–1908). Merged with Table Talk.

2 National Grocer. v.1–12, 1916–1929//. Merged with Grocer's Magazine (Boston).

1 National Provisioner.; American Meat Packer's Association, 1891–.

2 National Pure Food News. New York; v.1–2, 1913–1916//.

1 National Retail Grocer. Chicago; v.1–42, 1896–1939//?. Began as Retailers' Journal (1896–1928).

1 National Wine Merchant and Bewer Gazette. R.I.; 1894–1899.

2 Nation's Chefs. Chicago; Chefs of Cuisine Association, v.1–5, 1925–1930//. Began as Chef de Cuisine (1925–1927), 1928 as Chef de Cuisine Year Book. Continued as part of Hotel Bulletin.

2 Nation's Health. Chicago; New York; American Association of Industrial Physicians and Surgeons, v.1–9 1919–1927//. Began as Modern Medicine (1919–1921). Merged with American Journal of Public Health to form American Journal of Public Health and Nation's Health.

2 Natural Food and Farming.

2 Natural Vitamin Flour Bureau Bulletin. Chicago; v.1– 1942–.

1 New England Grocer and Tradesman. Cambridge, Mass.; v.1–102, 1877–1932//. Superseded by N.E. Grocery and Market Magazine.

2 New South Baker. Atlanta, Ga.; v.1– 1910–.

2 New York State Association of Retail Meat Dealers, Bulletin.

2 News Exchange of Nutrition and Health Education.; General Mills, v.1– 1946–.

1 Northwestern Miller. Minneapolis; v.1– 1873–. 1887–1899 as Weekly Northwestern Miller.

1 Northwestern Miller and American Baker. Minneapolis; v.1– 1924–.

2 Nutrition; Important Flashes of Nutrition News.; Quaker Oats Co.

2 Nutrition and Dental Health. St. Paul, Minn.; v.1– 1935–.

1 Nutrition and Health News. New York; v.1– 1931–. Began as Nutrition News (1931).

1 Nutrition News. Chicago; v.1– 1937–.

1 Nutrition News.; Chicago National Dairy Council, v.1– 1925–.

2 Nutrition News (Nutrition Surveys). New York; v.1– 1945–. Began as Nutrition News Letter (1945–1948?).

2 Nutrition News Bulletin.

2 Nutrition Notes. New York; Community Service Society of N.Y., Nutrition Bureau., v.1–20, 1930–1949//.

2 Nutrition Notes. UFFV Association

2 Nutrition Newsletter. Boston; Nutrition Foundation Inc.

Ranking

2 Nutrition Research. Los Angeles; Sunkist Research Staff, v.1– 1940–.
1 Oil Mill Gazetteer. Wharton, Tex.; National Oil Mill Superintendents' Association, v.1– 1900–.
2 Oil Mill Superintendents' Association, Report of the Proceedings, v.1–30, ?-1923//?.
2 Oil Miller and Cotton Ginner. Atlanta, Ga.; v.1–47, 1912–1936//. Began as Oil Miller (1912–1926). Merged with American Ginner and Cotton Oil Miller.
1 Orchard and Garden. New York; Little Silver, N.J.; v.1–14, 1879–1892//. Began as American Wine and Grape Grower (1879–1880), 1881–1885 as Wine and Fruit Grower.
1 Pacific Bottler. San Francisco; v.1–50, 1893–1933//. Merged with Western Brewing World.
1 Pacific Coast Packer. Los Angeles; v.1– 1909–.
1 Pacific Northwest Merchant, Grocer and Meat Dealer. Seattle; v.1– 1906–. Began as Pacific Northwest Grocer and Meat Dealer (1940–1945).
1 Pacific Wine, Brewing and Spirit Review. San Francisco; v.1–61, 1880–1935//. Began as San Francisco Merchant (1880–1889), 1889–1890 as Merchant and Viticulturist, 1890–1913 as Pacific Wine and Spirit Review.
1 Packages. Milwaukee, Wis.; v.1–32, 1898–1929//. Merged with United Barrel and Box to form Barrel and Box and Packages.
2 Packer. Chicago; Cincinnati, Ohio.
2 Packer. Kansas City.
1 Packer. New York ed.; v.1– 1901–. Began as New York Packer (1901–1946).
2 Packing House News. Tampa, Fla.; v.1–5, 1922–1926//. Began as Skinner Packing House News (1922– 1923).
2 Packing Institute, New York, Proceedings of the Annual Forum.
1 Peanut Journal and Nut World. Suffolk, Va.; Official Organ of Several U.S. Trade Associations, v.1– 1921–. Began as Peanut Journal (1921–1931).
2 Peanut Butter Manufacturers Association, Bulletin.
1 Philosophy of Health. Denver, Colo.; v.1–30, 1900–1929//. Began as Stuffed Club (1900–1915).
1 Planter and Sugar Manufacturer. New Orleans, La.; v.1–83, 1888–1929//. Began as Louisiana Planter and Sugar Manufacturer (1888–1924). Merged with Sugar (N.Y. 1914–.)
2 Potato Chipper, National Potato Chip Institute. Cleveland, Ohio; 1941–.
2 Poultry and Egg National Board, Nutrition Research Bulletin. Chicago; v.1– 1940–.
1 Practical Home Economics. East Stroudsburg, Penn.; v.5–34, 1927–1955//. Continues numbering of American Food Journal. Began as Food and Health Education (1927), 1927–1928 as Home Economist, 1928 as Home Economist and the American Food Journal, 1947–1955 as Practical Home Economics and Better Food. Superseded by Practical Home Economics Edition of Co-Ed.
1 Prix Courant. Montreal, Canada; v.1–48, 1887–1915; nsv.29–, 1916–.
1 Produce Guide. New York; v.1–71, 1896–1942//. Began as Fruit Man's Guide (1896–1930), 1930–1932 as Fruit and Produce Guide.
2 Produce Review and American Creamery. New York.
2 Producer-Consumer. Amarillo, Tex.; v.1–20, 1935–1952//.

Ranking

1 Progress in Nutrition. New York; v.1– 1938–.
2 Pure Products, Conducted Exclusively in the Interest of Science and Research as Applied to the General Food and Beverage Industries. New York; v.1–17, 1905–1921//.
1 Quick Frozen Foods. New York; v.1– 1938–. 1941–1952 as Quick Frozen Foods and the Locker Plant.
2 Retail Grocers' Journal.
2 Retail Merchant. Dallas, Tex.; Retail Grocer's Association of Texas, v.1–26, 1901–1914//. Superseded by Southwestern Retailer.
1 Retailer. Vancouver, Canada; Retail Merchant Association of Canada, v.1– 1908–.
2 Retail Merchants Journal. Omaha, Nebr.
2 Rice Industry. Houston, Tex.; v.1–13, 1900–1911//?.
1 Rice Journal. v.1– 1898–. Began as Rice Journal (1898–1934), 1935–1937 as Rice, Sugar and Coffee Journal, 1937–1938 as Rice and Sugar Journal. Divided into Rice Journal and Sugar Journal in 1938.
1 Roller Mill. Buffalo, N.Y.; v.1–30, 1882–1912//.
1 San Francisco Grocer. San Francisco; v.1–13, 1899–1906; nsv. 1–30, ?-1914//?.
2 School Feeding; A Management Magazine. Chicago; v.1–20, 1921–1931//. Began as School and College Cafeteria (1921–1926), 1926–1929 as School Feeding Management. Merged with Club Management and Catering Management to form Catering World.
2 School Lunch Journal. Denver, Colo.; American School Food Sciences Association, v.1– 1947–.
2 Self Service Grocer. New York; v.1– 1940–. Volume 1, no.2–3 issued with Voluntary and Cooperative Group Magazine.
2 Soft Drink Industry. Chicago; v.1–5, 1918–1922//.
2 Southeastern Grocer. Atlanta, Ga.
2 Southern California Grocers Journal. Los Angeles; v.1– 1914–.
2 Southern Fisherman. New Orleans, La.; v.1– 1940–. 1957 as Southern Fisherman and Seafood Merchandising. Absorbed Fish and Oil Industry in 1952 and Seafood Business in 1953.
2 Southern Food Processor. Atlanta, Ga.; v.1– 1940–. Began as Southern Canner and Packer (1940–1951).
2 Southern Baker. Houston, Tex.; 1931–.
2 Southern Food Journal. Dallas, Tex.
1 Southwestern Miller. Kansas City, Mo.; v.1–51, 1922–1972//. Continued by Milling & Baking News.
1 Southwestern Miller. St. Louis, Mo.; v.1–22, 1879–1892//?. ?Began as St. Louis Miller, 1879–1892?.
2 Spirits, Combined with American Wine and Liquor Journal. New York; v.1– 1933–. Began as American Wine and Liquor Journal (1933–?).
2 Successful Grocer. Chicago; Retail Butchers and Grocers Association of Cook County, v.1– 1922–. Began as International Grocer (1922–1935).
1 Sugar. Azucar. New York; v.1– 1914–. Began as Facts About Sugar (1914–1941), 1941–1956 as Sugar.

Ranking

1 Sugar Beet. Mason City, Ida.; Denver, Colo.; Ogden, Utah; Amalgamated Sugar Company, v.1–8, 1924–1931; s2 v.1– 1936–.
1 Sugar Beet. Philadelphia; v.1–32, 1880–1911//.
2 Sugar Beet Journal. Saginaw, Mich.; Farmers and Manufacturers Beet Sugar Association, v.1– 1935–.
1 Sugar Bulletin. New Orleans, La.; American Sugar Cane League of the U.S.A., v.1– 1922–. Began as the society's Bulletin (1922–1925).
2 Sugar Cane Press. Clewiston, Fla.; v.1– 1938–
2 Sugar Cossette. Salt Lake City, Utah; v.1–12, ?-1929//. Superseded by U & I Farm Messenger.
2 Sugar Facts. Chatham, Ontario; no.1–175, 1945–1953//?.
2 Sugar Index. New York; 1929–1938//.
2 Sugar Journal. Crowley and New Orleans, La.; v.1– 1938–.
2 Sugar Molecule. New York; Sugar Research Foundation, Inc., v.1– 1947–.
1 Sugar Planters' Journal. New Orleans, La.; v.1–41, 1870–1910//. Began as Sugar Bowl and Farm Journal (1870–1894). Merged with Modern Sugar Planter.
2 Sugar Press. Denver, Colo.; v.1– 1918–.
2 Sweets. Atlanta, Ga.; v.1–65, 1910–1941//?. Superseded by Southern Candy Jobber.
1 Table and Home Magazine. v.1–3, 1901–1903, nv.1–14, 1904–1918//.
1 Table Talk. Philadelphia and Cooperstown, N.Y.; v.1–31, 1885–1916; v.41–45, 1916–1920//.
2 Table Talk. New York; Consumers' Cooperative Services. Cooperative Cafeterias, v.1– 1940–.
1 Tea and Coffee Trade Journal. New York; v.1– 1901–. Began as Tea and Coffee Journal (1901), 1901–1903 as Tea, Coffee and Sugar.
1 Telefood Magazine. Chicago; v.1– 1935–.
2 Tomato Sauce.
2 Trade Journal for Canners, Packers, Grocers and Allied Interests. San Francisco; v.1–5, 1906–1909//?.
1 Trade Review and Grocer. Portland, Ore.
1 United Fresh Fruit and Vegetable Association, Bulletin. Washington, D.C.
1 Up to Date. Chicago; v.1–7, 1894–1898//?.
1 Vegetarian. New York; v.1–4, 1895–1899//?.
1 Vegetarian-Fruitarian-Humanitarian. Chicago; Vegetarian Society of America, National Vegetarian Society, etc., v.1–41, 1896–1941//. Superseded by Human Culture Digest. Began as Chicago Vegetarian (1896–1899), 1901–1903 as Vegetarian and Our Fellow Creatures, 1903–1925 as Vegetarian Magazine, 1925–1926 as Vegetarian Magazine and Fruitarian, 1926–1934 as Vegetarian and Fruitarian.
2 Voluntary and Co-operative Groups Magazine. New York; v.1–21, 1931–1951//. Began as Voluntary Chain (1931), 1932–1934 as Voluntary Chain Magazine, 1931–1934 as Voluntary Chain Institute.
2 Voluntary Chains. New York; American Institute of Food Institutions, v.1–4, 1929–1933//.
1 Wallerstein Laboratories, N.Y., Communications. 1937–. Began as Communications on the Science and Practice of Brewing.

Ranking

2 Welfare Federation of Cleveland, Nutrition Bulletin.
2 Welfare Federation of Cleveland, Nutrition Notes.
2 West Coast Brewer. San Francisco; California State Brewers Institute, v.1–17, 1935–1952//. Absorbed by Western Brewing and Distributing.
1 Western Baker. San Francisco; v.1– 1906–. Began as Pacific Coast Gazette (1906–1919), 1919 as Bakers and Confectioners Gazette. Supersedes Pacific Coast Baker-Confectioner Magazine.
2 Western Bottler. Los Angeles; v.1– 1937–.
1 Western Brewing and Distributing. Los Angeles; v.1– 1893–. Began as Western Brewing World (1893–1941).
1 Western Canner and Packer. San Francisco; v.1–50, 1909–1958//. Absorbed by Canner/Packer in 1958.
1 Western Confectioner, Ice Cream News. San Francisco; v.1– 1914–. Began as Western Confectioner (1914–1931).
2 Western Frozen Foods. Seattle; v.1–9, 1939–1948//. Merged with Western Locker.
1 Wholesale Grocery Chain Review. New York; v.1–31, 1900–1930//. Began as Wholesale Grocery Review (1900), 1927 as Chain Store Grocer, 1928–1929 as Chain Grocery Review.
1 Whole Sale Grocer News. Chicago; v.1– 1926–.
2 Wine and Liquor Retailer. New York; v.1– 1933–. Began as American Wine and Liquor Retailer (1933–1935).
1 Wine Review, Combined with Wine News. Los Angeles; v.1–18, 1933–1950//. Absorbed by Wines and Vines.
1 Wines and Vines. San Francisco; v.1– 1919–.
2 Yankee Beverage News.
2 Yankee Food Merchant. Boston; v.1– 1940–.
2 Yeast: Dried Yeasts and Their Derivatives.; Anheuser-Busch, v.1–3, 1948–1954//.

Additional Selected References

Beatty, William K. "The History of Nutrition: A Tour of the Literature." *Federation Proceedings* 37 (11) (Oct. 1977): 2511–2512.

Billick, Gloria. "References for the History of Human Nutrition in America, 1600 to the Present: A Selected Bibliography." *Journal of the NAL Associates* 5 (1980): 45–58.

"Celebrating the 50th Anniversary of the Institute of Food Technologists." *Food Technology* 43 (9) (1989). Entire issue.

Darby, William J. "Nutrition Science: An Overview of American Genius." *Nutrition Reviews* 47 (1) (1989): 1–14.

Erdman, John W., Jr. "Nutrition: Past, Present, and Future." *Food Technology* 43 (9) (1989): 220–227.

Hill, Fredric W., ed. "The American Institute of Nutrition: A History of the First 50

Years, 1928–1978, and the Proceedings of a Symposium Commemorating the 50th Anniversary of the *Journal of Nutrition*," *Journal of Nutrition* Vol. 108 (Bethesda, Md.: American Institute of Nutrition, 1978).

Holmes, Zoe Ann. "Historical and National Perspectives on Food Research." In Deacon, Ruth E. and Wallace E. Huffan, eds. *Human Resources Research, 1887–1987: Proceedings*. Ames: Iowa State University, 1986, pp. 43–57.

Sharrer, Terry G., comp. *1001 References for the History of American Food Technology*. Davis: Agricultural History Center, University of California, 1978.

Swan, Patricia. "A History of Nutrition Research in the United States with Emphasis on Agricultural Experiment Stations." In Deacon, Ruth E. and Wallace E. Huffan, eds. *Human Resources Research, 1887–1987: Proceedings*. Ames: Iowa State University, 1986, pp. 27–40.

"Symposium: History of Food Science and Technology." *Food Technology* 29 (1) (1975). Contains seven articles.

"Symposium: 200 Years of Food: A Historical Perspective." *Food Technology* 30 (6) (1976). Contains five articles.

Index

Authors and titles in the core list of monographs (pp. 61–139), the core list of journals (pp. 157–160), the reference titles (pp. 186–215), and the primary historical literature (pp. 229–287) are *not* included in this index.

WITHDRAWAL